D0186038

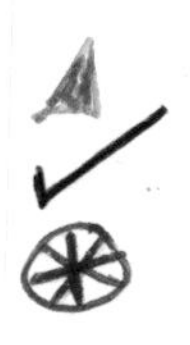

Pharmacology for Anaesthesiologists

Pharmacology for Anaesthesiologists

Edited by

JP Howard Fee MD, PhD, FCARCSI
Professor and Head
Department of Anaesthetics and Intensive Care Medicine
School of Medicine
Queen's University
Belfast, United Kingdom

James G Bovill MD, PhD, FCARCSI
Professor
Department of Anaesthesiology
Leiden University Medical Centre
Leiden, The Netherlands

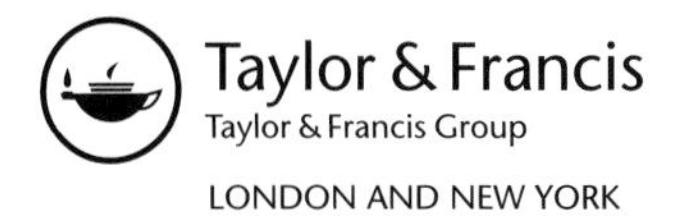

LONDON AND NEW YORK

First published in 2005 by Taylor & Francis, an imprint of the Taylor and Francis Group,
2 Park Square, Milton Park, Abingdon, Oxon OX14 4RN

Tel.: +44 (0) 20 7017 6000
Fax.: +44 (0) 20 7017 6699
E-mail: info.medicine@tandf.co.uk
Website: http://www.tandf.co.uk/medicine

A CIP record for this book is available from the British Library.

ISBN 1-84184-236-2

Distributed in North and South America by
Taylor & Francis
2000 NW Corporate Blvd
Boca Raton, FL 33431, USA

Within Continental USA
Tel.: 800 272 7737; Fax 800 374 3401
Outside Continental USA
Tel.: 561 994 0555; Fax: 561 361 6018
E-mail: orders@crcpress.com

Distributed in the rest of the world by
Thomson Publishing Services
Cheriton House
North Way
Andover, Hampshire SP10 5BE, UK
Tel.: +44 (0) 1264 332424
E-mail: salesorder.tandf@thomsonpublishingservices.co.uk

Composition by Wearset Ltd, Boldon, Tyne & Wear
Printed and bound in Great Britain by The Bath Press

Contents

Contributors

Amit Bedi
Department of Anaesthetics and Intensive Care Medicine
Royal Victoria Hospital
Belfast
United Kingdom

James G Bovill
Department of Anaesthesiology
Leiden University Medical Centre
Leiden
The Netherlands

Stephen J Cooper
Department of Mental Health
School of Medicine
Queen's University
Belfast
United Kingdom

JP Howard Fee
Department of Anaesthetics and Intensive Care Medicine
School of Medicine
Queen's University
Belfast
United Kingdom

CP Henney
Department of Anaesthesiology
Academic Medical Centre
Amsterdam
The Netherlands

John P Howe
Consultant Anaesthetist
Belfast City Hospital
Belfast
United Kingdom

W McCaughey
Department of Anaesthetics
Craigavon Area Hospital
Craigavon
United Kingdom

Ronan McMullan
Department of Medical Microbiology
Royal Victoria Hospital
Belfast
United Kingdom

T J McMurray
Postgraduate Dean
Northern Ireland Medical and Dental Training Agency
Belfast
United Kingdom

Rajinder K Mirakhur
Department of Anaesthetics and Intensive Care Medicine
School of Medicine
Queen's University
Belfast
United Kingdom

Vesna Novak-Jankovič
Institute of Anaesthesiology and Intensive Care
University of Ljubljana Medical Centre
Ljubljana
Slovenia

Martin Pfaffendorf
Department of Pharmacotherapy
Academic Medical Center
Amsterdam
The Netherlands

Adela Stecher
Institute of Anaesthesiology and Intensive Care
University of Ljubljana Medical Centre
Ljubljana
Slovenia

Harry B van Wezel
Department of Anaesthesiology
Academic Medical Center
Amsterdam
The Netherlands

Preface

Anaesthetists, uniquely, administer drugs intravenously and by inhalation which profoundly interfere with fundamental physiological functions such as breathing, cardiac output, blood pressure, the protective reflexes, and the perception of pain. The drugs used are often highly potent and potentially toxic. It is therefore entirely appropriate that anaesthetists are required to have a good working knowledge and understanding of pharmacological and physiological principles, and their application to anaesthesia and intensive care. As in other fields of medicine and biology, there have been marked advances in physiology and pharmacology in recent years, which seem to proceed at an ever increasing pace. Much of what was considered 'state of the art' ten years ago is now considered commonplace; a consequence is that textbooks rapidly become outdated.

This book and its companion on physiology were conceived primarily to provide up-to-date information to trainees in anaesthesiology and related specialities preparing for postgraduate examinations in these subjects. In addition to covering the core material for these examinations, topics not usually dealt with in textbooks for anaesthetists are also covered, since they can have at least an indirect relevance to the practising anaesthesiologist. These include immunosuppressive and antineoplastic drugs, drugs for epilepsy and psychiatric disorders in the pharmacology volume and immunology in the physiology volume. Although these drugs will seldom, if ever, be directly administered by anaesthetists, they do need to understand how their use by patients can impact on the conduction of anaesthesia. There is also a growing awareness of the impact of anaesthesia and surgery on the immune response, and its potential relevance for patients who have undergone or about to undergo organ transplantation. Alterations in the immune system can also have a direct, and sometimes dramatic effect during anaesthesia, e.g an anaphylactic reaction to an anaesthetic drug.

While we have attempted to produce volumes that are comprehensive and clinically relevant, they are not intended to be authoritative works of reference. Thus, we have been restrictive in the use of references, preferring instead to add additional reading lists, or references to recent reviews, at the end of individual chapters. We hope this will be useful for readers wishing to supplement the material covered in the volumes.

Satisfying the examiners, however, is not the end of the story. Postgraduate education is a continuing process, and we hope that this series will also be of benefit to established anaesthesiologists, and those in other related specialities, who want to keep up to date with recent developments in physiology and pharmacology.

As editors we are indebted to the individual authors for their valuable contributions to this series. We also wish to acknowledge the support of the publishers, Taylor & Francis Medical, and in particular the editorial support and encouragement provided by Maire Harris (who was very much involved in the conception of the volumes), Robert Peden, and Giovanna Ceroni.

Howard Fee
James Bovill

1

Principles of drug action

JG Bovill

Introduction • Receptors • Ion channels • Ligand-gated ion channels • G protein-coupled receptors • Receptors with intrinsic enzyme activity

INTRODUCTION

Most drugs produce their pharmacological actions through interactions with receptors, which are specialised proteins normally activated by endogenous transmitters or hormones, leading to an increase or decrease in transmembrane signalling. Transmembrane signalling is achieved by several different classes of integral membrane proteins, including ion channels and G protein-coupled receptors. In both cases, the major function of the protein is to recognise and transduce extracellular signals that can originate either by ligand binding or a change in transmembrane voltage. Signal transduction involves a conformational change in the protein. In the case of ion channels this results in opening of the channel and either an influx or efflux of ions into or out of the cell. In G protein-coupled receptors the conformational change alters the interaction between receptor and an intracellular G protein. Structurally, both classes of proteins have a membrane-spanning domain consisting of between five and seven helices. Other drugs interact with enzymes, e.g. cholinesterase, carbonic anhydrase, cyclooxygenase, and monoamine oxidase inhibitors. A few drugs act by virtue of their physicochemical properties, e.g. the reversal of heparine by protamine, while others inhibit transport systems. Examples of the latter are local anaesthetics that block Na^+ channels and the cardiac glycosides that inhibit active transport by Na^+/K^+ ATPase. Many of these mechanisms are dealt with in other chapters, and this chapter will concentrate on receptors and ion channels.

RECEPTORS

There are four main types of receptors:

1. Ligand-gated ion channels that contain a ligand binding site as part of the ion channel.
2. G protein-coupled receptors linked to a second messenger system by a guanine nucleotide protein.
3. Receptors with intrinsic enzyme activity directly linked to tyrosine kinase.
4. Nuclear receptors that alter DNA transcription.

Receptors stereospecifically bind molecules, known as ligands, with high affinity and specificity. Ligands may be *agonists* or *antagonists*. An agonist has affinity for the receptor and produces a response as a result of the ligand–receptor interaction. This ability to produce a response is known as efficacy or intrinsic activity. An antagonist binds to the receptor but lacks intrinsic activity, i.e. has zero efficacy. Antagonists usually have high affinity—indeed this is essential if they are to displace the agonist from the receptor. Ligands with negative efficacy are referred to as inverse agonists. These include certain compounds that bind to the $GABA_A$ benzodiazepine receptor and β adrenoceptors. Inverse agonists produce pharmacological effects opposite to those of the agonists, e.g. for benzodiazepines, they produce anxiety rather than relieving it.

The binding of an agonist (A) to a receptor (R) is a chemical process that can be assumed to obey the Law of Mass Action. The concentration of occupied receptors $[AR]$ is given by:

$$\frac{[AR]}{[R_T]} = \frac{[A]}{[A] + K_a}$$

where R_T is the total concentration of receptors and K_a is the dissociation constant, which is numerically equal to the free ligand concentration when half the receptors are occupied ($[AR]/[R_T] = 0.5$). If the magnitude of the response (E) is proportional to fractional receptor occupancy, then the response may be expressed as

$$\frac{E_A}{E_{max}} = \frac{[AR]}{[R_T]} = \frac{[A]}{[A] + K_a}$$

where E_{max} is the maximum possible response. The graph of E/E_{max} versus $[A]$ is a rectangular hyperbola (Figure 1.1a), but plotting E/E_{max} versus $\log[A]$ produces a sigmoid relationship (Figure 1.1b).

Agonists may be full agonists or partial agonists. A full agonist is able to cause a maximal response that corresponds to an activity of unity, whereas partial agonists cannot produce the maximum response so have intrinsic activities less than unity (Figure 1.2). Not all full agonists have equal efficacy—some may produce a maximum response when only 5% of the available receptors are occupied while less efficient agonists may need to occupy 30% or more of receptors to obtain a full response.

Competitive antagonists

Competitive antagonism occurs when the binding between the agonist and the antagonist is freely reversible, and can be fully overcome by sufficiently increasing the concentration of the agonist, i.e. the antagonism is *surmountable*. Increasing the concentration of the antagonist causes a displacement of the agonist concentration–response curve to the right (Figure 1.1b). Many clinically useful drugs are competitive antagonists of endogenous ligands, e.g. atropine, β-adrenoceptor antagonists, and antihistamines.

Non-competitive antagonists

A non-competitive antagonist prevents the agonist, at any concentration, from producing a maximum effect. Agonist concentration–response curves in the presence of increasing concentrations of a non-competitive antagonist are different that those produced by a competitive antagonist (Figure 1.3). Irreversible or *unsurmountable* binding often arises from covalent bonding between antagonist and receptor, e.g. the binding of phenoxybenzamine to α-adrenoceptors. Covalent bonds are very strong, requiring considerable energy to break. Since these compounds dissociate only very slowly or not at all from the receptor they often have very prolonged action, and their effects are usually unrelated to their plasma concentration. Non-competitive antagonism also occurs when the antagonist blocks some part of the chain of events that lead to the production of a response by an agonist. For example, hexamethonium acts by producing a non-competitive block of the action of acetylcholine on nicotinic receptors.

Stereoisomerism

Many drugs exhibit stereoselectivity, with actions dependent on their spatial configuration. Substances with the same elementary chemical composition but with the elements occupying different positions in space are called isomers. Structural isomers are compounds with the same numbers of chemical

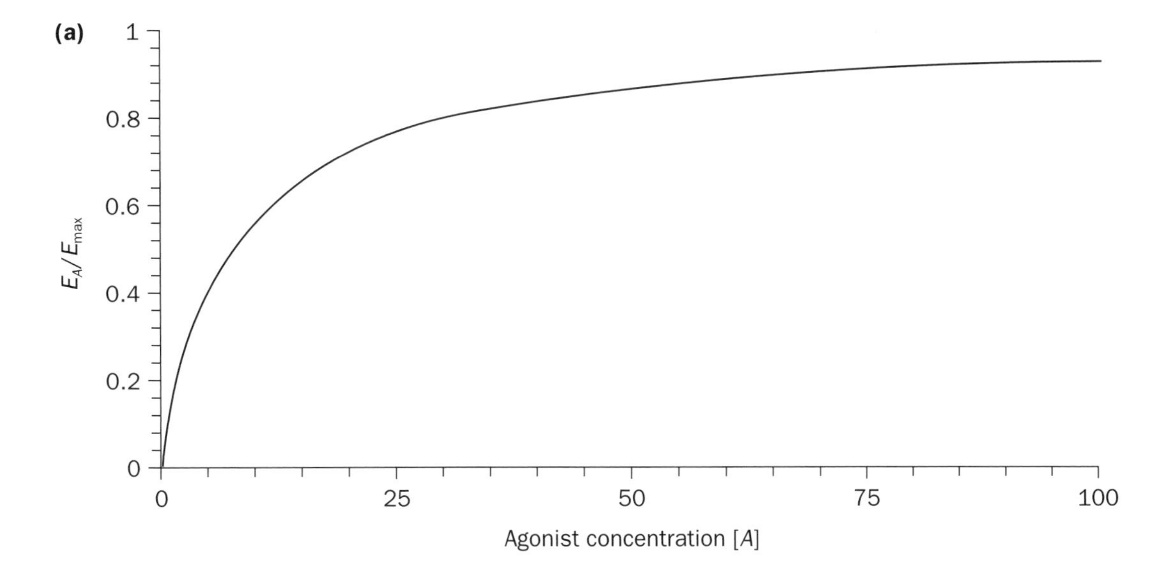

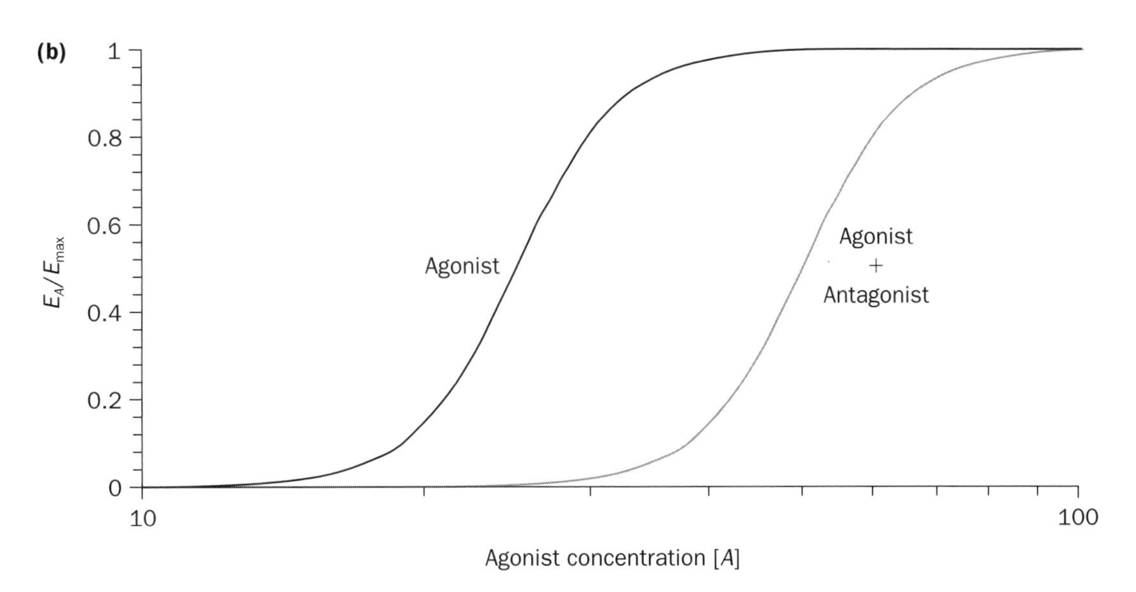

Figure 1.1 *(a) The graph of fractional receptor occupancy* (EA/E_{max}) *against agonist concentration* [A] *(linear scale for* [A]*) is a rectangular hyperbola. (b) Graphs of* E_A/E_{max} *as a function of agonist concentration* [A]*, in the absence and presence of a competitive antagonist. The antagonist shifts the agonist curve to the right. The graphs are plotted on a semilogorithmic axis for* [A]*, yielding sigmoid curves.*

elements that differ in their position and arrangement. As such, they are different chemical and biological substances. Examples are enflurane and isoflurane and the β-adrenoceptor antagonists, practolol and atenolol.

Optical isomers

Optical isomers are compounds differing only in their ability to rotate the plane of polarised light. The (+), or dextrorotatory (D), isomer rotates light to the right (clockwise), and the (–),

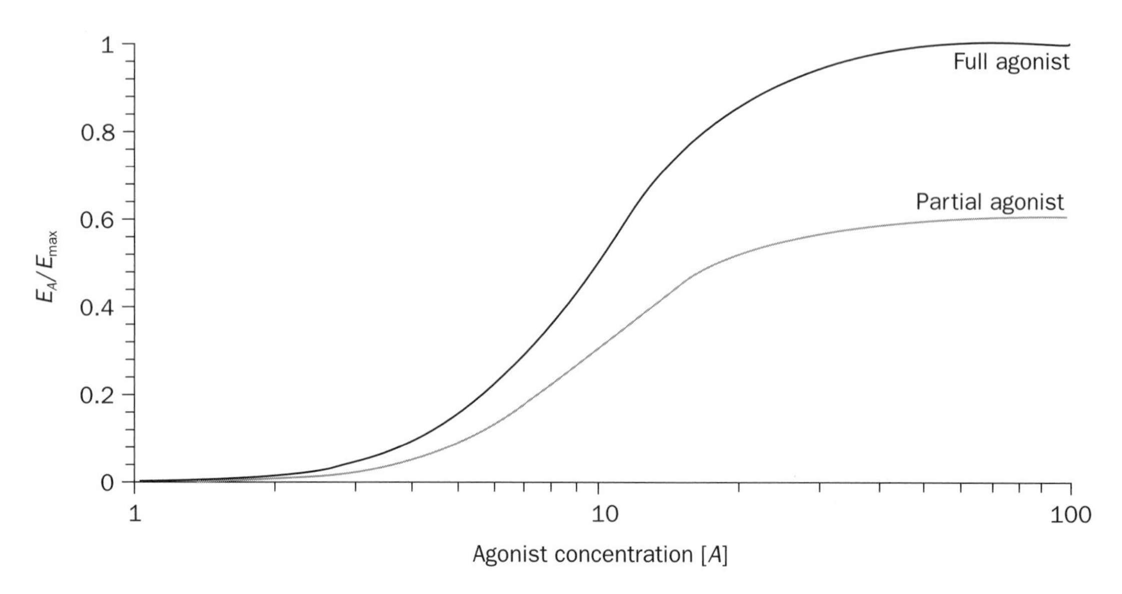

Figure 1.2 *Response curves for agonists and partial agonists.*

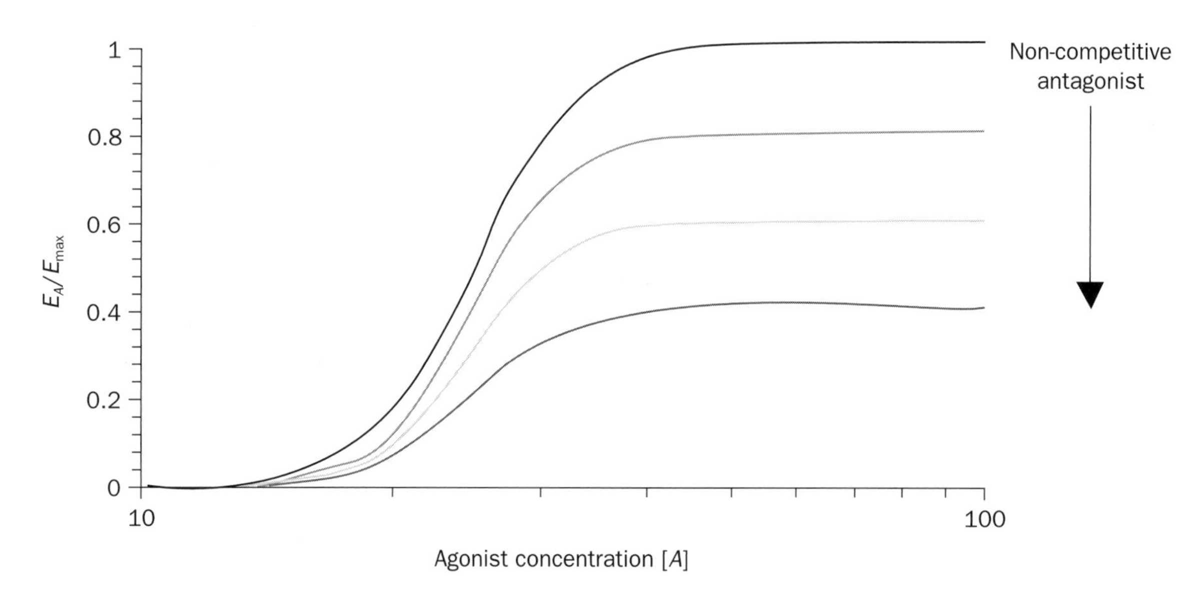

Figure 1.3 *Displacement of the agonist response curve by increasing concentrations of a non-competitive antagonist.*

or laevorotatory (L) isomer rotates light to the left (anticlockwise). Optical isomers or *enantiomers* (from the Greek 'opposite shape') arise when molecules contain an asymmetric or chiral centre (from the Greek for hand), arranged so that the molecules differ only as does the right hand from the left (i.e. they are non-superimposable mirror images, Figure 1.4). A 50:50 mixture of (+) and (–) enantiomers is a racemic mixture, which has no effect on polarised light. The commonest asymmetric centre is a carbon atom with four different groups attached. Enantiomers have identical chemical and physical properties but may have different physiological or pharmacological activities. Some drugs have more than one asymmetric centre. Labetalol has two chiral centres and is a mixture of two racemates, i.e. labetalol is a mixture of four stereoisomers. Differences in the pharmacological activities between enantiomers can be considerable. Thus (+)-lofentanil is a μ-opioid agonist while (–)-lofentanil is a μ antagonist.

In addition to the prefixes (+) and (–), or *d*- and *l*-, modern nomenclature uses the R,S system. For a chiral atom, the four substituents are assigned relative priorities according to atomic weights, the group with the highest sum of weights being given the highest priority. The molecule then is rotated so that it is viewed from the side opposite the group with the lowest priority and the symbol R, for *rectus* (right), is assigned if the remaining groups follow descending priorities in a clockwise order about the centre. If the order from highest to lowest is anticlockwise then the symbol S (for *sinister* or left) is assigned (Figure 1.4). Note that the R,S nomenclature for chirality (right- or left-handedness) does not necessarily correspond to the optical rotation of polarised light by a compound. For example, R(–)-ketamine and S(+)-ketamine but (R+)-bupivacaine and S(–)-bupivacaine.

Naturally occurring compounds are usually single enantiomers, e.g. L-morphine, L-hyoscine. Atropine is an exception. Although synthesised in the belladonna plant as L-atropine, it is partly converted in the extraction process to the D isomer (chiral inversion), and is administered as a racemic mixture. During this process its

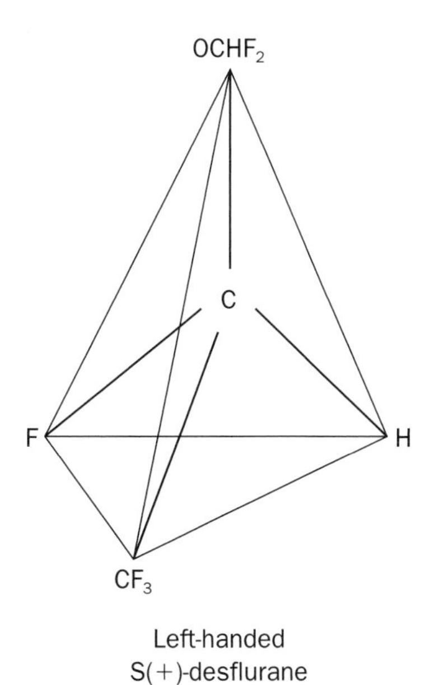

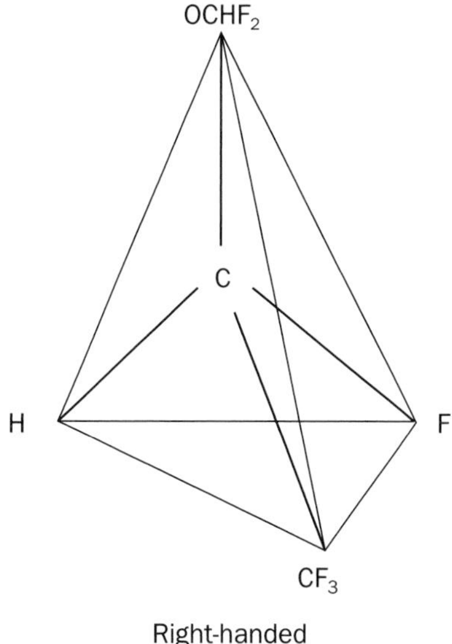

Figure 1.4 *The enantiomers of desflurane.*

anticholinergic activity is approximately halved since the D isomer has little activity. In contrast to biological synthesis, organic synthesis usually results in racemic mixtures. More than half of the drugs used in anaesthesia are chiral. Of the inhalational anaesthetics, only sevoflurane does not possess a chiral centre. Many amide local anaesthetics are chiral and, with the exception of ropivacaine, are used clinically as the racemic mixtures. The cardiotoxicity of bupivacaine is predominantly due to the R(+) isomer, which also has greater central nervous system (CNS) toxicity.

Geometric isomers

Geometric isomers form a second type of stereoisomerism (but not necessarily optical isomerism). They occur when there is restricted rotation in a molecule, either around a double bond or a rigid ring system. Stereoisomerism arising from the presence of a double bond is indicated by using Z (German *zusammen* meaning together) or E (German *entgegen* meaning opposite). These correspond to the older *cis* and *trans* designations. The two forms arise when the substituents are on the same side (Z or *cis*) or on the opposite sides (E or *trans*) of the double bond (Figure 1.5). Geometric isomers have different physicochemical and pharmacological properties. Mivacurium is a mixture of three geometrical isomers, *cis-cis*, *trans-trans*, and *cis-trans*. The *cis-cis* isomer has only about 10% of the potency of the other two isomers. *Cis*-atracurium is one of the 10 stereoisomers of atracurium.

ION CHANNELS

Ion channels are membrane-spanning proteins containing a central water-filled pore through which ions can traverse the cell membrane. When activated, there is a change in the ionic conductance, resulting in either membrane depolarisation or hyperpolarisation. Opening of the channel allows selected ions (Ca^{2+}, Na^+, K^+, or Cl^-) to flow down their electrical or chemical gradients. Because the rate of ion flow is very fast response times are short (often < 1 ms). Ion channels are found when speed is essential to the signalling process, as in nerve cells and pacemaker cells in the heart.

There are two types of ion channels, voltage-gated and ligand-gated. Voltage-gated ion channels, which open and close in response to changes in membrane potential, are named according to the ion they selectively control. Ligand-gated ion channels often have several ligand binding sites, e.g. $GABA_A$ and *N*-methyl-D-aspartate (NMDA) complexes. The ion currents generated by ligand-gated channels often provide the stimulus for the subsequent opening of voltage-gated ion channels.

Voltage-gated ion channels

Voltage-gated ion channels consist of motifs with six membrane-spanning α helices formed by predominantly hydrophobic amino acids. The fourth transmembrane helix contains positively charged amino acids, arginine and lysine, that act as the voltage sensor controlling gating of the channel. Rotational and longitudinal movement of this segment in response to a change in transmembrane potential causes the ion pore to open.

Sodium ion channels

The trigger for the opening of sodium channels is an increase in the intracellular potential to approximately –55 mV. The opening of the channel is very transient and within less than 1 ms it spontaneously closes and enters an inactivated state. It can only return to its resting state when the membrane potential returns to near the resting potential. Local anaesthetics act on Na^+ channels, binding tightly to the inactivated state, stabilising this form of the channel. The closed or resting state has the least affinity for local anaesthetics. This differential affinity explains the frequency-dependent neuronal block produced by local anaesthetics. Sodium channels are also an important target for class I anti-arrhythmic drugs.

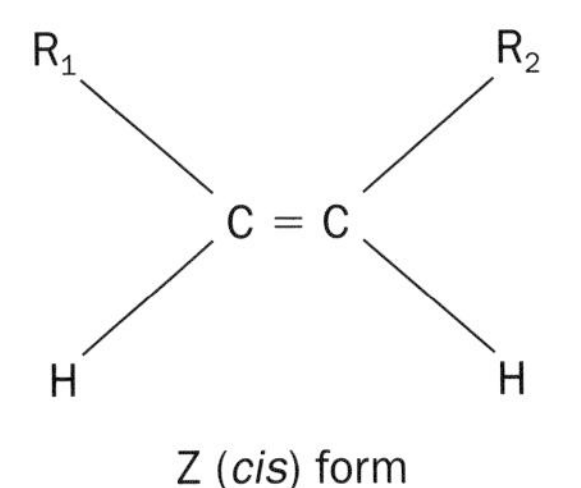

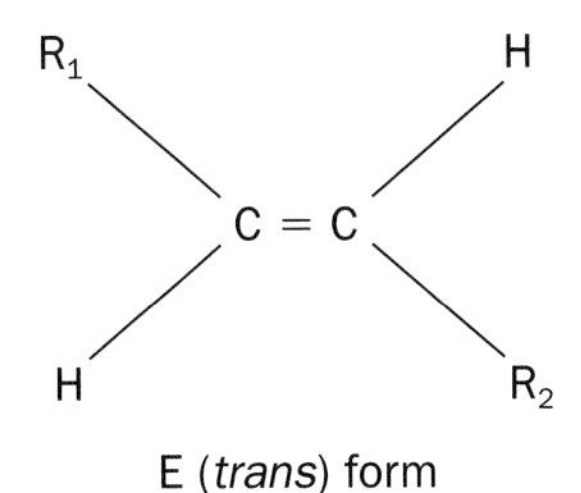

Figure 1.5 Cis *and* trans *isomerism.*

Potassium ion channels

Potassium ion channels are a very diverse family of membrane proteins, with numerous subtypes both in the CNS and peripheral tissues, in particular in the heart. On the basis of the amino acid sequence of the pore-forming α subunit, they are classified into two main superfamilies, the inward rectifier superfamily (which includes receptor-coupled, adenosine 5′-triphosphate (ATP)-sensitive and voltage-dependent channels) and the *Shaker*-related superfamily (which includes Ca^{2+}-dependent channels).

A particularly important potassium channel in terms of pharmacology is the ATP-sensitive K^+ channel, K_{ATP}, whose opening is inhibited by intracellular ATP. They occur in the myocardium, pancreatic β cells, vascular smooth muscle and skeletal muscle, and various neurones. Activation of K_{ATP} channels leads to shortening of the cardiac action potential, relaxation of vascular smooth muscle, and inhibition of both insulin secretion and neurotransmitter release. K_{ATP} channels are inhibited by sulphonylurea antidiabetics, such as glibenclamide and tolbutamide. They are activated by K_{ATP} channel opening drugs. To this group belongs cromakalin and its active enantiomer levcromakalin, bimakalin and celikalin, nicorandil, pinacidil, aprikalim, minoxidil, and diazoxide. They are used in treating various cardiovascular conditions as well as asthma, urinary incontinence, and certain skeletal muscle myopathies. Nicorandil, in addition to causing vasodilatation by activating K_{ATP} channels, is also an NO donor producing a nitrate-like action. In renal tubular cells, K_{ATP} channels contribute to potassium balance and K_{ATP} blocking drugs may have potential as potassium sparing diuretics. Glibenclamide, a sulphonylurea that inhibits K_{ATP} channels, induces significant sodium diuresis without urinary potassium loss.

Calcium ion channels

Calcium is involved in the regulation of a multitude of cellular physiological processes, and also functions as an intracellular second messenger. Intracellular calcium concentrations can be increased by:

- Entry through voltage- or ligand-gated calcium channels in the cell membrane.
- Ryanodine receptor- and IP_3 receptor-mediated calcium release from the sarcoplasmic reticulum.
- Na^+/Ca^{2+} exchange in the mitochondrial membrane.

Most of these sites are amenable to pharmacological manipulation, especially the calcium channels. To date, six distinct Ca^{2+} channel types have been defined, designated T, L, N, P, Q, and R. They have different voltage thresholds for activation and different kinetics for opening and closing, and also exhibit distinct selectivities for blocking compounds. Although these channels permit the passage of Na^+ and K^+, they are highly selective for Ca^{2+}, by a factor greater than 1000. The group of drugs known as calcium entry blockers selectively inhibit L-type channels. Mibefradil blocks both L- and T-type calcium channels, but is 10 times more potent at blocking T channels than L channels. It is selective for the coronary circulation but has no negative inotropic properties. None of the other calcium ion channels are targets for currently available drugs

LIGAND-GATED ION CHANNELS

The physiological stimulus for activation of ligand-gated ion channels is the binding of a neurotransmitter to a receptor on the channel protein, opening the channel and allowing ions to cross the cell membrane. This allows the membrane potential to change very rapidly (0.1–0.2 ms), transferring the chemically transmitted signal of a neurotransmitter into an electrical signal, which is then rapidly conducted along the nerve fibre of a second cell. Ligand-gated ion channels may be either excitatory or inhibitory. Excitatory receptors, e.g. nicotinic acetylcholine receptors, NMDA glutamate receptors and $5\text{-}HT_3$ receptors, when activated open channels that allow the passage of Na^+, K^+, or Ca^{2+} ions. This causes depolarisation of the postsynaptic membrane. GABA and glycine bind to ligand-gated chloride channels, causing hyperpolarisation of the postsynaptic membrane and inhibition. Members of the ligand-gated ion channel family are composed of four or five subunits, each consisting of four membrane-spanning α helices (Figure 1.6).

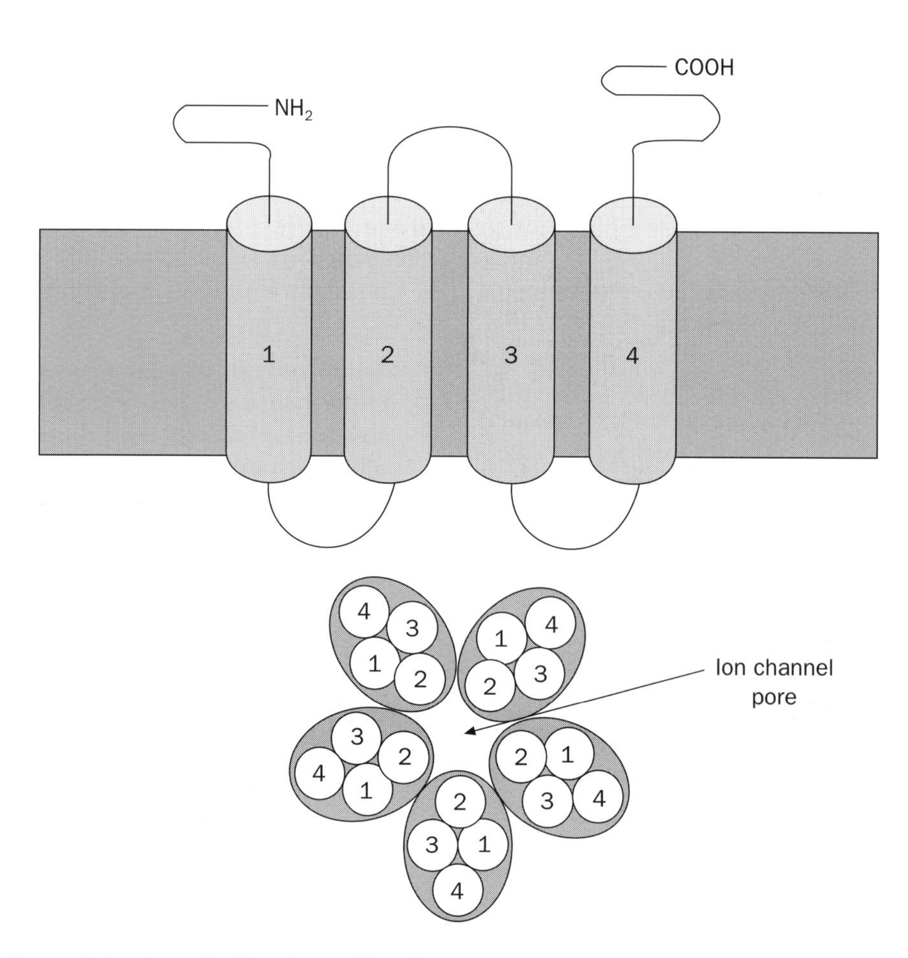

Figure 1.6 *General structure of a ligand-gated ion channel. They are formed by 4–5 subunits each consisting of four membrane-spanning hydrophobic α helices that form the central ion channel pore.*

Nicotinic acetylcholine receptors

Acetylcholine (ACh) is an example of an endogenous neurotransmitter that binds to more than one receptor type, the nicotinic acetylcholine receptor (nAChR) which preferentially binds nicotine and the muscarinic receptor which binds muscarine, a mushroom alkaloid. The latter is a G protein-coupled receptor while the nACh receptor is an excitatory ligand-gated ion channel that transports Na^+ ions. Nicotinic cholinergic receptors are found in the CNS, autonomic ganglia, and at the neuromuscular junction of skeletal muscles. They are a possible target for anaesthetics.

$GABA_A$ receptors

GABA (γ-aminobutyric acid) is the major inhibitory transmitter in the CNS and acts at either ionotropic $GABA_A$ or metabotropic (G protein-linked) $GABA_B$ receptors. Recently, a third class of ionotropic receptor, $GABA_C$, has been identified. $GABA_A$ and $GABA_B$ receptors are found pre- and postsynaptically on GABA and non-GABA terminals, including those containing NMDA receptors. Baclofen, the only currently available selective $GABA_B$ receptor agonist, is used to treat muscle spasticity. Binding of GABA to the $GABA_A$ receptor opens the ion pore, allowing Cl^- to enter the cell. This leads to membrane hyperpolarisation and a reduction in neuronal excitability. Many intravenous and inhalational

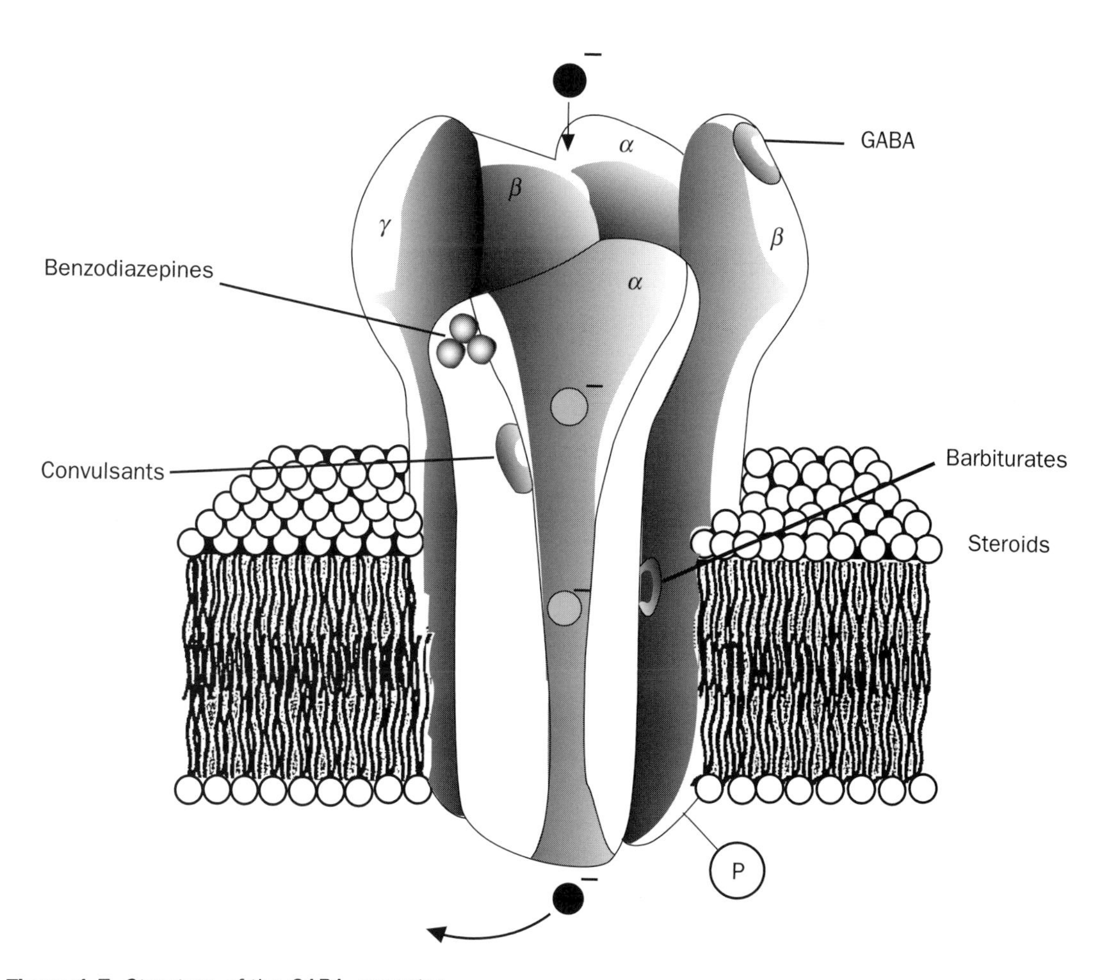

Figure 1.7 *Structure of the $GABA_A$ receptor.*

anaesthetics bind to the $GABA_A$ receptor and augment GABA-mediated neuronal inhibition.

Barbiturates and steroid anaesthetics bind to distinct sites on the $GABA_A$ receptor (Figure 1.7). They facilitate the response to GABA and mimic GABA by opening the receptor chloride channel in the absence of GABA. At least some of the anaesthetic properties of propofol are mediated via the $GABA_A$-receptor complex. Propofol binding to the $GABA_A$ receptor is at a site distinct from those for barbiturates, benzodiazepines, or steroids. Benzodiazepines bind to a distinct site on the $GABA_A$-receptor complex, often referred to as the benzodiazepine receptor. Benzodiazepines alone do not have any effect on chloride currents in the absence of GABA or GABA agonists. When GABA is present they increase chloride ion flux.

NMDA receptors

The amino acid L-glutamate activates three subtypes of excitatory amino acid ion channel receptors, alpha-amino-3-hydroxy-5-methylisoxazole-4-propionic acid (AMPA) receptors, NMDA receptors and, a non-NMDA receptor activated by kainite. A fourth family of glutamate receptors are the metabotropic (G protein-coupled) receptors. NMDA receptors are widely distributed throughout the brain and spinal cord, and have very widespread physiological functions, including sensory information processing, memory, and learning. They also have an important role in nociception, in particular, neuronal plasticity associated with chronic pain, tissue injury, and inflammatory states. Sustained afferent input to the dorsal horn produces a prolonged depolarisation so that the Mg^{2+} block on spinal NMDA receptors is removed, allowing NMDA activation and an influx of Ca^{2+}. NMDA receptors are involved in the phenomenon referred to as 'wind-up' where the responses of neurones increase with each subsequent stimulus (Figure 1.8). This is associated with facilitation of spinal nociceptive reflexes and hyperalgesia. Wind-up of dorsal horn nociceptive neurones is selectively reduced by NMDA antagonists, including ketamine.

NMDA receptors control an ion channel that permits entry of monovalent (mainly Na^+) and divalent (mainly Ca^{2+}) ions into the cell. Calcium flux is by far the most important. In addition to a binding site for L-glutamate, the NMDA receptor has binding sites for glycine, Mg^{2+}, and Zn^{2+}. A recognition site for phenylcyclidine and ketamine lies in the opening of the ion channel (Figure 1.9) and these drugs are non-competitive antagonists of the NMDA receptor.

The NMDA receptor is unique in that it is the only ligand-gated ion channel whose probability of opening depends upon the voltage across the membrane. The channel is inoperative when the neurone is in the resting state, with a negative intracellular membrane potential. This imposes a voltage-dependent Mg^{2+} block on the channel. Presynaptically released glutamate cannot activate any significant ion flow through the channel unless the postsynaptic membrane is sufficiently depolarised to remove this Mg^{2+} block. The gaseous anaesthetics, nitrous oxide and xenon, are also NMDA-receptor antagonists.

The 5-HT_3 receptor

The 5-HT_3 receptor is the only monoamine neurotransmitter receptor that functions as a ligand-gated ion channel, controlling the flux of Na^+ and K^+ ions. 5-HT_3 receptors are located on parasympathetic nerve terminals in the gastrointestinal tract, and high densities are found in areas of the brain associated with the emetic response, such as the area postrema. The antiemetic effects of 5-HT_3 antagonists, such as ondansetron, result from actions at these sites. 5-HT_3 receptors in the dorsal horn of the spinal cord have been implicated in nociception and development of new 5-HT_3 receptor-related compounds may have potential as non-opioid, non-addictive analgesics.

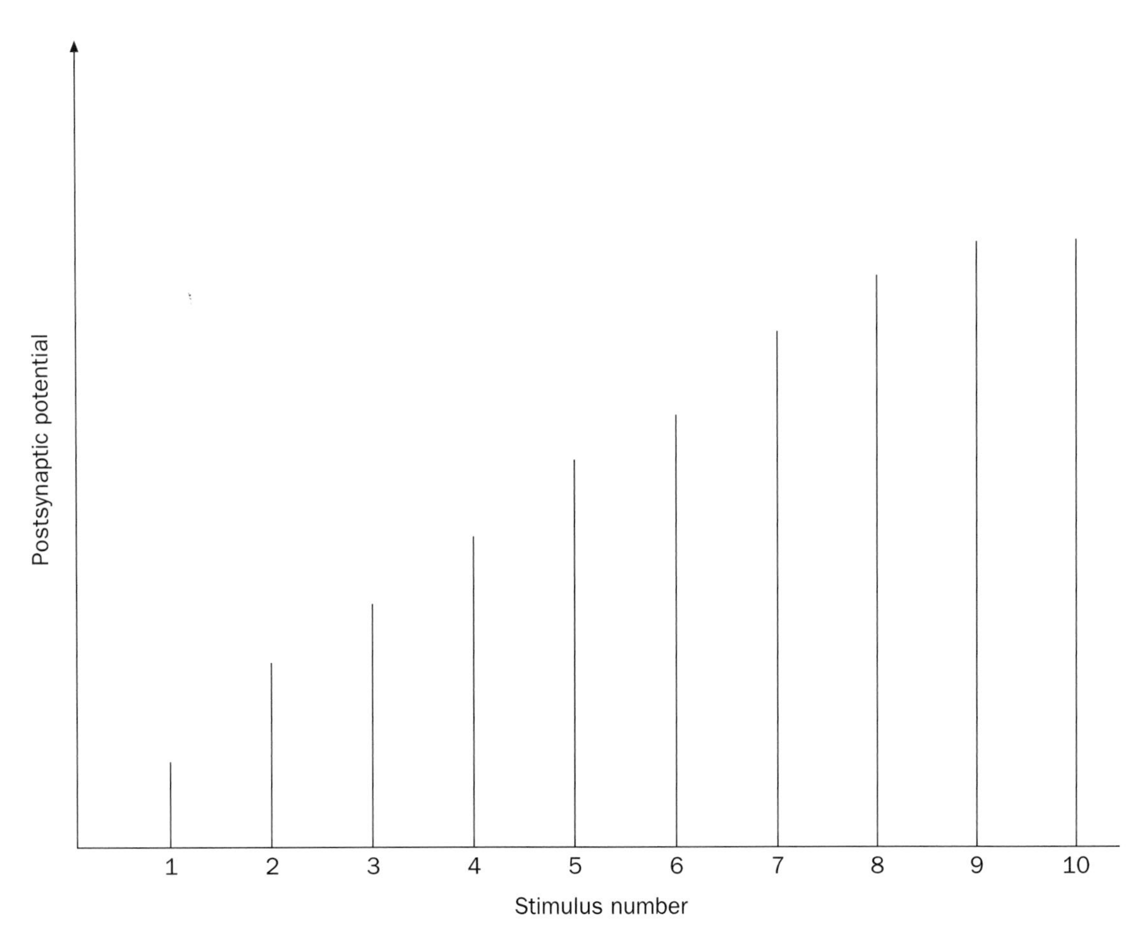

Figure 1.8 *An illustration of the phenomenon of 'wind-up'. With repetitive stimulation of dorsal horn neurones the postsynaptic potential steadily increases in amplitude with each successive stimulus. This facilitation is blocked by NMDA-receptor antagonists.*

G PROTEIN-COUPLED RECEPTORS

G protein-coupled receptors (guanine nucleotide proteins, hence the 'G' terminology) are the largest family of cell-surface proteins involved in intra- and intercellular communication, accepting stimuli as diverse as light, neurotransmitters, hormones, and odorant molecules. They are targeted by at least 50% of currently available therapeutic drugs. G protein-coupled receptors share similar structural and mechanistic features. They consist of seven α-helical transmembrane segments connected by three extracellular and three intracellular loops (Figure 1.10). The intracellular loops form a high affinity binding domain for guanosine 5′-triphosphate (GTP)-binding proteins (G proteins) composed of α, β, and γ subunits. When activated by an agonist the receptor in turn activates the G protein by increasing the rate of dissociation of a tightly bound molecule of guanosine 5′-diphosphate (GDP). Another guanine nucleotide, usually GTP, then binds to the α subunit. This causes the G protein subunits to dissociate from each other and from the receptor. Consequently, Gα and Gβγ subunits

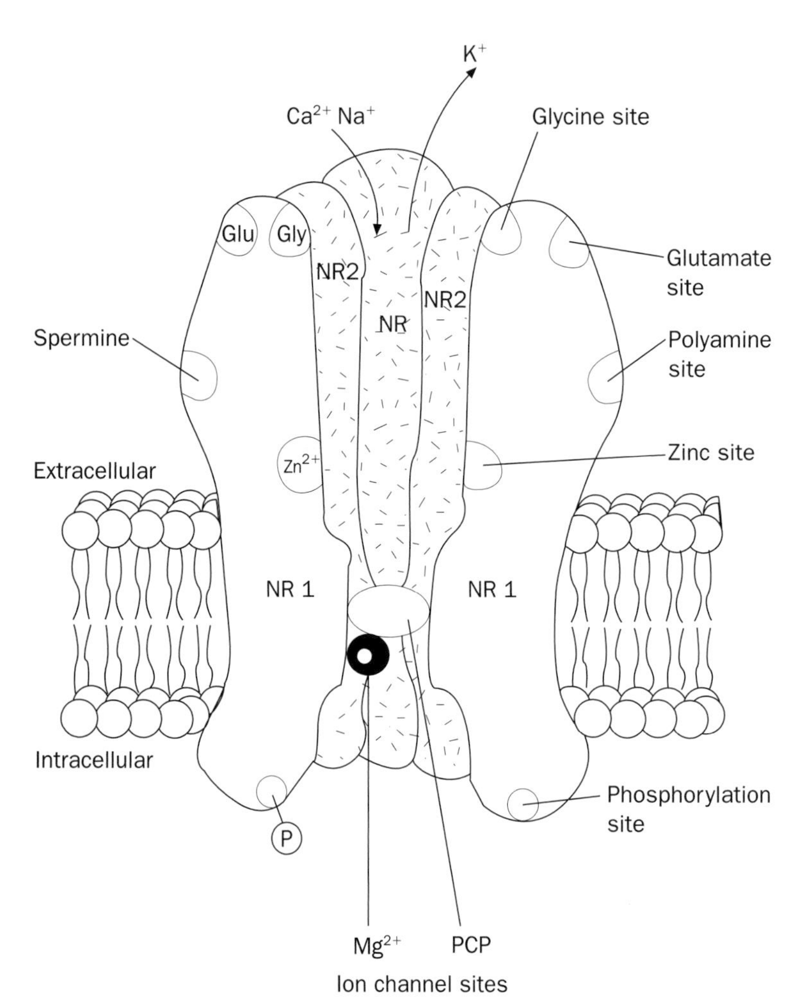

Figure 1.9 *The NMDA receptor, showing the sites of interaction for glutamate (Glu), glycine (Gly), polyamine, Zn^{2+} and Mg^{2+}. Glutamate requires the presence of glycine to open the receptor channel. Polyamine positively modulates, and Zn^{2+} and Mg^{2+} negatively modulate, the opening of the channel. Ketamine and phencyclidine bind to the site labelled PCP.*

separate and modulate the activity of various effector enzymes, thereby activating or inhibiting the production of a variety of second messengers, in addition to promoting increases in the intracellular concentration of Ca^{2+} and the opening or closing of a number of ion channels (Figure 1.11). Over 20 G proteins have been identified, the most important being G_s, G_i, G_o, and C_q (Table 1.1).

The adenylyl cyclase pathway

Activation of G_s or G_i proteins results in stimulation or inhibition, respectively, of adenylyl cyclase which catalyses the formation of cyclic adenosine monophosphate (cAMP) from ATP The cAMP binds to protein kinase A (PKA), which mediates the diverse cellular effects of cAMP by phosphorylating substrate enzymes, thereby increasing their activity. Among the responses mediated by cAMP are increases in contraction of cardiac and skeletal muscle and glycogenolysis in the liver by adrenaline (epinephrine). Because a single activated receptor can cause the conversion of up to 100 inactive G_s proteins to the active form, and each of these results in the synthesis of several hundred cAMP molecules, there is a very considerable signal amplification. For example, adrenaline concentrations as low as 10^{-10} M can stimulate the release of glucose sufficient to increase

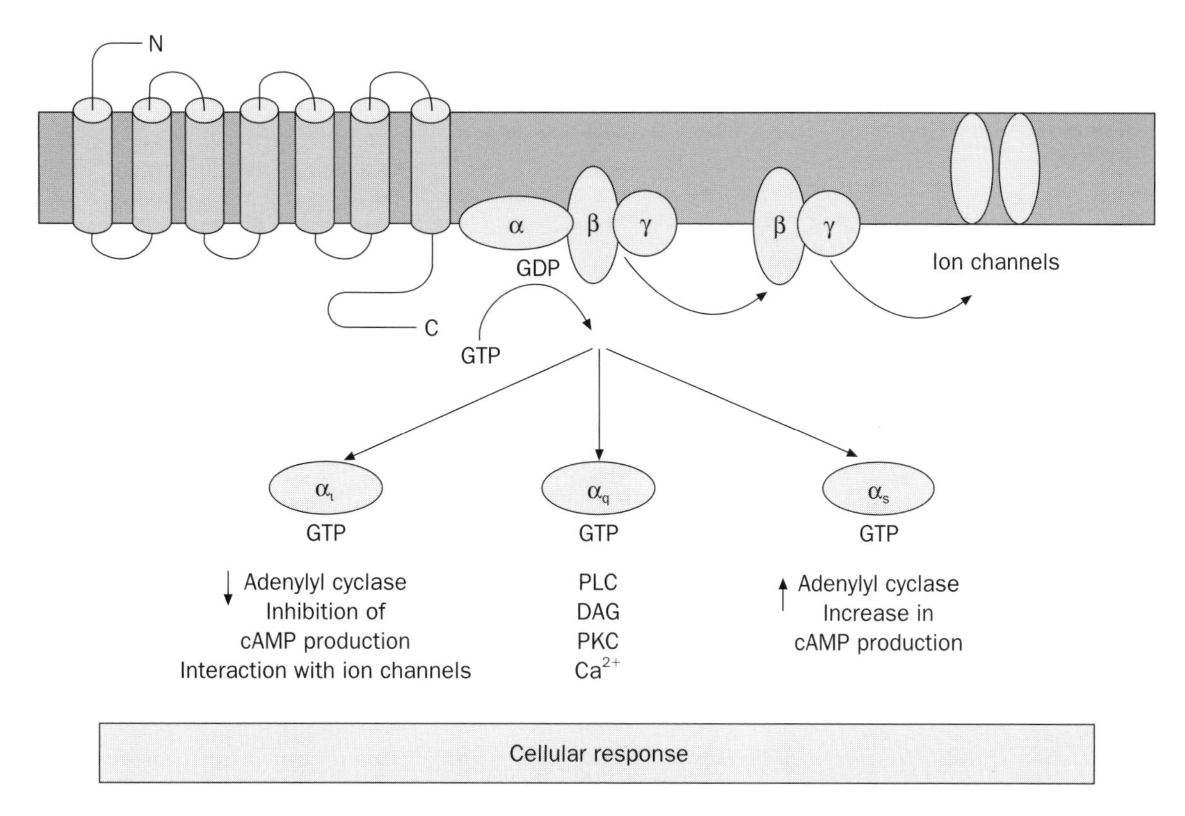

Figure 1.10 *Model of a G protein-coupled receptor with 7 membrane-spanning domains. Binding of an agonist to the receptor causes GDP to exchange with GTP. The α-GTP complex then dissociates from the receptor and the βγ complex and interacts with intercellular enzymes or ion channels. The βγ complex can activate an ion channel or possibly also interact with intercellular enzymes. GDP, guanine diphosphate; GTP, guanine triphosphate; cAMP, cyclic adenosine monophosphate; PKC, protein kinase C; PLC, phospholipase C; DAG, diacylglycerol.*

blood glucose by 50%. Activation of G_i protein-coupled receptors results in inhibition of adenylyl cyclase and a fall in the intracellular concentration of cAMP. For example, noradrenaline (norepinephrine) acting at β adrenoceptors (G_s-coupled) increases cAMP but when it acts on α_2 adrenoceptors (G_i-coupled) it decreases cellular cAMP.

The phospholipase C pathway

This pathway is activated by activation of receptors coupled to G_q proteins (Figure 1.10). Among neurotransmitters using this pathway are acetylcholine (muscarinic M_1, M_3, or M_5 receptors), noradrenaline ($\alpha_{1A\text{–}C}$ adrenoceptors), histamine (H_1 receptor), and serotonin (5-HT_{1C} and 5-HT_2 receptors). Activation of phospholipase C hydrolyses phosphatidylinositol 4,5-bisphosphate (PIP_2), one of several inositol phospholipids found in the plasma membrane. Hydrolysis of PIP_2 yields two second messengers, inositol 1,4,5-triphosphate (IP_3) and diacylglycerol (DAG). IP_3 interacts with IP_3-sensitive Ca^{2+} channels in the membrane of the endoplasmic reticulum, stimulating the release of stored calcium. The calcium binds to cytosolic calmodulin, which then activates other enzymes, e.g. myosin in muscle. Each calmodulin molecule binds four calcium ions in a cooperative fashion, so that a small change in cytosolic Ca^{2+}

Table 1.1 G protein-coupled receptors, their effector systems, and intracellular second messengers

G protein	*Effector*	*Second messenger*	*Receptor*
G_s	Adenylyl cyclase (+)	cAMP	Adrenergic (β_{1-3})
	Ca^{2+} channels (+)	$[Ca^{2+}]_i$	Dopamine (D_1, D_3, DA_1)
			Histamine (H_2)
			Adenosine (A_2)
			Serotonin (5-$HT_{4,6,7}$)
G_i	Adenylyl cyclase (–)	cAMP	Acetylcholine (M_2, M_4)
	K^+ channels (+)	Hyperpolarisation	Adrenergic (α_2)
			Dopamine (D_{2A}, D_3, D_4, DA_2)
			Adenosine (A_1)
			Histamine (H_3)
			Opioids (μ, δ, κ)
			Serotonin (5-$HT_{1A,1C}$)
			$GABA_B$
G_q/G_o	Phospholipase C (+)	IP_3, DAG	Acetylcholine (M_1, M_3, M_5)
			Adrenergic (α_1)
			Histamine (H_1)
			Adenosine (A_3)
			Dopamine (D_{2A})
			Serotonin (5-HT_2)
$G_?$	Phospholipase A_2	Arachidonic acid	Adrenergic (α_1)
			Adenosine (A_2)
			Serotonin (5-HT_{2A})

IP_3, inositol triphosphate; DAG, diacylglycerol; $[Ca^{2+}]_i$, intracellular Ca^{2+} concentration.

leads to a large change in the level of active calmodulin. This is another example of signal amplification.

The DAG produced by the hydrolysis of PIP_2 by PLC remains in the plasma membrane where it activates a family of membrane-associated protein kinases collectively termed protein kinase C (PKC). Activated PKC produces a variety of cellular responses, including the regulation of protein synthesis and key metabolic pathways.

In muscle cells and neurones a second mechanism exists for the release of intracellular Ca^{2+}, involving ryanodine receptors in the endoplasmic reticulum (ER) membrane. This pathway is activated by an action potential opening a plasma membrane voltage-gated Ca^{2+} channel, allowing a small influx of extracellular Ca^{2+}. Binding of Ca^{2+} to the ryanodine receptor triggers a massive release of Ca^{2+} from the ER stores.

The acetylcholine muscarinic receptor

Drugs acting at this receptor include muscarinic antagonists, such as atropine and anticholinesterases, e.g. neostigmine and edrophonium, which stimulate the receptor indirectly

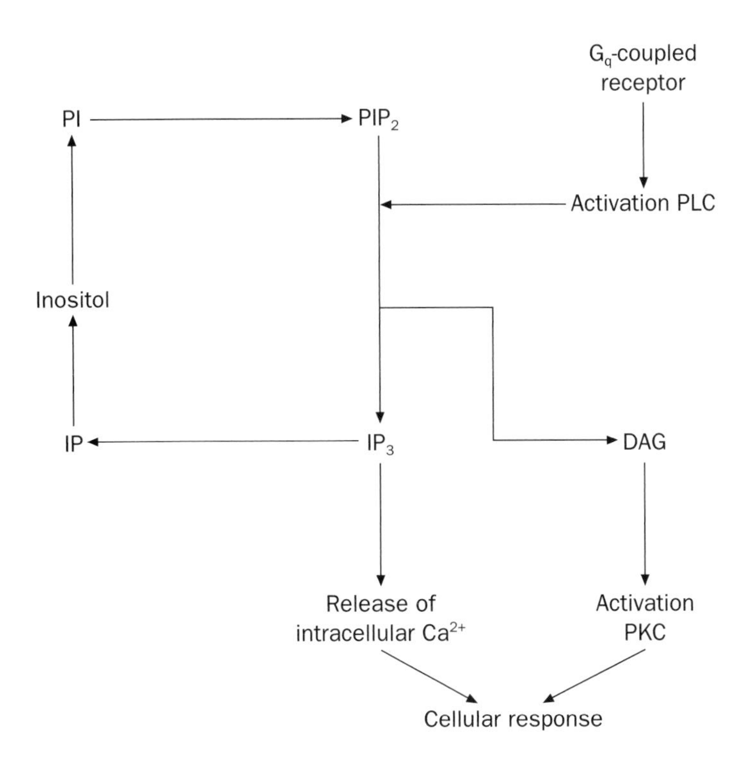

Figure 1.11 *Pathways involved in phospholipase C (PLC) cellular signalling. PKA, protein kinase A or cAMP-dependent protein kinases; PKC, protein kinase C; PI, phosphatidylinositol; PIP_2, phosphatidylinositol bis-phosphate; IP_3, inositol triphosphate; IP, inositol phosphate; DAG, diacylglycerol.*

by preventing the breakdown of acetylcholine. To date, five muscarinic acetylcholine receptor subtypes have been identified, M_1 to M_5. Muscarinic receptors are widely distributed throughout the CNS, in cardiac and smooth muscle and exocrine, endocrine and paracrine glands. The M_1, M_3 and M_5 receptors are coupled to G_o and G_q proteins and activate IP_3/DAG to mediate the release of Ca^{2+} from intercellular stores. This opens a calcium-gated K^+ channel and hyperpolarises the cell. The M_2 and M_4 muscarinic receptors activate G_i proteins to decrease cAMP. In the heart, M_2 receptor activation also opens inwardly rectifying K^+ channels, and this is responsible for the cardiac side effects of anticholinergic drugs.

Anticholinergic drugs, such as atropine, are non-selective antagonists at all five muscarinic receptors, although the increase in heart rate caused by atropine may be mediated selectively through M_2 receptor-mediated action on K^+ channels. Brain muscarinic signalling is important in the modulation of consciousness, and the actions of anaesthetic agents at these sites possibly contribute to the mechanisms of general anaesthesia (Durieux 1996). Muscarinic receptors in the spinal cord are involved in nociception and intrathecal administration of cholinergic agonists or anticholinesterases produces a potent antinociceptive effect.

Adrenergic receptors

Since Ahlquist first proposed the existence of two adrenoceptor subtypes, α and β, in 1948, the number of receptors has considerably expanded and at present nine distinct adrenoceptor subtypes have been identified. There are two subtypes of the α receptor (α_1 and α_2, with subfamilies of each of these) and three subtypes of the β receptor, β_1, β_2 and β_3. The adrenoceptors are G protein-coupled receptors, but second messenger and G protein linkage differ between the subtypes. α_1-Adrenoceptor activation increases phospholipase C via a G_q protein, resulting in an elevation in intracellular Ca^{2+}.α_2. Adrenoceptors are coupled to a G_i protein and inhibit adenylyl cyclase. The three β adrenoceptors mediate G_s protein-linked stimulation of adenylyl cyclase, although in cardiac muscle there is also a direct link between the G_s protein and a voltage-gated calcium channel. While many drugs act directly on adrenergic receptors, others act indirectly by influencing the synthesis, uptake, or metabolism of endogenous cathecholamines, e.g. monoamine oxidase inhibitors, tricyclic antidepressants, ephedrine.

The α_1 and β adrenoceptors are located on the postsynaptic junction of sympathetic nerve terminals innervating smooth muscles and endocrine glands or cardiac cells (β_1). Most vasoconstrictor responses to sympathetic stimulation are mediated by α_1 adrenoceptors. In general α_2 and β_2 receptors are located on prejunctional adrenergic neuronal membranes, and inhibit and facilitate, respectively, the release of noradrenaline. Prejunctional α_2 adrenoceptors also exist on cholinergic neurones and inhibit the release of acetylcholine. The three β-adrenoceptor subtypes have markedly different tissue distribution. The β_1 adrenoceptor is present mainly in the heart, where it is the target for β-adrenoceptor antagonists and agonist inotropic drugs. The β_2 adrenoceptor is found in skeletal muscle, the uterus and in bronchial smooth muscle, where β_2 agonists act as bronchodilators. The main location for the β_3 adrenoceptor is adipose tissue, where it seems to regulate energy metabolism and thermogenesis.

Dopamine receptors

Dopamine is a major neurotransmitter which acts on multiple receptors. It can activate both α and β adrenoceptors in addition to acting on specific dopamine receptors. These are widely distributed throughout the CNS and are also present in the renal tubules and renal and mesentric blood vessels, and many dopaminergic drugs are used in the treatment of Parkinson's disease, psychiatric disorders, as antiemetics, and for renal protection. Neuroleptic drugs, such as haloperidol and droperidol, are dopamine receptor antagonists.

Six CNS and two peripheral dopamine receptors have been identified by pharmacological means. The CNS receptors are designated 'D' and those in the periphery as 'DA'. Those in the CNS are postsynaptic receptors, belonging to two major classes, D_1 and D_2, but recent cloning experiments have expanded this number to D_3, D_4 and D_5. The new receptors appear to have restricted localisation to the limbic and frontal cortical areas of the brain. They all bind neuroleptic drugs, and the D_4 receptor has a notably high affinity for clozapine. Central D_1 and D_3 receptors and peripheral DA_1 receptors increase, while D_{2A}, D_3, D_4, and DA_2 receptors decrease cAMP. The antiemetic agent, metoclopramide, is a dopamine antagonist whose central effects are mediated via D_2 receptors in the chemotherapeutic trigger zone (CTZ) in the area postrema.

The effect of low concentrations of dopamine in enhancing urine output is due to its action on DA_1 receptors in the renal vasculature. Dopexamine, which is especially useful in preserving the mesentric circulation in shock states, is a DA_1 agonist with β_2-adrenoceptor agonist properties. Fenoldopam, a recently developed selective dopaminergic DA_1 receptor agonist, is a rapidly acting vasodilating agent. Unlike dopamine, it provides maximum dopaminergic effects without adrenergic stimulation.

Adenosine receptors

Adenosine belongs to a biologically important group of substances known as autacoids, that act on their cell of origin or on neighbouring cells. Adenosine is a purine nucleotide found throughout the body, but with highest concentrations in the CNS. It is a potent peripheral vasodilator in all vascular beds except the kidney and the placenta, where it produces vasoconstriction through A_2-receptor activation. In the heart, adenosine has antiarrhythmic properties possibly due to a shortening of the atrial action potential duration and membrane hyperpolarisation due to increased K^+ conductance. Adenosine interacts with at least four different G protein-coupled receptors, A_1, A_{2A}, A_{2B} and

A_3 receptors. These are also known collectively as purine P1 receptors. There are two other classes of purine receptors, P2X and P2Y, which are thought to be involved in nociception and especially visceral pain. The ligand for these receptors is ATP. The A_1 receptor is coupled to the inhibitory G_i protein and the A_2 receptor to the stimulatory G_s protein, and respectively inhibit or activate adenylyl cyclase, while the A_3 receptor mediates G protein-dependent activation of phospholipase C.

There is evidence that in cerebral ischaemia adenosine may have protective effects, since it inhibits the release of many excitatory neurotransmitters, such as glutamate, and it also stabilises the membrane potential. Unfortunately, adenosine has an extremely short half-life, but recently nucleoside (adenosine) transport inhibitors, e.g. draflazine, have been developed that prevent the endothelial uptake and breakdown of adenosine and prolong its beneficial effects. Nucleoside transport inhibitors also have myocardial protective properties and may have a role in organ preservation prior to transplantation. Adenosine also has an antinociceptive function and various adenosine analogues have antinociceptive activity, which correlates with their affinity for the A_1 receptors (Lipkowski and co-workers 1996).

5-HT (serotonin) receptors

Serotonin (5-HT, 5-hydroxytryptamine) is another neurotransmitter that binds to multiple types of receptors. At least 14 subtypes of 5-HT receptors have been described, belonging to seven families, 5-HT_1 to 5-HT_7, widely distributed throughout the CNS and the cardiovascular and gastrointestinal systems. Apart from 5-HT_3 (a ligand-gated ion channel), 5-HT receptors are G protein-coupled receptors. 5-HT_{1A} and 5-HT_{1D} receptors are 'autoreceptors' that control the release of 5-HT and other neurotransmitters. A class of second-generation anxiolytics, the azapirones (buspirone, ipsapirone, gepirone), are selective agonists or partial agonists at the 5-HT_{1A} receptor. They cause minimal sedation, and do not appear to have potential for drug abuse or dependence. Ketanserin is the prototype 5-HT_2 antagonist. It potently blocks 5-HT_{2A} receptors and has no significant effect on other 5-HT receptors. However, ketanserin also has high affinity for α adrenoceptors and histamine H_1 receptors. The physiological function of the 5-HT_4 receptor is as yet unknown but may be involved in the regulation of gastrointestinal (GI) functions. The only available 5-HT_4 agonist is cisapride, which activates excitatory presynaptic 5-HT_4 receptors of cholinergic neurones in the GI tract, increasing the release of ACh from the nerve terminals. Cisapride is thus a prokinetic drug and is used to increase GI contractions and propulsion. Cisapride has been associated with acquired long QT syndrome and ventricular arrhythmias, such as *torsades de pointes*, which produces sudden cardiac death. These cardiotoxic effects, which may be due to blockade of one or more types of K^+ channel currents, are potentiated by inhibitors of the cytochrome P-450 enzymes responsible for cisapride metabolism, such as macrolide antibiotics. This leads to elevated blood concentrations of cisapride. For this reason cisapride has been withdrawn in the UK and Ireland.

Alterations in 5-HT neurotransmission may be involved in a variety of neuropsychiatric disorders, including depression and generalised anxiety disorders. Many of the drugs used in their treatment in some way alter the serotonergic system. Tricyclics sensitise postsynaptic neurones to 5-HT, monoamine oxidase inhibitors (MAOIs) increase the availability of 5-HT, while the selective serotonin reuptake inhibitors (SSRIs), e.g. fluoxetine, sertraline, increase the efficacy of 5-HT neurones by desensitising 5-HT autoreceptors located on 5-HT nerve terminals. Some of the newer drugs used in the treatment of schizophrenia, such as clozapine and risperidone, are combined $5\text{-HT}_{2A/2C}$ and dopamine D_2-receptor antagonists. Clozapine also has a high affinity for 5-HT_6 and 5-HT_7 receptors, but it is unclear whether this contributes to its clinical actions. The appetite suppressant drugs, fluoxetine and D-fenfluramine, alter feeding behaviour by increasing extracellular brain 5-HT levels and also by acting directly at 5-HT_{2C} receptors and possibly at other 5-HT receptors.

Methysergide, used for the prophylactic treatment of migraine and other vascular headaches, is a 5-$HT_{2A/2C}$ antagonist, although it is not selective and also blocks 5-HT_1 receptors. It inhibits the vasoconstrictor and pressor effects of 5-HT. The newest and most effective drug for the treatment of acute migraine attacks is sumatriptan, a selective 5-HT_{1D} receptor agonist. Its antimigraine effect is thought to be due to constriction of intracranial blood vessels, restoring vascular tone and/or blockade of neural transmission and neurogenic inflammation. Unlike most other antimigraine drugs, it inhibits rather than enhances the emetic symptoms normally associated with a migraine attack.

RECEPTORS WITH INTRINSIC ENZYME ACTIVITY

This is a large group of ligand-activated receptors that pass through the plasma membrane of the cell only once. Ligand binding on the extracellular domain causes an activation of the cytosolic domain, which possesses the intrinsic enzyme activity. These receptors fall into two main classes, protein kinases that phosphorylase either tyrosine or serine residues in their target proteins and whose endogenous ligands include insulin and a variety of other growth-related factors, and guanylyl cyclase. Ligand binding to kinase receptors initiates multiple intracellular events with both immediate, e.g. activation of PLC, and long-term, e.g. cell growth, consequences.

The other family of receptors with intrinsic enzyme activity is the membrane-bound receptors linked to guanylyl cyclase. This family includes cell membrane receptors activated by atrial, cardiac or brain natriuretic factors and cytosolic receptors associated with nitric oxide. These receptors catalyse the formation of cGMP from cGTP. cGMP acts as a second messenger and can either act directly on target molecules, e.g. ion channels, or it can activate cGMP-dependent phosphorylation of many proteins, resulting in a wide variety of metabolic changes. Activation of soluble guanylyl cyclase to produce cGMP is one of the primary ways in which nitric oxide, now recognised as an important cellular messenger, mediates cellular and intracellular communication.

Intracellular receptors

In addition to plasma membrane receptors, some cells also have receptors on the membrane of the nucleus or soluble receptors in the cytosol. Examples are steroids, thyroid hormones, and vitamins A and D, which exert their effects by binding to intracellular receptors that control specific gene transcription and expression. The steroid receptor in its inactive form is present in the cytoplasm associated with other proteins. Binding of a steroid molecule results in dissociation of the receptor, exposing a specific recognition site for binding to DNA. The activated hormone-receptor complex then enters the nucleus where it binds to specific regions of DNA called the hormone response elements. This initiates the transcription of genetic material resulting in new protein production. When the receptor is not occupied by a steroid it has a negative regulatory function to prevent the gene from being transcripted, so no proteins are produced. One of the characteristics of hormone and drug effects mediated by intracellular receptors is a comparatively slow response time (minutes to hours) because of this requirement of new protein synthesis. Conversely, the effects persist after withdrawal of the agonist.

FURTHER READING

Durieux ME. Muscarinic signalling in the central nervous system. *Anesthesiology* 1996;84:173–89.

Lipkowski AW, Maszcz-Yuska I. Peptide, N-methyl-D-aspartate and adenosine receptors as analgesic targets. *Curr Opin Anaesthesiol* 1996;9:443–8.

2

Principles of pharmacokinetics and pharmacodynamics

JG Bovill

Introduction • Transfer of drugs across membranes • Factors affecting transmembrane transfer • Lipid solubility • Drug absorption • Drug metabolism and excretion • Drug disposition • Non-compartmental or model-independent approaches to pharmacokinetics • Pharmacodynamics of drug action • Pharmacokinetic-pharmacodynamic models

INTRODUCTION

Pharmacokinetics and pharmacodynamics form the two major branches of pharmacology. Pharmacokinetics is the study of drug disposition and deals with the processes of absorption, distribution, metabolism and elimination. Pharmacodynamics is concerned with the relationship between the concentration of a drug and its effect. Put another way, pharmacodynamics is what a drug does to the body while pharmacokinetics is what the body does to a drug. This chapter will cover the general principles relating to these processes, and develop some of the principles that describe their kinetics and dynamics.

TRANSFER OF DRUGS ACROSS MEMBRANES

To reach their site of action, most drugs must traverse one or more cellular membranes to reach their target organ. Non-polar substances dissolve readily in the lipid layers of cell membranes, and can cross the membranes by passive diffusion, although other mechanisms, such as facilitated diffusion and active transport, apply to some drugs. *Polar compounds* are those containing chemical bonds in which the shared electrons are unevenly shared between adjacent atoms, i.e. the electrons are polarised. A common polar compound is the water molecule. Polar compounds are only soluble in polar solvents, while unionised, non-polar molecules are poorly soluble in water, but are soluble in non-polar solvents, such as lipids. The rate of transfer is also related to the nature of the membrane. The basement membrane upon which the endothelial cells of the brain capillaries are attached, and through which drugs must pass to reach the brain, is tightly applied to the underlying astrocyte cells. The endothelial cells are also tightly bound together so that this membrane (the *blood–brain barrier*) is a more formidable obstacle than those at other sites in the body.

Passive diffusion

Drug transfer by simple diffusion represents the free passage of a drug down its concentration gradient, without the expenditure of energy. Only unionised molecules with a molecular weight < 500 Da that are not bound to plasma proteins can transfer by passive diffusion. The net transfer of the molecule is governed by the Fick equation:

$$\frac{dQ}{dt} = \frac{K \cdot A \cdot \Delta C}{D}$$

where dQ/dt is the rate of diffusion, K is the diffusion constant (which depends on the physicochemical characteristics of the drug), A is the surface area of the membrane, D its thickness, and ΔC is the concentration gradient across the membrane.

Facilitated diffusion

Facilitated diffusion is a mechanism of transmembrane transfer that is carrier mediated but not energy-dependent. The carrier molecule is usually a transmembrane protein, which binds molecules and releases them on the other side of the membrane. It is an important mechanism for endogenous substances, such as glucose.

Active transport

Active transport is a carrier-mediated process that requires energy to move molecules against an electrochemical or concentration gradient. It is more important in elimination or secretory processes than for absorption. Only a few drugs, such as α-methyldopa and 5-fluorouacil, are transferred by active transport.

FACTORS AFFECTING TRANSMEMBRANE TRANSFER

The ability of a drug to penetrate cell membranes is determined by its chemical structure and its physicochemical properties, in particular the degree of ionisation, protein binding and lipid affinity. Lipid-soluble drugs diffuse easily across membranes, whereas water-soluble ones pass through at slower rates.

Ionisation

Drugs cross biological membranes most readily in the unionised state. The unionised drug is 1000–10 000 times more lipid-soluble than the ionised form and thus is able to penetrate the cell membrane more easily. Chemical compounds in solution are acids, bases or neutral. The Brønsted-Lowry definition of an acid is a species that donates protons (H^+ ions) while bases are proton acceptors. Strong acids and bases in solution dissociate almost completely into their conjugate base and H^+. Weak acids and weak bases do not completely dissociate in solution, and exist in both ionised and unionised states. Most drugs are either weak acids or weak bases. For an acid, dissociation in solution is represented by:

$$\underset{\text{Unionised}}{HA} \rightleftharpoons \underset{\text{Ionised}}{H^+ + A^-}$$

The dissociation constant, K_a:

$$K_a = \frac{[H^+][A^-]}{[HA]}$$

is a measure of the strength of an acid. Because K_a has a very small numerical value, it is usually converted to pKa, the negative logarithm to the base 10 of K_a, analogous to pH ($pKa = -\log_{10} K_a$). Rearranging the above equation and converting to logarithmic form gives the *Henderson-Hasselbalch Equation*, which describes the relationship between the unionised and ionised forms of a drug and the pH of the solution:

$$pK_a - pH = \log_{10}\frac{[HA]}{[A^-]} = \log_{10}\frac{[\text{Unionised}]}{[\text{Ionised}]}$$

When $pK_a = pH$, there will be equal fractions of ionised and unionised drug. This is sometimes used as an alternative definition of pK_a, i.e. the pH of a solution in which a substance is 50% ionised and 50% unionised. When $pH > pK_a$ the ionised form of weak acids predominates.

For a base

$$BH^+ \rightleftharpoons H^+ + B$$
$$\text{Ionised} \quad \text{Unionised}$$

and the Henderson-Hasselbalch equation is:

$$pH - pK_a = \log_{10}\frac{[B]}{[BH^+]} = \log_{10}\frac{[\text{Unionised}]}{[\text{Ionised}]}$$

A base exists predominantly as the ionised form at pH $<pK_a$ and in the unionised form when pH >pKa. Rearrangement of the Henderson-Hasselbalch equation gives the expressions for the fraction of unionised drug as a function of pH and pKa:

$$F_n = \frac{10^{pH - pKa}}{1 + 10^{pH - pKa}} \text{ for a base and}$$

$$F_n = \frac{10^{pKa - pH}}{1 + 10^{pKa - pH}} \text{ for an acid.}$$

These are shown graphically in Figure 2.1.

Ion trapping

Ionisation determines the partitioning of drugs across membranes. Unionised molecules can easily cross and reach an equilibrium across a membrane, while the ionised form cannot cross. When the pH is different in the compartments separated by the membrane the total (ionised + unionised) concentration will be different on each side. An acidic drug will become concentrated in a compartment with a high pH and a basic drug in one with a low pH. This is known as ion-trapping, and occurs in the stomach, kidneys, and across the placenta. Urinary acidification accelerates the excretion of weak bases, such as pethidine, while alkalinisation increases the excretion of acidic drugs, such as aspirin. As an example consider pethidine (pKa 8.6) with an unbound plasma concentration of 100 (arbitrary units). At pH 7.4 only 6% of the pethidine will be unionised so that at equilibrium the concentration of unionised pethidine in the urine will be 6 units. In urine at pH 6.5 only 0.8% of the pethidine will be unionised so that the total concentration in the urine will be 744 units.

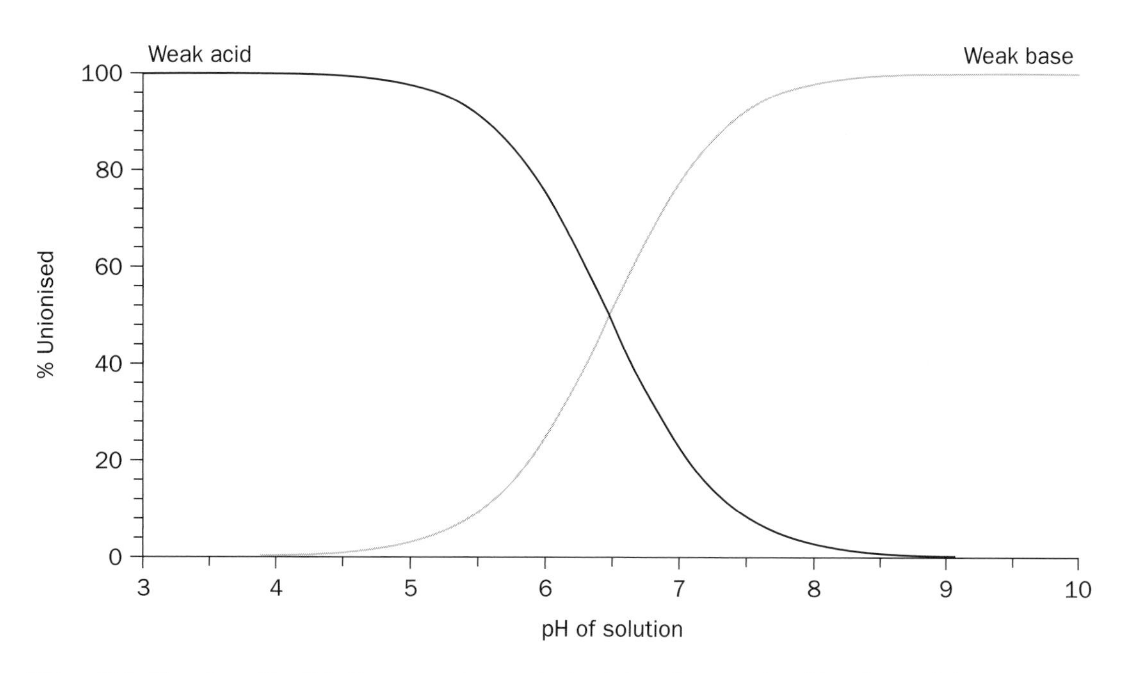

Figure 2.1 *Changes with pH in the percentage unionised drug for a weak acid and a weak base.*

This illustrates the potential for increasing the excretion of pethidine. In reality, less than this theoretical amount will be excreted since equilibrium is not reached due to continuing urine flow.

Protein binding

Most drugs are bound to plasma proteins. Acidic drugs tend to have a high affinity for albumin while basic drugs have a high affinity for lipoproteins and α_1-acid glycoprotein (AAG). AAG is an acute phase reactant whose concentration is raised as a response to trauma, myocardial infarction, malignancy and inflammatory diseases, such as ulcerative colitis and rheumatoid arthritis. The degree of protein binding is expressed as the percentage of the drug that is bound to plasma proteins. The free fraction is the ratio of the concentration of free (unbound) drug to the total (free and bound) concentration. Most drug assays measure total drug concentration.

The rate of diffusion of a drug to the site of action, and thus its effect, is proportional to the free drug concentration, not the total concentration. The binding reaction is usually reversible. In tissues where the concentration of free drug is low, the drug–protein complex dissociates. For most drugs, the concentration resulting from therapeutic doses is much lower than the binding capacity of plasma proteins, so that the bound fraction is independent of the drug concentration. For some drugs, e.g. warfarin, tolbutamide, aspirin, and some sulphonamides, binding sites approach saturation at therapeutic concentrations. For them, a relatively small increase in total concentration can result in a disproportionate increase in unbound drug and consequently therapeutic effect or toxicity. When two or more drugs of this type, e.g. aspirin and warfarin, are given concurrently, they will compete for scarce binding sites and the unbound fraction of both will be increased. The consequences of these disturbances will usually only be significant for drugs which are highly protein-bound. For example, for a drug that is only 40% bound, a 20% decrease in binding capacity will increase the unbound fraction from 60% to 68%, an increase of 11%. For a drug that is 95% bound the concentration of free drug will increase from 5% to 24%, an increase of 480%. However, the extra 'free' drug will be 'diluted' in the body water so that the increase in free drug concentration will be less than expected. The net result is to mitigate the consequences of the initial displacement reaction.

LIPID SOLUBILITY

Since cell membranes are lipid structures lipid solubility plays an important role in drug transport across these membranes. The lipid solubility of a drug is determined by several factors, including chemical structure. The poor lipid solubility of morphine is related to the presence of two hydroxyl (–OH) groups that confer polar characteristics to the molecule. Polar molecules have poor lipid solubility. Substitution of the hydroxyl groups with acetyl ($CH_3.CO.O–$) groups produces diamorphine (heroin), a non-polar, lipid-soluble drug. In the laboratory, lipid solubility is estimated by measuring the partitioning of a drug between an organic solvent and an aqueous buffer phase. Unfortunately, there is no organic solvent that fully resembles cell membranes, but good correlations are found between rates of passage across biological membranes and partitioning into non-polar solvents, such as *n*-octanol or *n*-heptane. The measurements are made first at a pH at which the drug will be fully ionised, e.g. pH 2 for bases and then at a pH at which the drug will be fully unionised (pH 10). At any intermediate pH, when the drug will be partially ionised, lipid solubility can be calculated by the formula:

$$\lambda = \frac{1}{1 + 10^{\mathrm{pH-pKa}}} \cdot \lambda_i + \frac{1}{1 + 10^{\mathrm{pKa-pH}}} \cdot \lambda_{ni}$$

where λ is the partition coefficient at the chosen pH and λ_i and λ_{ni} are the partition coefficients of the fully ionised and fully unionised drug.

DRUG ABSORPTION

When a drug is given intravenously, all the drug immediately enters the systemic circulation (the drug is 100% *bioavailable*). However, for administration by other routes, bioavailability to the systemic circulation is potentially slower, less complete and less predictable. Bioavailability is measured by administering the same dose of the drug, on separate occasions, orally and intravenously and measuring plasma concentrations. The bioavailability is given by:

$$\text{Bioavailability} = \frac{AUC_{oral}}{AUC_{IV}} \times 100\%$$

where AUC_{oral} and AUC_{IV} are the areas under the respective concentration–time curves.

Enteral

Many drugs given orally are susceptible to degradation or modification at the low pH in the stomach. Absorption from the stomach is notoriously variable and is highly dependent on the way in which a drug is formulated. Acidic drugs will be completely unionised at gastric pH (2–3) and readily absorbed whereas basic drugs will be predominantly ionised and are poorly absorbed from the stomach. In the small intestine, where the pH is 6–7, basic drugs will be better absorbed than acidic drugs. After absorption through the gastric or intestinal mucosa, drugs pass via the portal vein to the liver. For drugs that undergo extensive hepatic metabolism, only a proportion of the drug presented to the liver will enter the systemic circulation. This is known as *first pass* or *presystemic metabolism*. Alternative routes, such as sublingual, rectal or transdermal, avoid presystemic metabolism.

Sublingual

The sublingual surface area is relatively small but has a rich blood supply. The major advantage of this route is avoidance of intestinal destruction and hepatic first pass metabolism. However, absorption can be highly variable; critical factors are the residence time of the drug in the mouth and saliva flow. Premature swallowing or excessive saliva production preclude efficient absorption. Nitroglycerin, nifedipine, propranolol, and buprenorphine are all available as sublingual preparations.

Rectal

The venous drainage of the lower part of the rectum drains directly into the systemic venous system. Drugs given rectally can thus partly avoid hepatic first pass metabolism. The rectal route is valuable for drugs which cause gastric irritation or erosions, e.g. non-steroidal anti-inflammatory analgesics (NSAIDs), or in patients with nausea and vomiting. To facilitate rectal absorption drugs must be formulated either as a suppository, a gelatine capsule, or as an enema.

Transdermal

Transdermal delivery is suitable for small, generally lipophilic, potent molecules that require low input rates to achieve effective plasma concentrations. There may be a slow rate of increase of concentration if the drug forms a depot in the skin. Depot formation will also result in a slow decrease in concentration when the system is removed from the skin. These disadvantages can be overcome by the use of iontophoresis, by which the molecules are actively carried across the skin by a small electrical current. This provides a faster and more controllable transfer of drug.

Intramuscular/Subcutaneous

The capillary walls in subcutaneous tissues and muscle offer little impedence to drug absorption, even for drugs that are polar and ionised. For example, gentamycin, which is water-soluble and ionised is poorly absorbed from the gastrointestinal tract but is rapidly and completely absorbed after intramuscular injection. The rate of absorption of drug from muscular or subcutaneous tissues is, however, heavily dependent on regional blood flow. A patient who is peripherally vasoconstricted due to hypovolaemia or hypothermia will absorb drug poorly when administered intramuscularly or subcutaneously, e.g. one needs to be careful when administering morphine by this route to a patient in shock. Absorption can be deliberately slowed by dissolving the drug in an emulsion or converting water-soluble drugs into water insoluble complexes, e.g. insulin–zinc complexes. These sustained release forms have a smoother onset and longer duration of action, avoiding the necessity and discomfort of repeated injections.

Inhalation

The alveolar–capillary membrane is normally very thin, has a huge surface area, and a large blood supply. Drugs given by this route, such as bronchodilators and pulmonary steroids, are rapidly absorbed into the bloodstream. This is also the route for administering the inhalational anaesthetics.

DRUG METABOLISM AND EXCRETION

The principal objective of drug metabolism is to make a drug available for excretion by urine or bile. The renal and biliary systems can excrete water-soluble molecules, whereas water-insoluble drugs must first be converted to a soluble form before they can be excreted. Drug metabolism, therefore, is principally, but not exclusively, of importance for drugs that are non-polar. Metabolism usually results in inactivation of the drug but there are exceptions, e.g. diazepam is metabolised to an active metabolite desmethyldiazepam, which has a much longer duration of action than the parent compound.

The liver is the principal site of drug metabolism. Hepatic drug metabolism is usually classified into two distinct phases. *Phase I* reactions are oxidation, reduction or hydrolysis. One of the most important systems that catalyse oxidation are the haem-containing cytochrome P-450 enzymes. *Phase II* reactions consist of a conjugation reaction, i.e. attachment of a substituent group, to either the parent molecule or the product of phase I metabolism. The most common substituents are glucuronic acid, glycine, glutamine, sulphate or acetate. Conjugates are more water-soluble than the parent compound and thus can be removed by renal or biliary excretion. For some drugs, e.g. morphine, phase II conjugation is the primary means of biotransformation.

Excretion

When a drug or its metabolite is rendered suitably polar it is usually excreted either in the urine or in the bile. Renal excretion occurs either by filtration at the glomerulus, by secretion into the proximal tubule or by diffusion into the distal tubule. Glomerular filtration is a passive process that permits free passage of non protein-bound drugs or drug metabolites into the tubular lumen. Drugs that are non-polar at the pH of the urine tend to be reabsorbed in the proximal tubule whereas polar compounds are 'trapped' within the tubule and excreted into the urine. Proximal tubular secretion, on the other hand, is an active process involving carrier systems. Competition between drugs for the carrier transport mechanisms is used therapeutically. For example probenacid prolongs the duration of action of penicillin by competing for a common secretory mechanism in the proximal tubule. In the distal tubule, diffusion is the principal mechanism whereby non-polar drugs are either secreted into or reabsorbed from the tubular lumen. The pH of the urine influences the reasorption of drugs since this determines the degree of ionisation.

Biliary excretion is of major importance for the excretion of drugs and metabolites that are predominantly ionised, e.g. muscle relaxants or antibiotics. Some drugs that are excreted in the bile as conjugates may subsequently be reabsorbed from the bowel following hydrolysis by bacterial flora in the bowel lumen (*enterohepatic recirculation*).

DRUG DISPOSITION

Most drugs have linear pharmacokinetics, i.e. the rate of decrease at any time is directly proportional to the amount present at that time; this is known as a 'first order' process. Such a process is termed *exponential decay*. First order exponential processes for a simple one-compartment system can be expressed mathematically as:

$$C(t) = C_0 e^{-kt}$$

where $C(t)$ is the concentration of drug at time t, C_0 is the concentration at time $t = 0$, and k is a constant known as the rate constant. During any period equal to one *half-life* ($t_{1/2}$) the drug concentration falls to half the value at the beginning of the period. A half-life has units of time and thus is easier to visualise than rate constants, which have units of reciprocal time, e.g. $\min^{-1}$. Taking logarithms of both sides in the equation above and rearranging gives:

$$t = \frac{1}{k} \ln\left(\frac{C}{C_0}\right).$$

When $C(t)$ is half C_0 then $t = t_{1/2}$ and $C/C_0 = \frac{1}{2}$, so that:

$$t_{\frac{1}{2}} = \frac{\ln 2}{k} = \frac{0.693}{k}.$$

Half-life is a composite parameter depending on the efficiency of drug elimination (Cl) and its distribution volume (V_D). For a one-compartment system,

$$t_{\frac{1}{2}} = \ln.2 * \frac{V_D}{Cl}.$$

Thus, as Cl increases, the half-life will decrease and an increase in the volume of distribution, e.g. in the elderly, will increase half-life.

Non-linear pharmacokinetics

Non-linear pharmacokinetics are much less common than linear kinetics. They occur when drug concentrations are sufficiently high to saturate the ability of the liver enzymes to metabolise the drug. This occurs with ethanol, therapeutic concentrations of phenytoin and salicylates, or when high doses of barbiturates are used for cerebral protection. The kinetics of conventional doses of thiopentone are linear. With non-linear pharmacokinetics, the amount of drug eliminated per unit time is constant rather than a constant fraction of the amount in the body, as is the case for the linear situation. Non-linear kinetics are also referred to as zero order or saturation kinetics. The rate of drug decline is governed by the Michaelis-Menton equation:

$$dC/dt = -\frac{V_m \cdot C}{K_m + C}$$

where dC/dt is the rate of decline in concentration, V_m is the theoretical maximum rate of elimination, and K_m is the Michaelis constant, which is equal to the concentration at which dC/dt is half V_m. When C is much smaller than K_m the equation reduces to:

$$\frac{dC}{dt} = -\frac{V_m}{K_m} C$$

which is the equation of first order elimination, equivalent to the post-distributive or terminal phase in a multicompartment linear model. When C is considerably greater than K_m the equation reduces to:

$$\frac{dC}{dt} = -V_m$$

and the rate of elimination is constant and independent of drug concentration (Figure 2.2).

Compartmental pharmacokinetic models

Compartmental models are commonly used in pharmacokinetics to explain drug disposition.

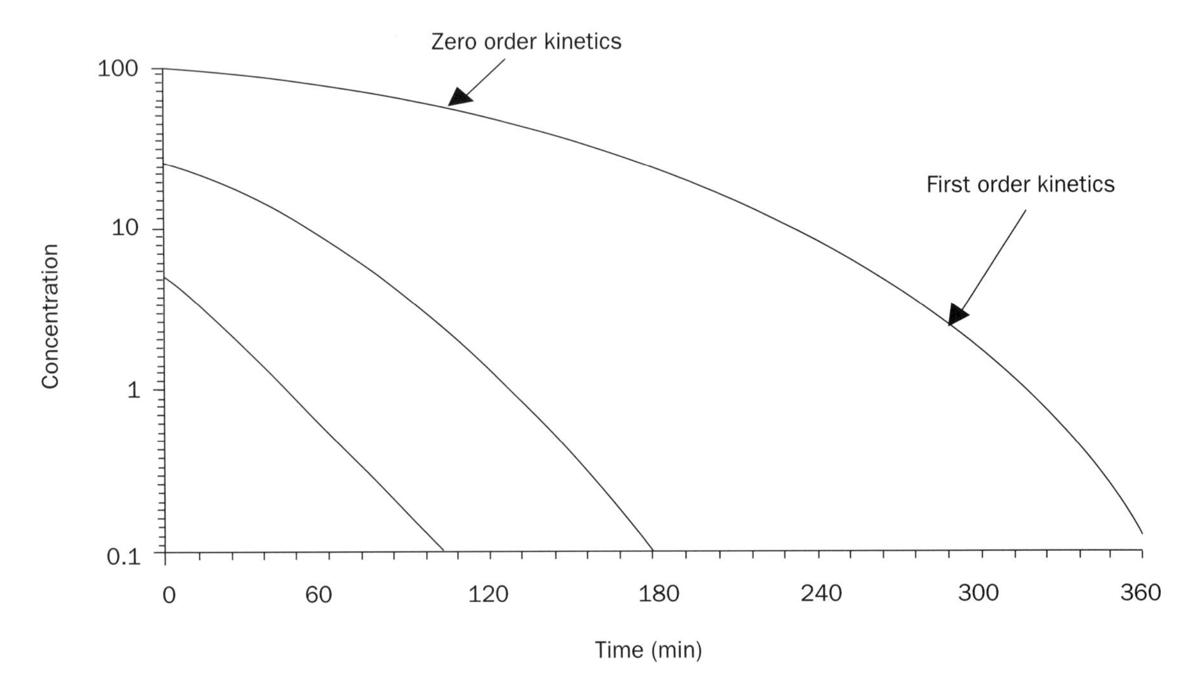

Figure 2.2 *Changes in drug concentration following three oral doses of a drug that exhibits non-linear pharmacokinetics.*

The models consist of interconnected compartments, with the drug moving between them at rates proportional to the concentration gradient, i.e. a first order process. A model with only one compartment describes the behaviour of few substances, e.g. indocyanine green and possibly warfarin, that are almost totally confined to the circulation and do not diffuse into the tissues. For most drugs, two or three compartments are required to adequately describe their disposition.

If we measure the plasma concentration of a drug following administration as a rapid intravenous bolus the data will follow a polyexponential curve (Figure 2.3). This can be modelled by assuming that the body consists of several interconnecting compartments, with drug being administered into and eliminated from a central compartment (Figure 2.4). For drugs that are metabolised in the blood and tissues, such as atracurium or remifentanil, the model can be adapted to allow elimination from one of the peripheral compartments. An underlying assumption of simple compartmental models is that the compartments are well-stirred and homogenous so that there is instantaneous mixing of the administered drug. Although this never happens in reality the model is nonetheless useful. More complex models are needed to account for non-instantaneous mixing, lung retention, and other effects.

From the moment that a drug is introduced into the body two simultaneous processes begin, distribution and elimination. Distribution refers to the transfer along concentration gradients between the central and the peripheral compartments. The rates of drug distribution between the compartments is given by the intercompartment transfer rate constants, $k_{i,j}$, where the subscripts give the direction of drug movement, i.e. from compartment i to compartment j. The rate constants havee dimensions of reciprocal time (min^{-1} or h^{-1}) and express the fractional change in concentration per unit time. Thus if the amount of drug in compartment 1 is X then $X \cdot k_{12}$ of drug will leave compartment 1 for compartment 2 per unit time. Applying the conservation principle

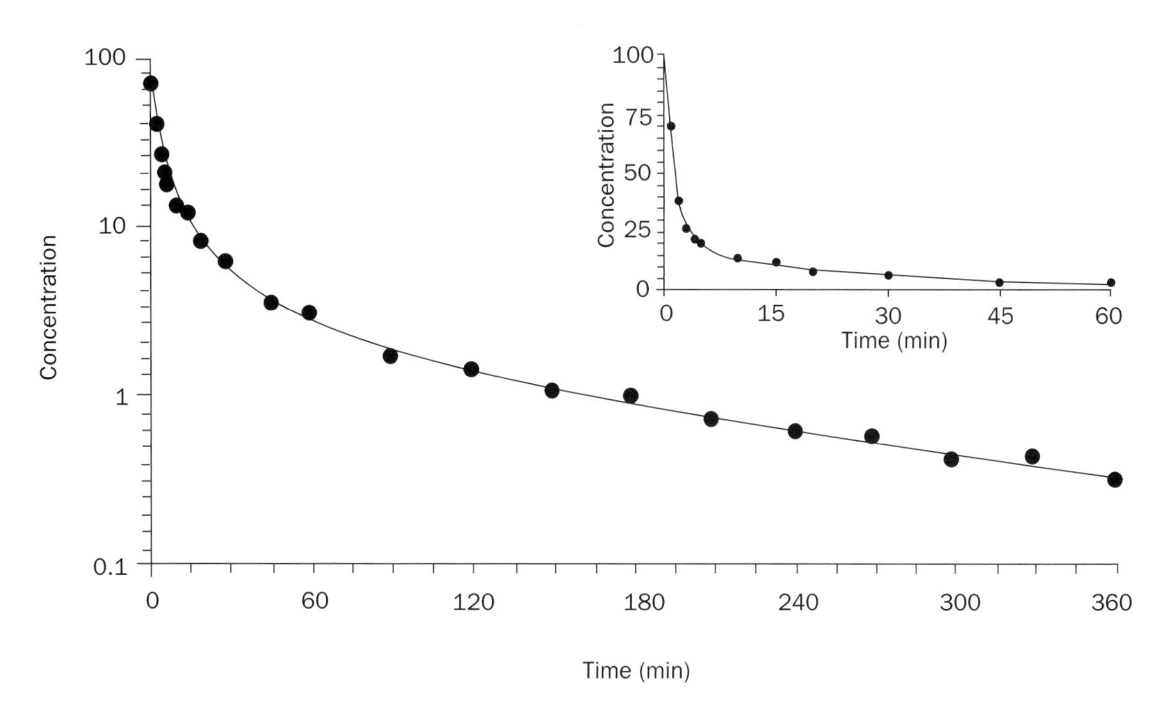

Figure 2.3 *Plot of concentration against time for a drug with polyexponential characteristics. The closed circles represent measured concentrations and the solid line the fitted polyexponential model. The main plot has a semi-logarithmic concentration axis, the insert shows the same data plotted on a linear scale.*

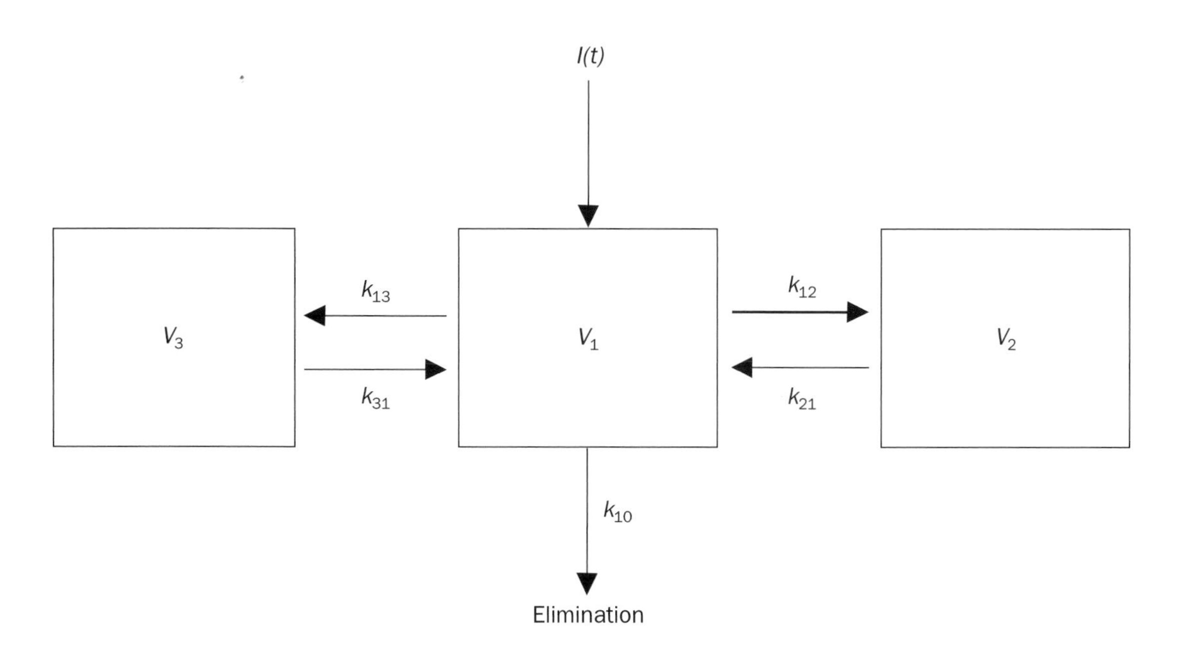

Figure 2.4 *Schematic of a three-compartment model.*

(rate in minus rate out equals rate of change of content), the rate of change of drug in each compartment can be described by a series of simultaneous differential equations (2 or 3 equations depending on whether there are two or three compartments in the model). For the three-compartment model these are:

$$\frac{dX_1}{dt} = -(k_{12} + k_{13} + k_{10})\, X_1 + k_{21}\, X_2 + k_{31}\, X_3 + I(t)$$

$$\frac{dX_2}{dt} = -k_{21}\, X_2 + k_{12}\, X_1$$

$$\frac{dX_3}{dt} = -k_{31}\, X_3 + k_{13}\, X_1$$

$I(t)$ is the input function; for a single bolus dose it equals the dose only at $t = 0$, at all other times $I(t) = 0$. The solution of these equations leads to a tri-exponential equation describing how the concentration of drug in the central compartment changes with time.

$$C(t) = Ae^{-\alpha t} + Be^{-\beta t} + Ce^{-\gamma t} \qquad (1)$$

For a two-compartment model C = 0 and the equation is bi-exponential. The exponents α, β and γ are related to the intercompartmental transfer rate constants by complex formulae. They are related to the half-lives for each of the distribution and terminal phases by the relationship:

$$t^{\alpha}_{\frac{1}{2}} = \frac{0.693}{\alpha};\; t^{\beta}_{\frac{1}{2}} = \frac{0.693}{\beta};\; t^{\gamma}_{\frac{1}{2}} = \frac{0.693}{\gamma}.$$

Note that the terminal rate constant, γ, is not the same as the elimination transfer rate, k_{10}.

As time progresses each of the three exponential terms in this equation decreases. However, since by definition $\alpha > \beta > \gamma$, the first two terms will decrease faster than the third term and at some time will approach zero and the equation reduces to $C(t) = Ce^{-\gamma t}$. If the decay curve is plotted on semilogarithmic axes (concentration logarithmic, time linear) this post-distribution phase will be a straight line, with zero time intercept 'C' and slope $-\gamma$. Subtracting ('stripping') this terminal portion from the rest of the curve leaves a bi-exponential curve from which, by the same processes, we can obtain B and β. Repeating the process yields estimates for A and α (Figure 2.5). For obvious reasons this process is referred to as curve stripping or the method of residuals. Note, however, that the results of graphical stripping will only yield rough estimates, that can then be used as starting estimates for a non-linear regression program, which will produce more accurate value of the parameters.

Volumes of distribution and clearance

Clearance (Cl) and volumes of distribution (V_D) are fundamental concepts in pharmacokinetics. Clearance is defined as the volume of plasma or blood cleared of the drug per unit time, and has the dimensions of volume per unit time (e.g. $mL \cdot min^{-1}$ or $L \cdot h^{-1}$). An alternative, and theoretically more useful, definition is the rate of drug elimination per unit drug concentration, and equals the product of the elimination constant and the volume of the compartment. The clearance from the central compartment is thus $V_1 \cdot k_{10}$. Since $e^0 = 1$, at $t = 0$ equation 1 reduces to $C(0) = A + B + C$, which is the initial concentration in V_1. Hence, $V_1 = \text{Dose}/(A + B + C)$. The clearance between compartments in one direction must equal the clearance in the reverse direction, i.e. $V_1 \cdot k_{12} = V_2 \cdot k_{21}$ and $V_1 \cdot k_{13} = V_3 \cdot k_{31}$. This enables us to calculate V_2 and V_3.

$$V_2 = \frac{V_1 \cdot k_{12}}{k_{21}};\; V_3 = \frac{V_1 \cdot k_{13}}{k_{31}}$$

Clearance can be calculated from the area under the concentration–time curve (AUC; area under the curve) following bolus administration; $Cl = \text{Dose}/\text{AUC}$. This can be used for any form of intravenous administration and does not rely on compartmental analysis.

The volume of distribution of a drug can be considered as the sum of the volumes of all the tissues into which it becomes distributed. A few compounds, such as indocyanine green, are tightly bound to plasma proteins and are there-

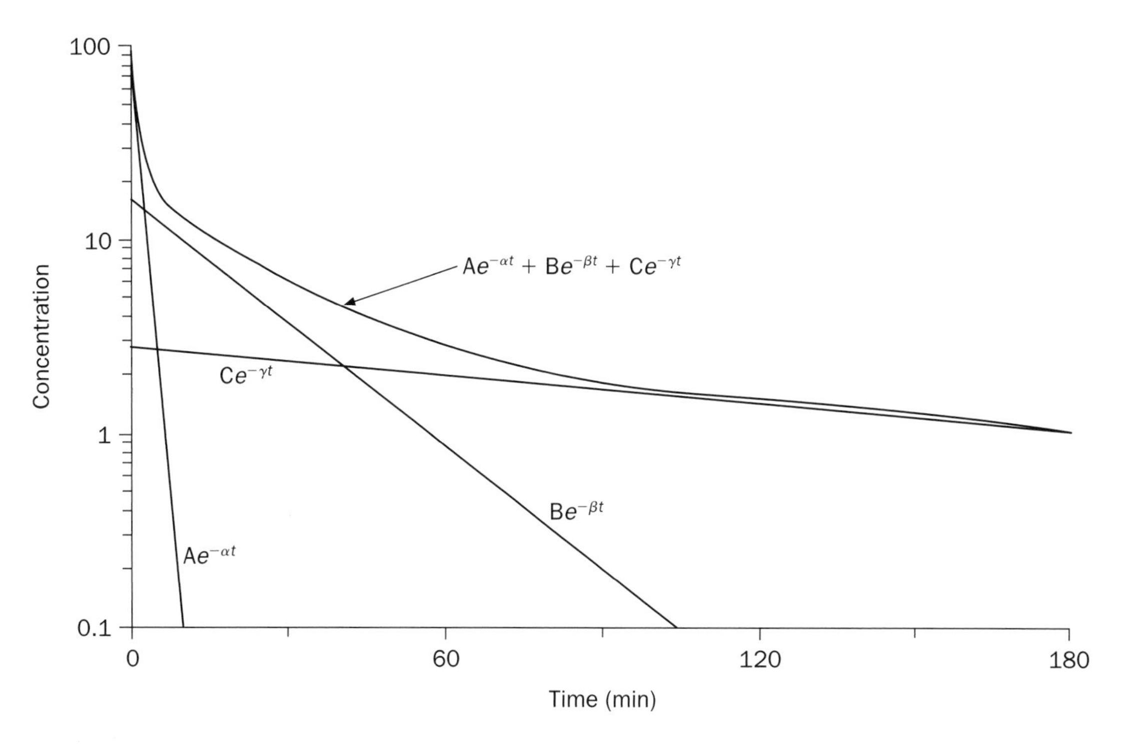

Figure 2.5 *Plasma concentration decay (semilogarithmic plot) of a drug with three compartment characteristics, illustrating that the disposition equation,* $C(t) = Ae^{-\alpha t} + Be^{-\beta t} + Ce^{-\gamma t}$, *is the sum of three exponential functions, with y-axis intercepts A, B, and C, and slopes* $-\alpha$, $-\beta$, *and* $-\gamma$.

fore confined to the circulating blood. They thus distribute into a space that corresponds to the plasma volume. Highly polar drugs, such as some non-depolarising muscle relaxants, are largely confined to the extracellular water (approximately 12 L for a 70 kg individual) and the drug will be diluted by this volume. However, if the volume in which a non-polar drug is evenly dispersed is simply considered as the amount of drug in the body divided by the concentration, one arrives at a volume of distribution that for many drugs is considerably in excess of total body volume. For example, the V_D of propofol is 200–700 litres. The reason for this is that drugs bind to proteins not only in the blood but even more extensively in the tissues. This bound drug is effectively 'lost' when one measures volume, and for this reason the calculated volume is referred to as an *apparent volume of distribution*, i.e. a hypothetical volume into which a drug would have to be dispersed to produce the observed blood concentration.

The apparent volume of distribution allows one to estimate the amount of drug in the body at any time after administration based on the concentration (amount = concentration × volume). If the plasma concentration of a drug with a V_D of 500 litres is 10 ng·mL^{-1}, the amount in the body will be 500 000 mL X·10 ng or 5 mg. Most pharmacokinetic texts describe several volumes of distribution, e.g. V_{Darea} and V_{DSS}. Following a single rapid intravenous injection, V_{Darea} can be calculated by:

$$V_{Darea} = \frac{\text{Dose}}{\text{AUC} \cdot \gamma} = \frac{Cl}{\gamma}$$

(remember Cl = Dose/AUC). This definition is clearly dependent on clearance and indeed is only a true measure of distribution volume when Cl is zero. For this reason V_{DSS}, the volume of distribution at steady state, is preferred since it avoids the use of distribution-sensitive terms. V_{DSS} is simply the sum of the individual compartment volumes:

$$V_{DSS} = V_1 + V_2 + V_3.$$

This definition remains model-dependent, but V_{DSS} can be calculated using a non-compartmental approach, which does not require any assumptions about the pharmacokinetic model concerned (see below).

Despite the lack of anatomical identity the concept of apparent volume of distribution does have value. It can be considered as the volume from which a drug must be cleared. Thus, for a drug with a large V_D, the plasma concentration during the terminal phase will decline slower than one with a smaller V_D and similar clearance. This can be seen by rearranging the equation above:

$$T^{\gamma}\tfrac{1}{2} = \frac{\ln 2}{\gamma} = \frac{\ln 2 \cdot V_D}{Cl}$$

V_{SS} is directly proportional to the free fraction in the plasma (f_p) and indirectly proportional to the free fraction of the drug in the tissues (f_t) according to the formula:

$$V_{SS} = V_p + V_t\left[\frac{f_p}{f_t}\right]$$

where V_p and V_t are the respective plasma and tissues volumes. The greater the degree of protein binding, the less of the drug will be available to leave the plasma space and hence the smaller the volume of distribution will be. Drugs that are highly bound to plasma proteins but less bound to tissue ($f_P/f_t > 1$) have volumes of distributions that are greater than plasma volume but less than the volume of total body water. Conversely, for drugs that are more extensively tissue bound than plasma bound ($f_P/f_t < 1$) V_{SS} will be greater than the volume of total body water. For alfentanil, which has high protein binding (91%) and moderate lipid solubility and therefore low tissue binding, V_{SS} is about 30 litres. By contrast, for fentanyl, which is less protein bound (85%) and highly lipophilic, V_{SS} is of the order of 300–400 litres.

Intravenous infusions

By setting the input function, $I(t)$, in the differential equations on p. 28 to a constant rather than zero the equations can be solved to yield the disposition function for an intravenous infusion. With a fixed rate infusion, the plasma concentration will gradually increase towards a steady state concentration, C_{SS}. Since C_{SS} is constant, the amount of drug entering the body via the infusion at steady state must equal that being eliminated, (i.e. the clearance). Thus the infusion rate, R, e.g. mg min^{-1}, needed to reach C_{SS} is $R = C_{SS} \cdot Cl$. It will take approximately 4 to 5 terminal half-lives to reach 95% C_{SS}. Note that if the infusion rate is doubled C_{SS} will also double, but the time taken to reach C_{SS} remains the same, i.e. it is independent of the infusion rate (Figure 2.6).

The rate of decline in plasma concentration after stopping an intravenous infusion is not the same as after a bolus injection of the same drug. With a single bolus the peripheral compartments are initially empty so that the drug can rapidly distribute into them from the central compartment. During an infusion the peripheral compartments gradually fill up so that when the infusion is stopped the contribution made by distribution to the fall in plasma concentration will be correspondingly less (Figure 2.7). To use engineering terminology, the peripheral compartment acts as a 'sink'. When the plasma concentration falls below that in the peripheral compartment the latter will then act as a 'source', releasing the drug slowly back into the plasma, slowing the decline in concentration.

The time needed to reach C_{SS} is one of the few instances where the concept of a half-life is useful in anaesthesia. Strictly speaking, the concept of half-life is only applicable to a drug which can be represented by a one-compartment model, when plasma concentrations will decline mono-exponentially. For drugs that

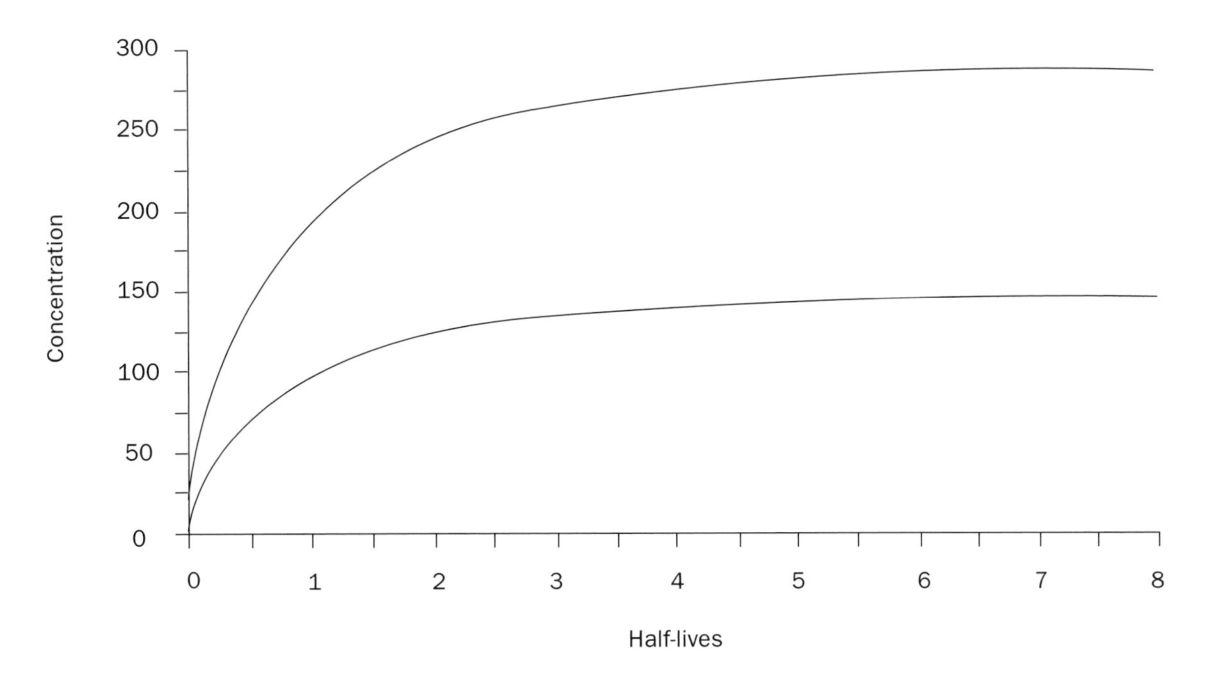

Figure 2.6 *Changes in plasma concentration during two fixed-rate intravenous infusions. The infusion rate producing the upper curve is double the rate for the lower curve. Note that the time to reach C_{SS} does not depend on the infusion rate.*

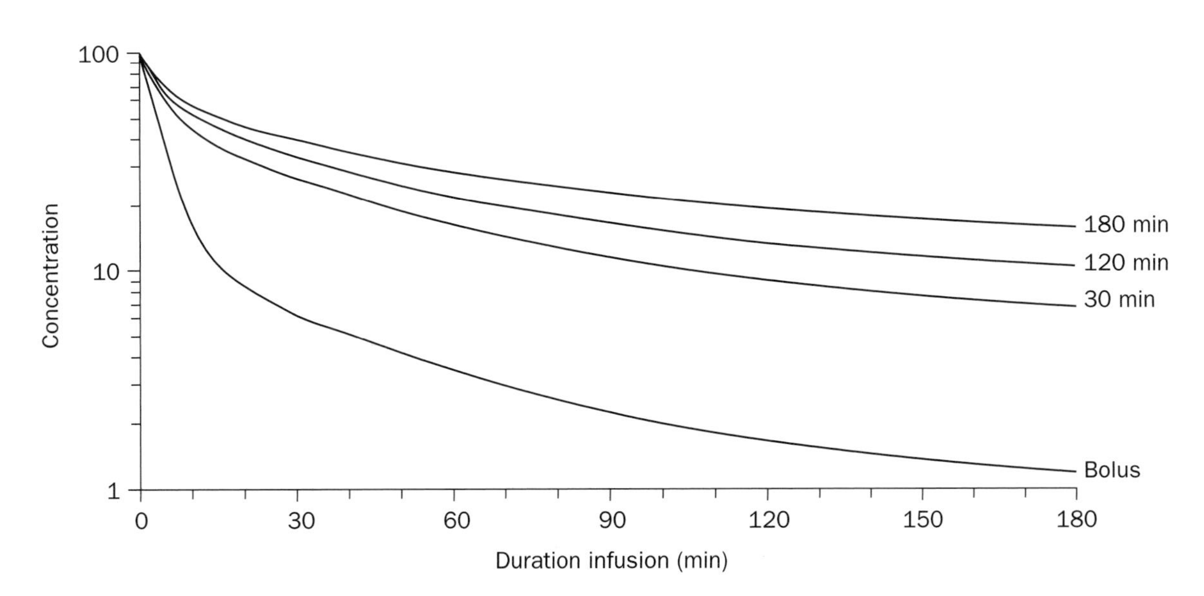

Figure 2.7 *Decline in the plasma concentration following cessation of intravenous infusions of different durations. The plasma concentrations at termination of the infusion have been normalised to 100.*

confer multicompartment characteristics, two or more half-lives may be calculated. Half-lives provide virtually no insight about the rate of decline in concentration and thus the conventional clinical interpretation of them as predicting the rate of recovery following drug administration is simplistic and wrong. To overcome the limited clinical usefulness of the elimination half-life for drugs with multi- compartment kinetics, Hughes and co-workers (1992) devised the concept of '*context-sensitive half-time*', the time required for plasma drug concentration to decrease by 50%. Context-sensitive half-time, unlike a half-life, is not a constant but is a function of infusion duration (Figure 2.8). This function represents the complex interactions between the rate constants governing transfer of drugs between the different compartments.

NON-COMPARTMENTAL OR MODEL-INDEPENDENT APPROACHES TO PHARMACOKINETICS

Non-compartmental analysis uses techniques derived from statistical moment theory to

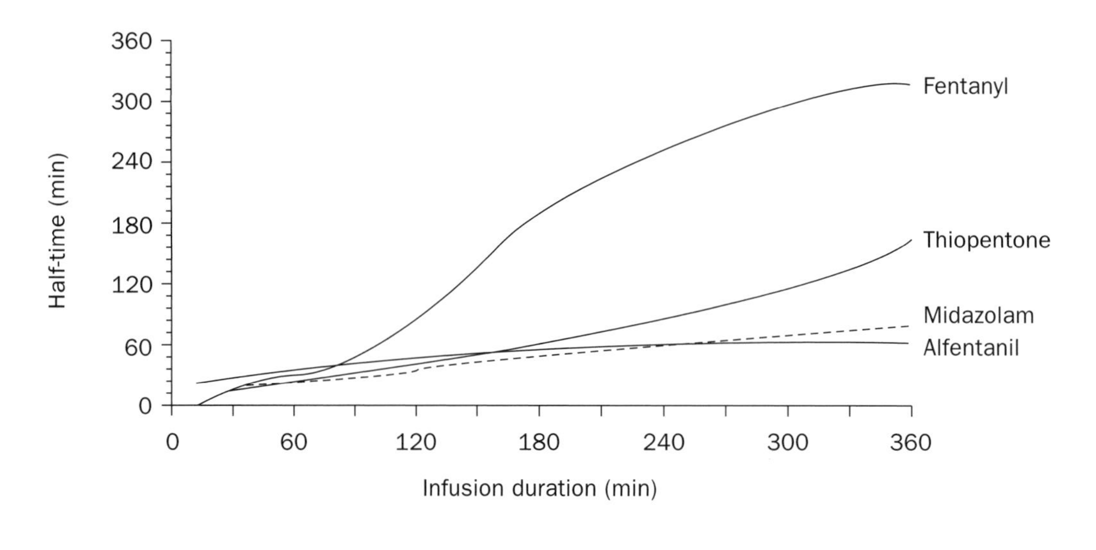

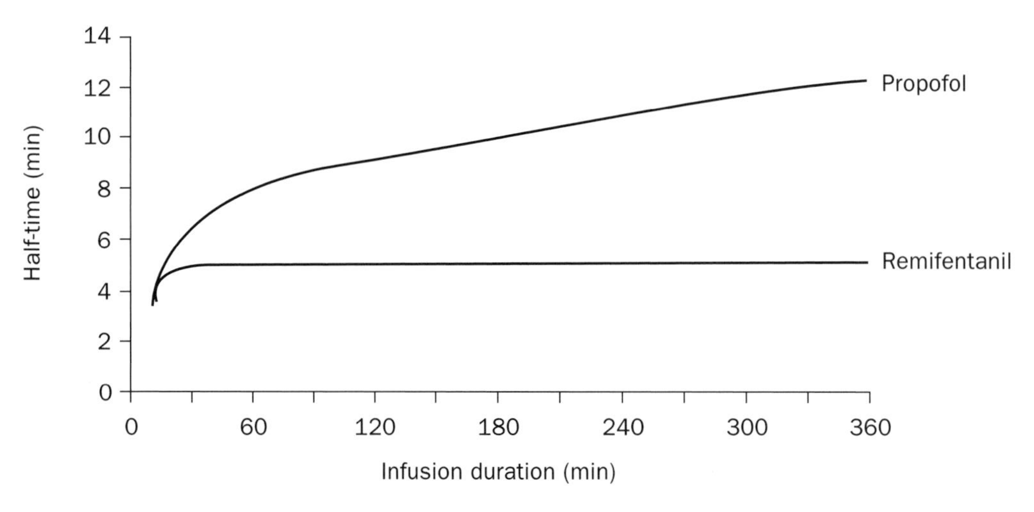

Figure 2.8 *Context-sensitive half-times for some intravenous anaesthetic drugs. Note the different half-time scale for the two panels.*

describe the disposition of a drug in the body. The area under the concentration–time curve (AUC) following a single injection is analogous to the *zero* moment and the area under the curve of $C(t) \cdot t$ against time (AUMC) is analogous to the *first* moment. The ratio AUMC:AUC is the mean residence time (MRT), the average time taken by drug molecules to leave the system. The MRT is equivalent to the time constant of a one-compartment model, and indicates the time taken for 62.5% of a dose to be eliminated from the body, i.e. $t_{\frac{1}{2}} = 0.693 \cdot \text{MRT}$, since concentration decreases by 62.5% in two time constants. The apparent volume of distribution at steady state (V_{SS}) is calculated as $V_{SS} = Cl \cdot \text{MRT}$.

PHARMACODYNAMICS OF DRUG ACTION

Pharmacodynamics deals with the relation between drug concentration (C) and effect (E). The relationship, expressed as a fraction of the maximum effect (E_{max}), is given by the sigmoid E_{max} equation:

$$E = E_{max} \cdot \frac{C^{\gamma}}{C^{\gamma} + EC_{50}^{\gamma}}$$

where γ is a dimensionless parameter that determines the slope of the concentration response curve and EC_{50} is the concentration producing 50% of the maximum effect. Drugs with a high value of γ have steep concentration–response curves. Clinically this means that a small increase in concentration (or a small additional dose) can result in a marked increase in clinical response. While this is of benefit during anaesthesia, in other circumstances it can increase the risk of side effects. A small additional bolus of an opioid in the postoperative period may result in respiratory depression. The graph of the above equation is sigmoid shaped, except when $\gamma = 1$, when it is a rectangular hyperbola. If the graph is redrawn, plotting log concentration against effect, one obtains the traditional sigmoid concentration–response curve (Figure 2.9). Plotting concentrations logarithmically has other advantages. The response to a wide concentration range is more readily displayed, and the relationship between concentration and response is approximately linear between about 25% and 75% of the maximum response. Some drugs have an inhibitory effect, e.g. reduction in heart rate by a β adrenoceptor antagonist. In the inhibitory E_{max} model, the effect of the drug is subtracted from the response when no drug is present (E_0):

$$E = E_0 - E_{max} \cdot \frac{C^{\gamma}}{C^{\gamma} + EC_{50}^{\gamma}}$$

The potency of a drug is characterised by the EC_{50}; the more potent the lower the EC_{50}. Thus, in Figure 2.9 drug A is more potent than drug B. Note that potency is defined as the dependency of effect on concentration. Traditionally, potency has been related to dose rather than concentration, i.e. based on ED_{50} (dose producing 50% of maximum effect). However, the dose–effect relationship involves both pharmacokinetic and pharmacodynamic components, while the concentration–effect relationship involves only pharmacodynamics.

Agonists, partial agonists and antagonists

An agonist is a drug that can cause a maximum response at sufficiently high concentrations (drugs A and B, Figure 2.9). Pure antagonists cause no response at all. Some drugs, termed *partial agonists*, cause responses that are less than that produced by full agonists, even at very high concentrations (drug C, Figure 2.9). Inverse agonists produce opposite effects to those of an agonist. For example, inverse agonists at the benzodiazepine receptor produce anxiety rather than anxiolysis. The degree to which a drug can activate a biological system is characterised by a parameter called 'intrinsic activity' or efficacy. Full agonists have an intrinsic activity value of 1 and partial agonists a value between 0 and 1. An antagonist has high affinity for a receptor but zero intrinsic efficacy.

Partial agonists, because they can compete with agonists (and competitive antagonists),

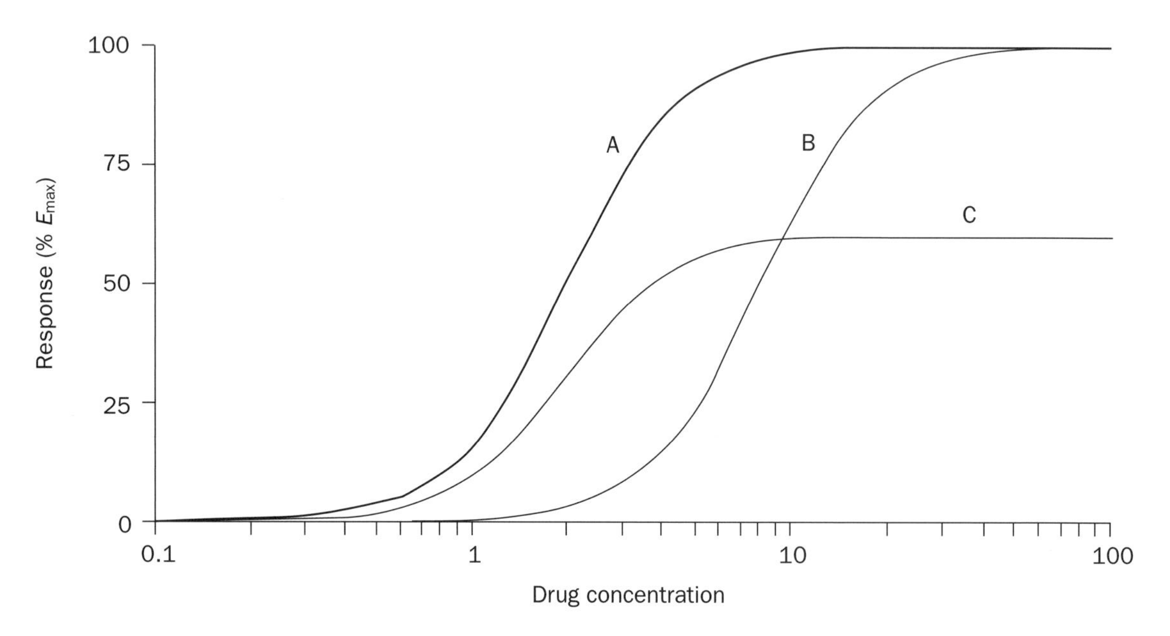

Figure 2.9 *Plasma concentration–response curves for full agonists (A and B) and for a partial agonist (C). Drug A is more potent than drug B (EC_{50} of A is lower than EC_{50} of B).*

can produce either agonist or antagonist effects. In low concentrations they produce agonist effects and in the presence of small concentrations of a full agonist the effect will be additive. When the concentration of the full agonist is high, addition of a partial agonist may displace the full agonist from the receptor. Since the response produced by the partial agonist is less than that of the full agonist, the final effect will be a reduction of the response, and the partial agonist acts as an antagonist (Figure 2.10). For example nalorphine, a partial opioid agonist, can be used to reverse the effects of a full opioid agonist, such as fentanyl.

Antagonists

Reversible competitive antagonism is the most common and most important type of drug antagonism. Competitive antagonists compete with the agonist for receptor binding sites, and are characterised by a progressive shift to the right of the agonist concentration–response curve with increasing concentration of the antagonist, without changing the slope of the curve or the maximum response. Many clinically useful drugs are competitive antagonists of endogenous substances, e.g. atropine and β adrenoceptor antagonists. A non-competitive antagonist prevents the agonist, at any concentration, from producing a maximum effect (Figure 2.11). This may arise from irreversible binding of the antagonist with the receptor, although this is not always the case. An example of a non-competitive, irreversible antagonist is phenoxybenzamine. Since these compounds dissociate only very slowly or not at all from the receptor they often have very prolonged action, and their effects are usually unrelated to their plasma concentration.

PHARMACOKINETIC-PHARMACODYNAMIC MODELS

While drug concentrations are readily measured in blood or plasma, this is not the site of action for most drugs. A drug's pharmacological effect is related to the concentration at its

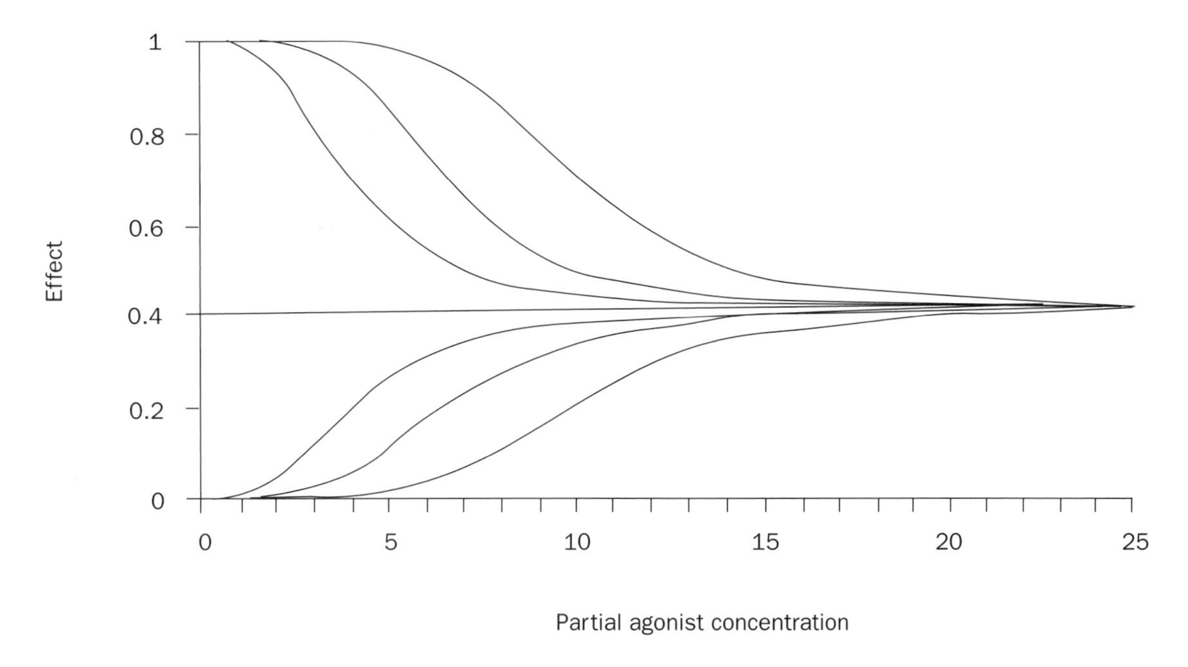

Figure 2.10 *Hypothetical concentration–response (AUC) curves for the combined effects of a partial agonist, with a maximum effect (intrinsic activity) of 0.4, and a full agonist. The lower curve shows the response when increasing concentrations of the partial agonist are added to a low concentration of the full agonist; the combined response increases asymptotically to the* E_{max} *of the partial agonist. When increasing concentrations of the partial agonist are added to a high concentration of the full agonist, the combined response decreases asymptotically to the* E_{max} *of the partial agonist.*

site of action, known as the *effect site* or the *biophase*. Since it takes a finite time for the drug to reach the effect site, there will be a delay between the time course of drug effect and plasma drug concentration. The delay is determined mainly by the drug's physicochemical properties, such as pKa and lipid solubility. The delay can be characterised using pharmacokinetic-pharmacodynamic models, which use mathematical functions to describe the relationship between drug concentration and effect. They use a link between the pharmacodynamic (or effect) response and the pharmacokinetic response by postulating an effect compartment linked to the central compartment by first order processes (Figure 2.12). The effect site compartment has negligible volume (usually taken as 1/1000 or 1/10000 of V_1) and receives only a negligible amount of the drug. This also means that negligible drug returns from the effect compartment to the plasma and thus adding the effect compartment does not change the pharmacokinetic model. The output from the effect compartment is a first order rate constant (k_{e0}) that characterises the temporal aspect of equilibrium between plasma concentration and drug effect. The time course of effect site concentration is a function of k_{e0} and the pharmacokinetic parameters that describe C_p. As for other pharmacokinetic rate constants, k_{e0} can easily be converted to a half-life:

$$t_{\frac{1}{2}}k_{e0} = \frac{\ln 2}{k_{e0}} = \frac{0.693}{k_{e0}}$$

The changes in plasma and effect site concentrations following an intravenous bolus of propofol is shown in Figure 2.13. If the plasma concentration of a drug were instantaneously increased to a higher steady state concentration,

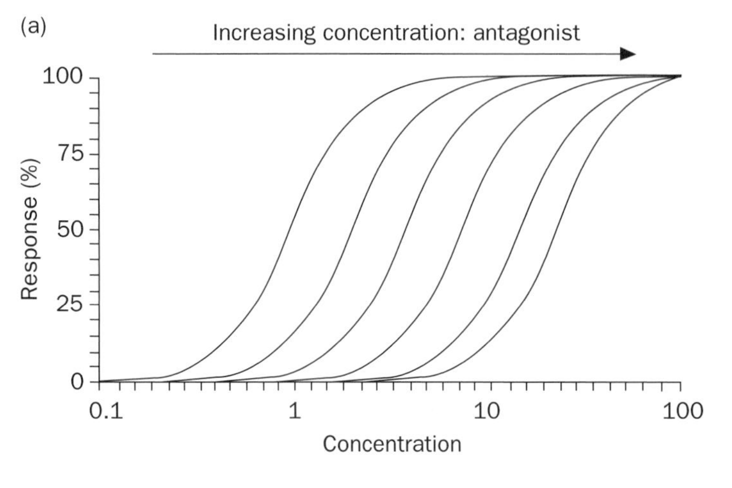

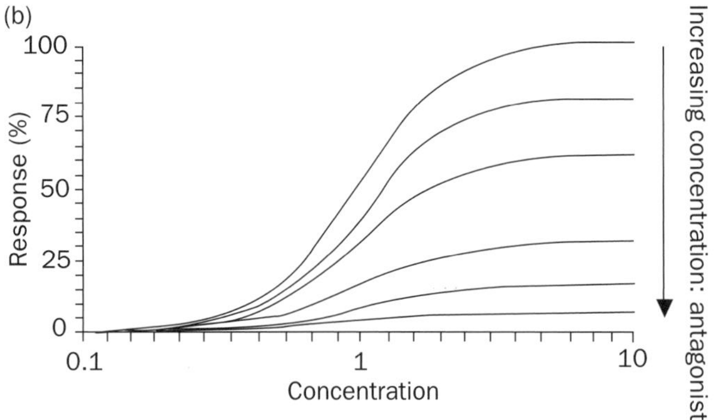

Figure 2.11 *(a) Effect of increasing doses of a competitive and (b) non-competitive antagonist on the concentration–response (AUC) curves of an agonist.*

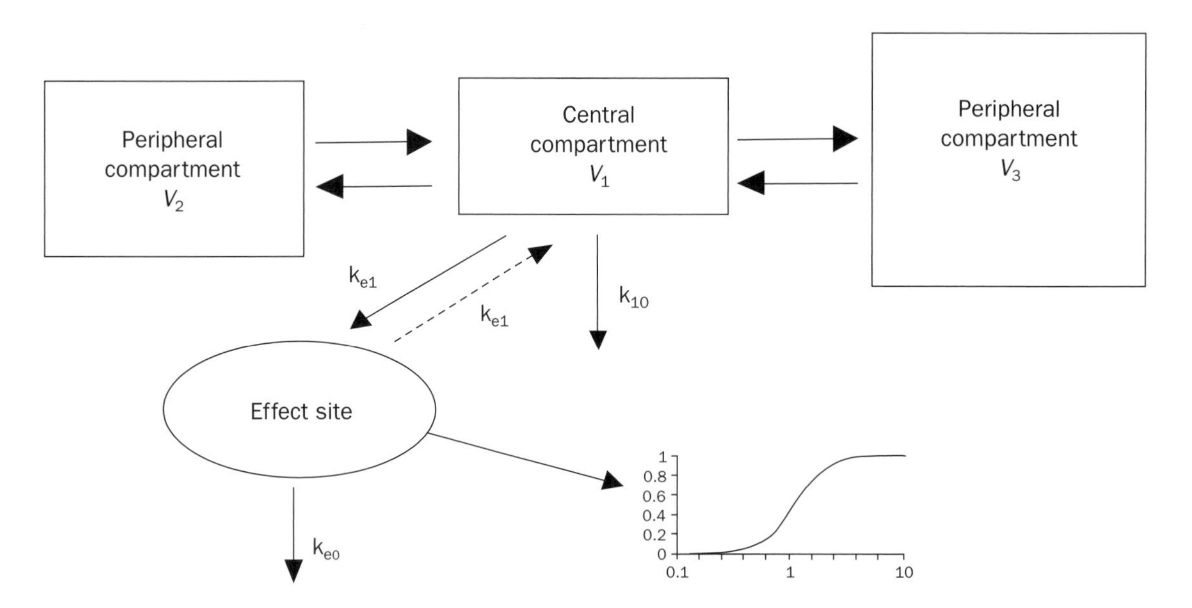

Figure 2.12 *Three-compartment pharmacokinetic model with a linked effect compartment.*

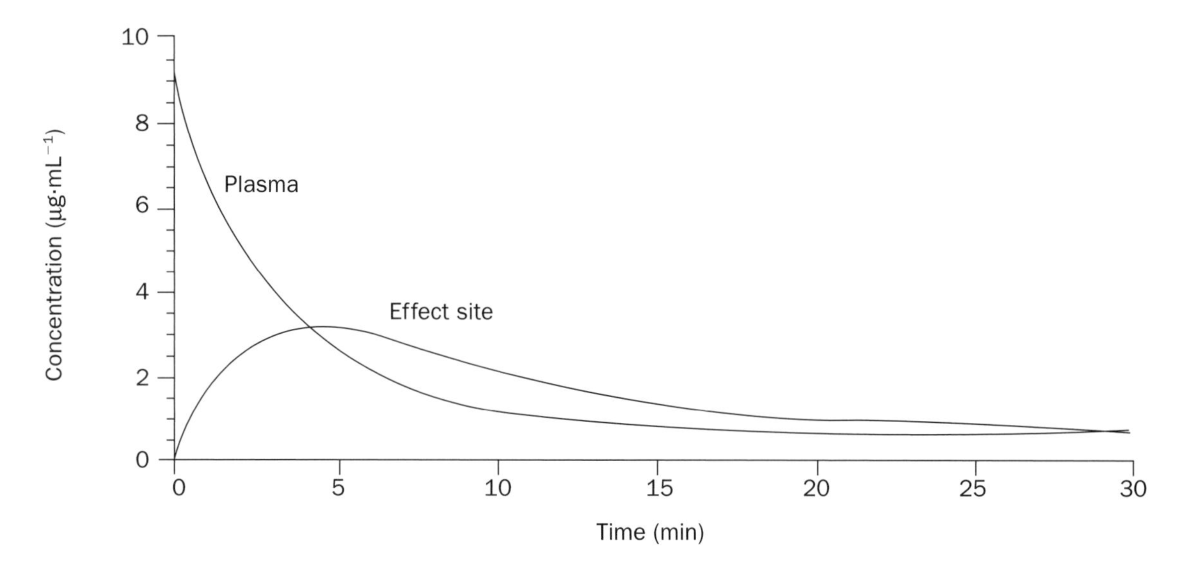

Figure 2.13 *The relationship between plasma (C_p) and effect site concentrations (C_e) following a single intravenous bolus of a drug.*

then it would takes 4–5 times the $t_{1/2}k_{e0}$ for the effect site concentration to reach 90–95% of its steady state concentration. Pharmacokinetic-dynamic models are a powerful tool in pharmacology and their use in the early stages of new drug development has almost become as mandatory as conventional pharmacokinetic analysis.

FURTHER READING

Hughes MA, Glass PS, Jacobs JR. Context-sensitive half-time in multicompartment pharmacokinetic models for intravenous anesthetic drugs. *Anesthesiology* 1992;76:334–41.

3

Inhalational agents

JPH Fee

Introduction • Uptake characteristics • Potency: Minimum alveolar concentration (MAC) • Individual agents • Gases

INTRODUCTION

The era of modern general anaesthesia dawned in 1846 with the first administration of diethyl ether by William Morton to a patient in Massachusetts General Hospital. One year later it was followed by Simpson's demonstration of the effects of chloroform in Edinburgh. Since that time the dominance of the inhalation route of administration as a means of providing general anaesthesia combined with safe control of the airway has not been seriously challenged.

For about one hundred years, and longer in some parts of the world, diethyl ether and chloroform had no rivals. This was despite major drawbacks, the main ones being the flammability and slow onset of diethyl ether, and the hepatotoxicity and cardiac arrhythmias induced by chloroform. New discoveries in organic fluorine chemistry at the end of World War II paved the way for the synthesis of modern fluorinated anaesthetic alkanes and ethers.

A large number of volatile drugs are capable of inducing general anaesthesia but only a small number come near to the 'ideal' (Table 3.1). All modern agents are non-flammable under normal clinical conditions. An in-depth understanding of the uptake characteristics, potency and metabolism of these agents is essential if they are to be administered safely and efficiently. Whilst the pharmacokinetic properties are important, the clinical effects of particular agents are, to a considerable extent, dependent on the skill of the anaesthetist, and the age and condition of the patient. All volatile anaesthetic drugs must be administered through regularly serviced, temperature-compensated vaporisers or injection systems calibrated for low (≤1 litre/minute) and high fresh gas flows. Similarly, gases must be given and stored in accordance with national regulations, including those on environmental pollution, and health and safety.

No volatile anaesthetic drug should be given to a patient with known or suspected malignant hyperpyrexia syndrome.

UPTAKE CHARACTERISTICS

Solubility

All inhaled anaesthetic drugs must be soluble in blood and brain in order to pass across the alveolar–capillary membrane and the blood–brain barrier. The term used to quantify solubility is *partition coefficient*. For anaesthetic purposes this is defined as 'the ratio of the concentration of dissolved gas/vapour in the blood to the concentration in the alveoli at

Table 3.1 The ideal inhalation agent

Blood/gas solubility	Low
MAC	<10%
Cardiovascular system	Minimally depressant
	Cardiostable
Respiratory	Minimally depressant
	Non-irritant
	Mild bronchodilator effect
Metabolism	Minimal biotransformation
	Inactive, non-toxic metabolites
Administration	Easy
	Suitable for low and high flow systems
Cost	Low
Soda-lime	No interactions with volatile agents or gases
	No binding
	No degradation products
Tolerability	Non-pungent
	Pleasant to breathe
Preservatives	Not required
Stability	UV light
	Plastics
	Metals

MAC, minimum alveolar concentration.

equilibrium'. The actual values vary between drugs, but values in blood and brain are much lower than those in fat (Table 3.2).

The blood/gas solubility values for modern anaesthetic drugs vary fourfold from the least (N_2O, 0.47) to the most soluble (halothane, 2.4). The most soluble drugs have the slowest induction and recovery characteristics. This seeming paradox occurs because the induction and recovery times are not related to the mass of drug that is absorbed into the bloodstream but to the relative tensions (or partial pressures) of the inhaled drug in the alveoli and the brain. For practical purposes it is usual to define the *relevant tensions* as those between alveoli and blood. Thus, by measuring inspired and expired concentrations of inhaled agent it is possible to identify the point at which equilibrium between alveoli and blood (hence brain) is approached (Figure 3.1). Depending on the potency of the agent (see below) this marks the point at which anaesthesia is induced. Equilibrium is achieved rapidly with less-soluble drugs since the mass of drug that must pass across the alveolar membrane to achieve equilibrium is small. A number of other factors are also relevant in this context, e.g. cardiac output, concentration, alveolar ventilation.

Cardiac output

Any decrease in cardiac output will allow the tension of the inhaled agent in the blood to increase more rapidly. This occurs because transit time through the pulmonary circulation is slowed. In this way, equilibrium between the tensions in alveoli and blood is accelerated.

Table 3.2 Characteristics of drugs used for anaesthesia

Characteristic *Drug*	*Blood/Gas*	*Brain/Blood*	*Oil/Gas*	*Boiling point (°C; STP)*	*Metabolism (%)*	*Preservatives*	*MAC (adults)*		*Inhalational induction time*	*Airway Irritability*[a]
							100% O_2	*70% N_2O*		
High solubility										
Ether	12.1	1.1	65	34.6	–	–	2.0	–	Slow	Very marked
Intermediate solubility										
Halothane	2.4	2.6	224	50.2	20–25	Required	0.78	0.29	Fairly fast	Minimal
Enflurane	1.9	2.6	98	56.5	2	None	1.63	0.57	Fairly fast	Some
Isoflurane	1.46	3.7	98	48.5	0.2	None	1.2	0.50	Rapid	Marked
Sevoflurane	0.65	1.7	53	58.5	3.0	None	1.8	0.60 (64%)	Very rapid	Minimal
Low solubility										
Nitrous oxide	0.47	1.1	1.4	–89	None	None	104	–	–	None
Desflurane	0.42	1.3	18.7	23.5	0.02	None	6.5	2.8 (60%)	Rapid	Marked

[a] Airway irritability during induction also depends on the inspired concentration and the presence of pre-existing airway disease.

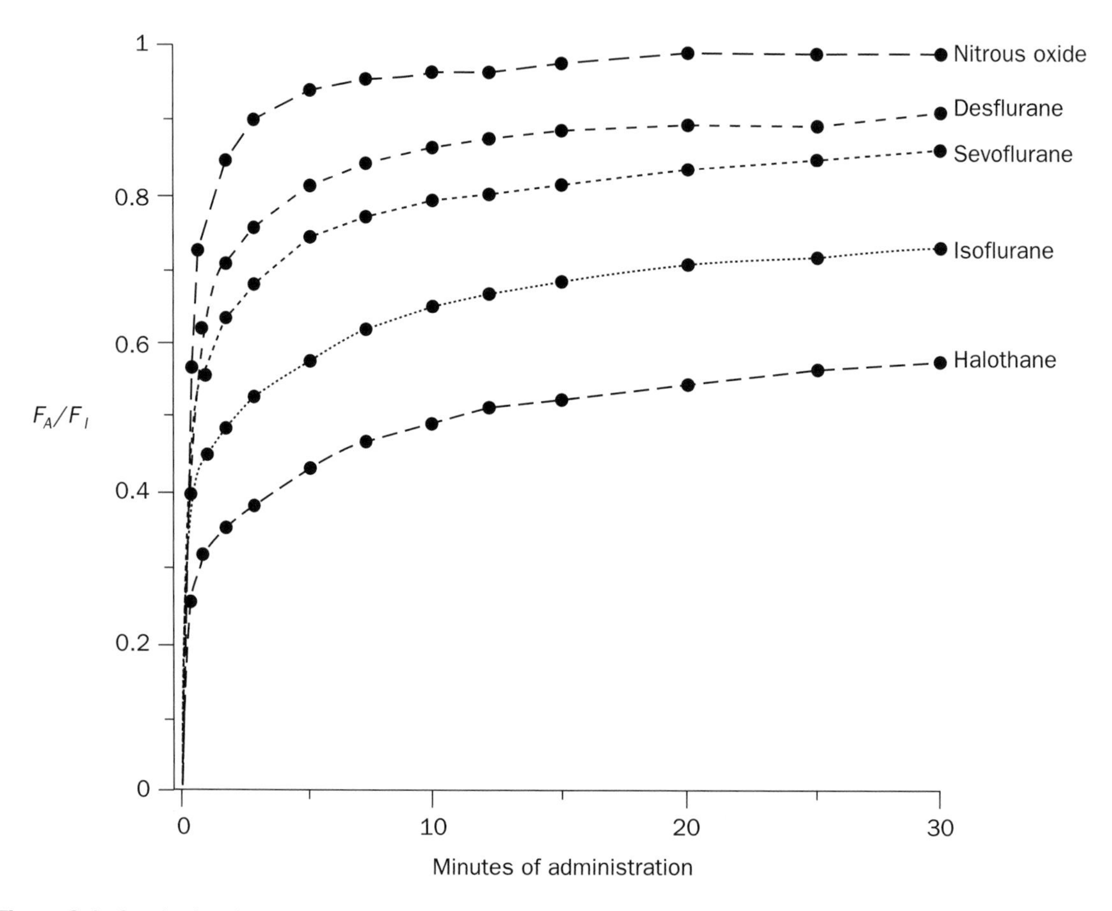

Figure 3.1 *Graph showing the ratio between inspired (F_I) and alveolar (F_A) end-tidal concentrations of the agents shown. The least soluble agents approach equilibrium ($F_A/F_I=1$) the most rapidly.*

Also, since both inhalation and intravenous anaesthetic drugs tend to reduce cardiac output, they facilitate the uptake of volatile agents. It follows that any inhaled anaesthetic drug must be given with great caution to patients in shocked states, e.g. hypovolaemia, arrhythmias, myocardial infarction.

The tensions of inhaled anaesthetics in tissues with a high blood flow—brain, heart, kidney (vessel rich group)—equilibrate quickly with the tensions in blood. The converse is true in tissues having low blood flows, e.g. fat, bone. Muscle occupies an intermediate position.

Concentration

The rate at which the alveolar concentration of a vapour or gas approaches the inspired concentration is directly proportional to its inspired concentration. This is sometimes referred to as the '*concentration effect*'. It states that the higher the inspired anaesthetic concentration, the more rapid the rise in alveolar concentration and hence the more quickly equilibrium is attained between tensions in the alveoli and the brain. In practice, it is necessary to strike a balance to avoid irritation of the airway, or other unwanted phenomena, due to excessively high inspired concentrations of vapour.

Alveolar ventilation

An increase in alveolar ventilation will cause an increase in the alveolar concentration of inhaled agent when semi-closed or open breathing circuits are employed. The effect is most noticeable with a highly soluble anaesthetic, such as diethyl ether. With modern, relatively insoluble agents, such as isoflurane and desflurane, the effects of changes in alveolar ventilation are less pronounced.

The 'second gas effect'

This term is generally used to describe the increase in the rate of uptake of a volatile anaesthetic which occurs when it is given concurrently with nitrous oxide. The phenomenon depends on the rapid uptake of a large volume of gas from the lungs thereby increasing the alveolar concentration of the volatile agent. In addition, the rapid uptake of a large volume of gas into blood from the alveoli results in an increase in alveolar ventilation. In these ways, the second gas (nitrous oxide) enhances the uptake of the first (volatile agent).

POTENCY: MINIMUM ALVEOLAR CONCENTRATION (MAC)

The stability of modern volatile agents is the result of the heavy fluorination of the ether molecule. The effect is most pronounced for CF_3 and CF_2 moieties. In the case of desflurane, of the eight available binding sites for halogens, six are occupied by fluorine atoms. Similarly, sevoflurane has seven fluorine atoms out of a possible ten. The lack of hydrogen atoms reduces both flammability and potency.

In order to compare the anaesthetic, haemodynamic, and other effects of these agents, it is necessary to have a measure of potency so that equivalent doses of the agents may be administered. Eger in 1974 coined the term *minimum alveolar ventilation* (MAC) to describe the potency of inhaled anaesthetics. MAC is defined as:

> . . . the minimum concentration of an anaesthetic at 1 atmosphere ambient pressure that produces immobility in 50% of patients or animals exposed to a standardised noxious stimulus.

Although at first sight this definition does not appear to be clinically useful, multiples of MAC are employed in clinical trials to allow doses of different inhaled agents to be standardised and the effects compared. The term 'MAC hours' (MAC × duration of exposure in hours) is widely used as a measure of total dosage over time, and is especially useful in toxicity and pollution studies. In gas mixtures, MAC values are broadly additive so that, e.g. 0.5 MAC N_2O combined with 0.5 MAC isoflurane is equipotent with 1 MAC isoflurane alone.

The MAC_{awake} value is commonly taken as the concentration midway between the concentration when a patient just becomes able to open their eyes on command, and the value at which this response is just suppressed in 50% of patients. MAC_{awake} values are typically 50% of the MAC values. This value may be used as a guide to the minimum concentration necessary to avoid awareness in paralysed patients (see below).

Factors affecting MAC

Patient factors

MAC values for a particular volatile anaesthetic are highest in neonates and lowest in the elderly although the explanation for this is not clear. MAC values are unaffected by gender, duration of exposure, and acid–base status. MAC is reduced by induced hypotension, hypothermia and hypoxia.

Drugs

Opioids, benzodiazepines, α_2-adrenergic agonists (clonidine, dexmedetomidine) and other gaseous or volatile anaesthetics all reduce the MAC value of a particular agent.

Muscle relaxants

An advantage of using muscle relaxants is that they allow lower inspired concentrations of volatile agents to be used. In practice, anaesthetists generally use 1.5–2.5 MAC of volatile agents to provide anaesthesia in non-paralysed patients, depending on the presence of other drugs and the age and condition of the patient. When a muscle relaxant is given, the values may be some 50% less.

Anaesthetic dose (AD)

The clinical usefulness of MAC is questionable since, by definition, 50% of those receiving that concentration move in response to noxious stimulation. The median anaesthetic doses (ADs) required to prevent movement in 50% (AD_{50}) and 95% (AD_{95}) of patients are a later development and range from 5% to 40% greater than the MAC value. Again, these values are of only limited practical value.

INDIVIDUAL AGENTS

The pharmacodynamic effects of all volatile agents on body systems may be modified by surgical stimulation depending on the depth of anaesthesia. The pharmacological properties of the drugs described below are those of the agents in the absence of surgical stimulation unless otherwise stated.

Isoflurane

```
    F       Cl  F
    |       |   |
F—C—O—C—C—F
    |       |   |
    H       H   F
```

Isoflurane was discovered by Terrell in 1965. It is a halogenated methyl ethyl ether and is a structural isomer of enflurane (Figure 3.2). It became commercially available in the UK in 1982.

Physical characteristics (Table 3.2)

Isoflurane is a clear, colourless liquid with a slightly pungent smell. It is non-flammable in oxygen, air and nitrous oxide under all normal conditions. It does not require a preservative and is stable in the presence of ultraviolet light. Under certain conditions it may interact with 'dried out' soda-lime or Baralyme to produce carbon monoxide. Any risk of this can be avoided by using calcium hydroxide absorbents which do not contain strong alkalis. With a blood/gas solubility coefficient of 1.4 it occupies an intermediate position between the highly insoluble agents, desflurane (0.42) and sevoflurane (0.6), and the more soluble agents enflurane (1.9) and halothane (2.4).

In theory, induction should be rapid, but in practice the inspired vapour concentration must be increased slowly to avoid airway irritation. MAC is 1.15% in 100% oxygen and 0.56% in 30% oxygen, making it less potent than halothane (0.75% and 0.29% at these oxygen concentrations). Isoflurane is the most potent of all the currently available anaesthetic ethers. Recovery from isoflurane anaesthesia is rapid and clear and the drug is suitable for use in day surgery.

Cardiovascular system

Isoflurane has a dose-dependent depressant effect on the myocardium. *In vitro* studies indicate that it reduces myocardial contractility to a similar extent as halothane. *In vivo*, isoflurane appears to be less of a cardiovascular depressant than other volatile agents.

Cardiac output

In young and elderly adult patients both systemic arterial blood pressure and peripheral vascular resistance are reduced (Figure 3.3). Unlike the elderly, cardiac index is only slightly affected in young patients due to a compensatory rise in heart rate (Figure 3.4). In older patients this mechanism is less efficient and both cardiac index and systemic blood pressure (systolic, diastolic and mean) values decrease significantly from baseline (Figures 3.3, 3.4). It is difficult, however, to interpret heart rate changes in the clinical situation since other factors may come into play: concomitant cardioactive medication; surgical stimulation; choice of muscle relaxant; use of opioids, etc.

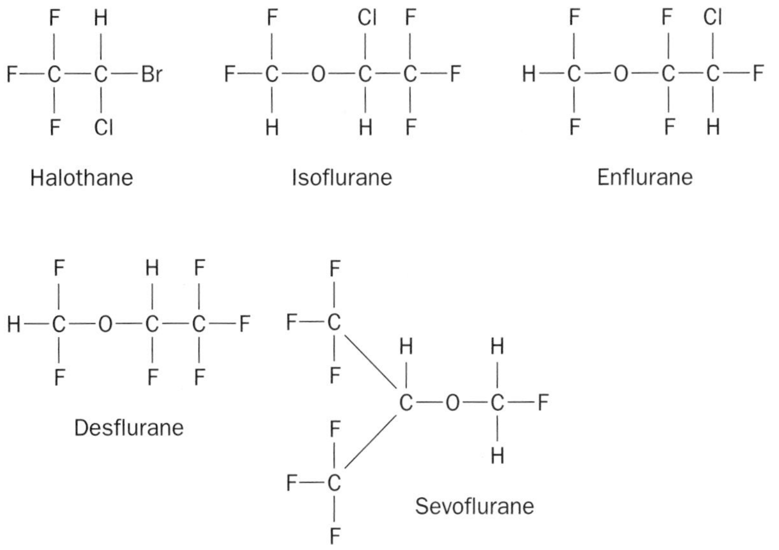

```
   F  H           F       Cl  F            F       F  Cl
   |  |           |       |   |            |       |  |
F—C—C—Br      F—C—O—C—C—F          H—C—O—C—C—F
   |  |           |       |   |            |       |  |
   F  Cl          H       H   F            F       F  H

 Halothane        Isoflurane             Enflurane

   F       H  F
   |       |  |
H—C—O—C—C—F
   |       |  |
   F       F  F

 Desflurane
```

Sevoflurane

Figure 3.2 Structural formulae of volatile anaesthetic agents in current use.

Arrhythmias

In contrast to halothane, cardiac arrhythmias are uncommon with isoflurane and it does not sensitise the heart to the effects of catecholamines.

Blood pressure

There is a dose-dependent decrease in systemic blood pressure during isoflurane anaesthesia. This is mainly the result of a marked reduction in peripheral vascular resistance. In contrast, the decrease in arterial blood pressure during halothane anaesthesia appears to be mainly the result of a reduction in myocardial contractility. Isoflurane, in common with other volatile agents, has little effect on pulmonary artery pressure or pulmonary vascular resistance.

Coronary circulation

Because of its marked vasodilatory properties it has been suggested that isoflurane might not be suitable for patients with coronary artery disease. This seeming paradox arises because of the inability of diseased arteries to dilate further during isoflurane anaesthesia whilst at the same time normal, non-diseased vessels in other areas dilate. In this way it has been proposed that normal vascular beds can 'steal' blood from diseased vessel beds, thereby worsening oxygen lack and ischaemia in those areas of myocardium—the 'coronary steal' phenomenon. Although studies in dogs appeared to support the theory, the findings cannot be directly applied to humans on account of major anatomical differences in the coronary circulations. There is no evidence that the risks associated with the careful administration of isoflurane to patients with coronary artery disease exceed those of other volatile agents.

Respiratory system

Isoflurane has a dose-dependent depressant effect on breathing. The evidence suggests that isoflurane has a greater respiratory depressant effect than halothane. The tidal volume decreases without an increase in respiratory rate. In volunteers, $P\text{CO}_2$ increases in a dose-dependent manner during isoflurane anaesthesia with the increase being greater with isoflurane than halothane but less than enflurane. All volatile agents impair the ventilatory response to carbon dioxide. Again, the effect is greater with isoflurane than with halothane. Bronchomotor tone is reduced during isoflurane anaesthesia.

Central nervous system

Isoflurane has no epileptogenic potential in humans and there is no clinical or EEG evidence of convulsive activity during isoflurane

Table 3.3 Comparative physical properties of nitrous oxide, xenon and nitric oxide

Physical property	*Nitrous oxide* (N_2O)	*Xenon* (Xe)	*Nitric oxide* (NO)
Molecular weight	44	54	30
Boiling point (°C)	–88.6	–108	–152
Critical temperature (°C)	36.4	16.6	–93.0
Critical pressure (bar)	72.5	58.4	64.85
Density (gas) (15°C)	1.850 $kg{\cdot}m^{-3}$	5.52 $g{\cdot}L^{-1}$	1.253 $kg{\cdot}m^{-3}$
Viscosity (gas)	0.0147 m*Pa*·s (25°C)	0.0227 m*Pa*·s (20°C)	0.018 m*Pa*·s (0°C)
Blood/gas solubility	0.47	0.14	–
Oil/gas solubility	1.4	1.8	–
MAC (%)	104	70	–

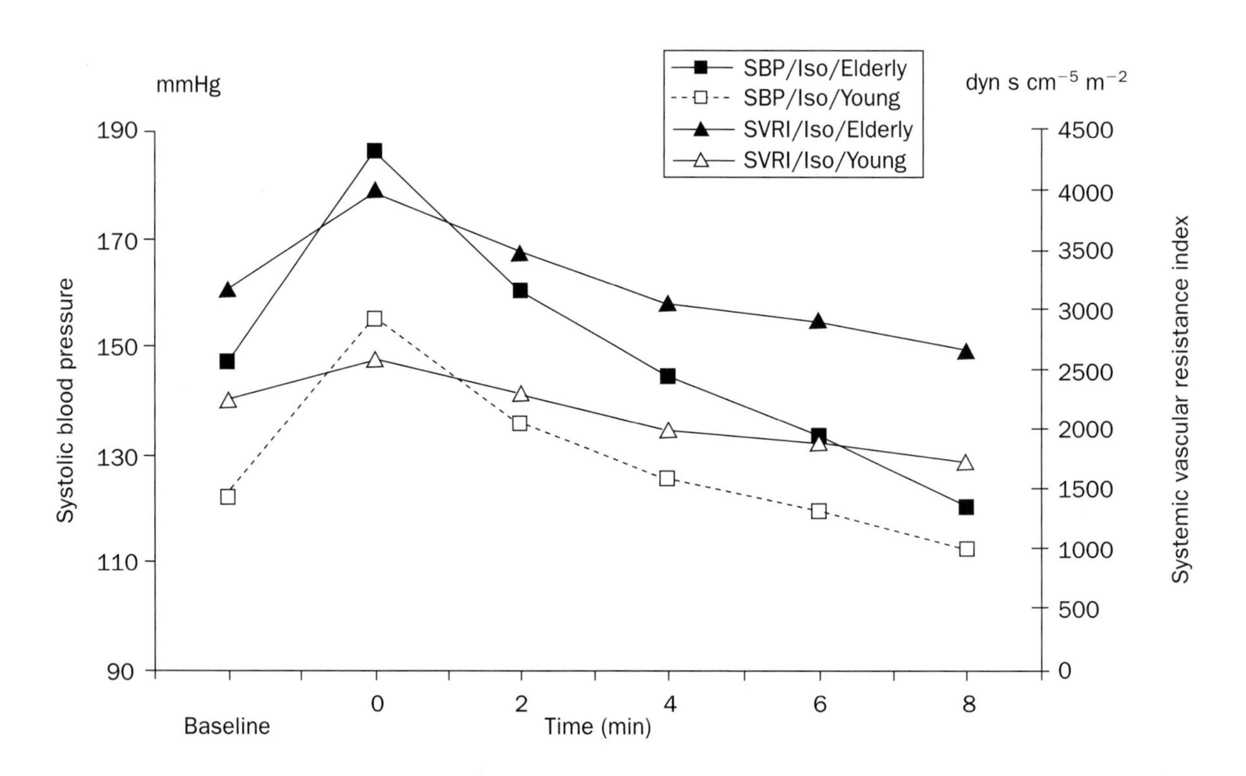

Figure 3.3 *Graph showing mean values for systolic blood pressure (SBP) and systemic vascular resistance index (SVRI) in young (n = 20) and elderly (n = 20) patients during induction of anaesthesia with isoflurane (1 MAC) in 100% oxygen. (Data from McKinney MS, Fee JPH, Clarke RSJ.* British Journal of Anaesthesia *1993;71:696–701.)*

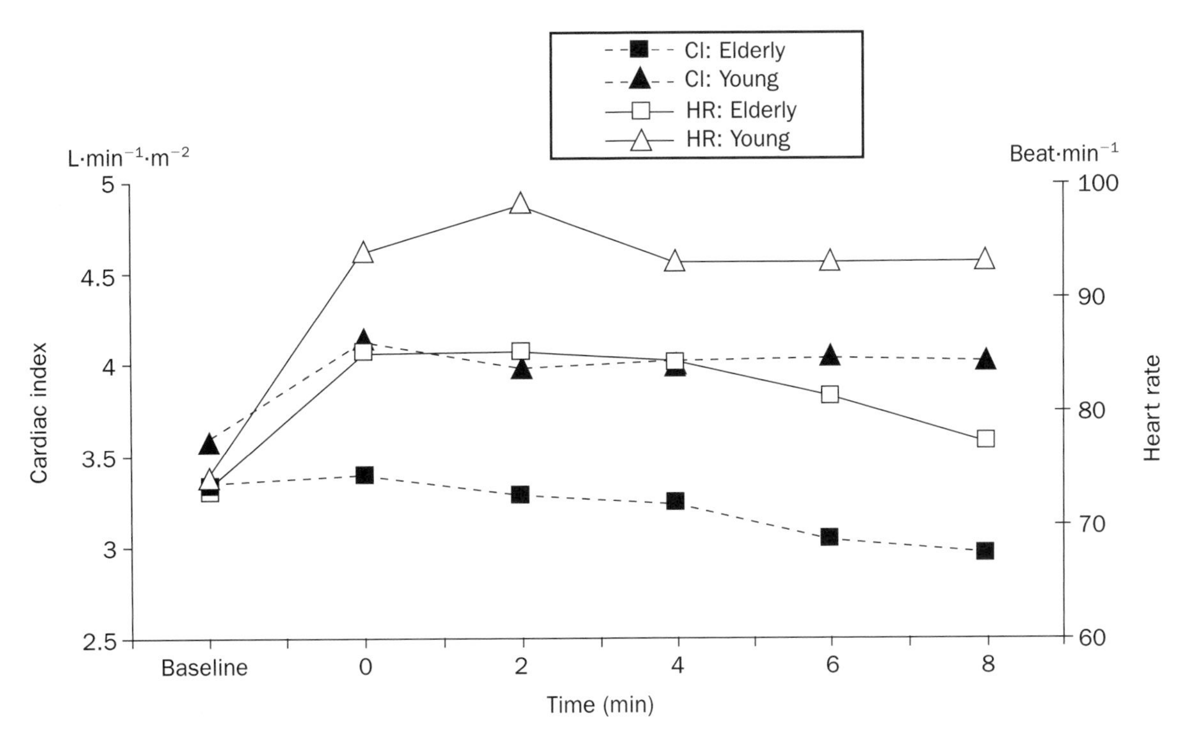

Figure 3.4 *Graph showing mean values for cardiac index (CI) and heart rate (HR) in young (n = 20) and elderly (n = 20) patients during induction of anaesthesia with isoflurane (1 MAC) in 100% oxygen. (Data from McKinney MS, Fee JPH, Clarke RSJ.* British Journal of Anaesthesia *1993;71:696–701.)*

anaesthesia. Marked cerebral vasodilation occurs with an increase in intracranial pressure. This can be mitigated by hyperventilation even in the presence of a space-occupying lesion.

Liver

Hepatic toxicity after isoflurane is uncommon. There is some evidence that volatile anaesthetic agents share a common immunological mechanism for hepatic damage but the exact aetiological role of autoantibodies in volatile agent induced hepatitis remains uncertain. The potential for liver injury appears to be related to the extent to which the agents are metabolised. With less than 0.2% of inhaled isoflurane subject to metabolism it is not surprising that it should have negligible toxic effects on the liver. In common with the other agents isoflurane is oxidized by cytochrome P-450 2E1 suggesting that metabolism may be increased by isoniazid.

In animal studies, volatile anaesthetics reduce portal venous blood flow. However, the hepatic arterial buffer effect is preserved during isoflurane anaesthesia (unlike halothane) with the net effect being no overall change in hepatic blood flow.

Muscle

Isoflurane depresses the contractility of skeletal muscle. It potentiates non-depolarising muscle relaxants and allows the use of lower doses of these than would otherwise be the case. The rapid elimination of isoflurane assists in the reversal of muscle block and may reduce the likelihood of partial reversal.

Kidney

Isoflurane, like other volatile agents, causes a transient reduction in renal blood flow, glomerular filtration rate and urinary output, but there is no evidence that these changes are harmful to the healthy kidney. Similarly, there is no evidence that isoflurane has any undesirable effects on the transplanted kidney. In keeping with its limited biotransformation only very small amounts of inorganic fluoride are produced; the peak plasma concentration has been reported as less than 5 μmol·L^{-1} although during prolonged anaesthesia higher concentrations are known to occur.

Uterus

When used in a concentration of approximately 0.75% for anaesthesia for Caesarean section, isoflurane would appear not to cause increased maternal blood loss or unacceptable neonatal depression.

Sevoflurane

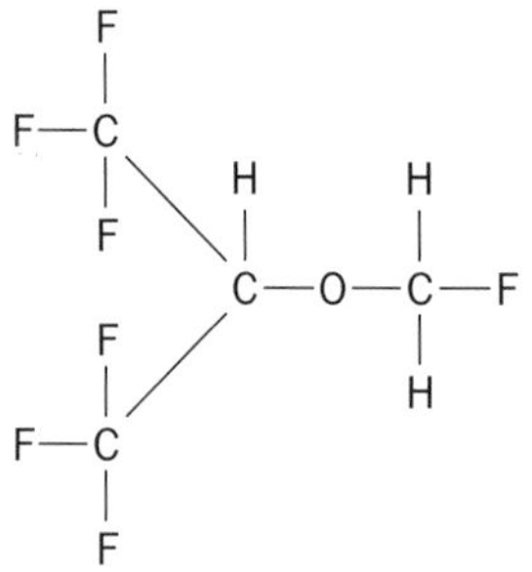

```
       F
       |
    F—C
       |\     H     H
       F \    |     |
           C—O—C—F
       F  /         |
       | /          H
    F—C
       |
       F
```

Physical characteristics (Table 3.2)

Sevoflurane is a fluorinated methyl isopropyl ether (Figure 3.2). It was first released for clinical use in Japan in 1990 and it is now available in many other countries worldwide. Being relatively insoluble (blood/gas solubility coefficient, 0.68) it has the potential to provide rapid anaesthetic induction and recovery. Unlike isoflurane it is non-irritant to the airway and can be given in high concentrations for anaesthetic induction. Its MAC ranges from 3.3 in infants to 2.5 in older children and 1.8 in adults. Its low solubility, lack of airway irritability, and moderate potency make it particularly useful for 'gas induction' in children. Other physical characteristics are shown in Table 3.2.

Degradation of strong alkali

Soon after its introduction to clinical practice there were reports of the degradation of sevoflurane by a strong base (KOH and/or NaOH). This was shown to be associated with the formation of a substance, compound A, in carbon dioxide absorbers containing soda lime or baralyme. Although nephrotoxic in rats, the toxic potential of compound A in healthy patients appears slight. Various factors influence the amount of compound A produced including canister temperature, the degree of hydration of the carbon dioxide absorbent, the fresh gas flow rate, and most importantly, the amount of a strong base, particularly KOH, in the absorbent. A practical and effective way of minimising compound A production in clinical practice is to remove the strong bases from the carbon dioxide absorbent. In these circumstances, neither barium nor calcium hydroxide will catalyse proton removal from sevoflurane. Studies with a calcium hydroxide absorbent, which does not contain strong bases, confirm the absence of sevoflurane degradation when this absorbent is employed. Another carbon dioxide absorbent, lithium hydroxide, reduces compound A production but it is too expensive and difficult to handle for routine clinical use.

Cardiovascular system

Sevoflurane, in common with all volatile agents, reduces cardiac output and systemic blood pressure. It does so mainly through a reduction in peripheral vascular resistance. Although it is a systemic vasodilator it does not appear to produce significant dilatation of small coronary vessels and there is no possibility of coronary 'steal' as hypothesised for isoflurane. A small increase in heart rate may be observed. This is less pronounced than with isoflurane and desflurane and is almost certainly the result of reflex activity secondary to the reduction in peripheral vascular resistance. Sevoflurane is associated with a stable heart rhythm and does not predispose the heart to sensitisation by catecholamines. In children, halothane causes a greater decrease in heart rate, myocardial contractility and cardiac output than sevoflurane at all concentrations. For these reasons sevoflurane is advocated for use in outpatient dental anaesthesia, especially in children.

Respiratory system

Like other volatile agents, sevoflurane causes dose-related respiratory depression. In healthy patients this results in a decrease in tidal volume and an increase in respiratory rate with a net decrease in minute ventilation. At anaesthetic concentrations the degree of depression is greater than that seen with halothane or isoflurane. There is a decline in the slope of the carbon dioxide response curve. Sevoflurane produces the same degree of bronchodilation as isoflurane and enflurane.

Central nervous system

Sevoflurane has a dose-dependent effect on cerebral blood flow and intracranial pressure; cerebral autoregulation is preserved (this is not the case with isoflurane). During hypocarbia, in the absence of nitrous oxide, 1 MAC does not increase intracranial pressure (ICP). It reduces the cerebral metabolic rate for oxygen ($CMRO_2$) by approximately 50% at concentrations approaching 2 MAC. This is similar to the reduction observed during isoflurane anaesthesia.

Agitation

Agitation in the early postoperative period has been noted in young children. It would appear that this is more common with sevoflurane than with isoflurane or total intravenous anaesthesia techniques. Although self-limiting, the agitation may be minimised by premedication with midazolam or similar benzodiazepine. It is thought that sevoflurane may, under certain circumstances, be proconvulsant and seizure-like activity has been observed on the electroencephalogram (EEG) during deep sevoflurane anaesthesia. The effect can be offset by adding nitrous oxide to the anaesthetic mixture, or by hyperventilating the patient.

Metabolism and toxicity

Approximately 5% of a given dose of sevoflurane is metabolised, a higher proportion than with isoflurane or enflurane. As with other volatile agents, cytochrome P-450 2E1 appears to be the specific isoform involved. Sevoflurane is broken down to organic and inorganic fluorides and hexafluoroisopropanol. These compounds are excreted as fluoride ions in the urine and as conjugates in the bile. Despite the relatively high proportion of drug metabolised, hepatitis is unlikely since the putative metabolic pathway does not include a reactive metabolite with potential to bind to lipid or protein. Serum inorganic fluoride concentrations of greater than 50 $\mu mol \cdot L^{-1}$ have been detected following administration of sevoflurane but nephrotoxicity is unlikely in healthy patients. Peak values of around 30 $\mu mol \cdot L^{-1}$ appear to be the norm and during prolonged administration values usually remain within the 50 $\mu mol \cdot L^{-1}$ threshold. It seems that the nephrotoxic potential of fluoride is related to the intrarenal production of the ion. This may explain why sevoflurane, unlike methoxyflurane, does not impair renal function despite occasional high serum fluoride concentrations. Patients who are dehydrated or whose renal function is otherwise compromised may be susceptible to the renal effects of sevoflurane.

Gastrointestinal tract

A higher incidence of nausea and vomiting has been reported after sevoflurane anaesthesia than when a target-controlled propofol infusion is used.

Applied pharmacology

For inhalational induction of anaesthesia in children, 6% sevoflurane in 50% nitrous oxide and oxygen is probably optimal. However, some anaesthetists consider it to be inferior to halothane for the management of the irritable or constricted airway and for anaesthesia for bronchoscopy. Sevoflurane is preferred for dental procedures as there is a lower risk of cardiac arrhythmias than with halothane, especially in children. In children with congenital heart disease, whereas the cardiac index is reduced by halothane it is preserved with sevoflurane. In adults, 8% sevoflurane is well tolerated and, provides rapid induction of anaesthesia without adversely affecting haemodynamic stability.

Desflurane

```
      F       H   F
      |       |   |
  H — C — O — C — C — F
      |       |   |
      F       F   F
```

Desflurane was synthesised by Terrell in the early 1960s and was the 653rd of a series of compounds which were evaluated for their anaesthetic potential. Desflurane was slow to become available commercially mainly because of problems with vaporisation (B.P. 23.5°C).

Physical characteristics (Table 3.2)

Desflurane is a fluorinated methyl ethyl ether identical to isoflurane except for the substitution of a chlorine by a fluorine atom (Figure 3.2). It is the least soluble of all the volatile anaesthetics with a similar blood/gas solubility to nitrous oxide (0.42). It is non-flammable under all clinical conditions. The vapour pressure of desflurane approaches 1 atm at 23°C making controlled administration impossible with a conventional vaporiser. A desflurane vaporiser is an electronically controlled pressurised device that delivers an accurately metered dose of vaporised desflurane into a stream of fresh gases passing through it. The MAC of desflurane (6.5% in adults) is the highest of any modern fluorinated agent but in common with these the value decreases in the elderly and in other circumstances (see below).

Cardiovascular system

The effects of desflurane are similar to those of isoflurane although possibly less pronounced at equi-MAC concentrations. There is a dose-dependent reduction in myocardial contractility, cardiac output, arterial blood pressure, and systemic vascular resistance. The possibility of coronary 'steal' is of negligible clinical significance.

Unlike isoflurane, desflurane may stimulate the sympathetic nervous system at concentrations above 1 MAC. Sudden and unexpected increases in arterial blood pressure and heart rate have been reported in some patients, accompanied by increases in plasma catecholamine and vasopressin concentrations and increased plasma renin activity. These 'pressor' effects may increase morbidity or mortality in susceptible patients. The mechanism of sympathetic activation is unclear but does not appear to be baroreceptor-mediated. Clonidine, esmolol, fentanyl and propofol partially block the response but lignocaine (lignocaine) is ineffective.

Respiratory system

At induction, high concentrations are irritant and may provoke coughing or breath-holding. Desflurane does not have a marked bronchodilator effect and in cigarette smokers it is associated with significant bronchoconstriction. In clinical practice, both humidification of inspired gases and opioids are thought to reduce airway irritability but even at moderate concentrations (2 MAC), desflurane is more likely to cause coughing than sevoflurane. In common with other volatile agents, desflurane causes dose-related respiratory depression. Tidal volume is reduced and respiratory rate increases, initially. As inspired concentrations of desflurane increase, the trend is to hypoventilation and hypercarbia and apnoea is to be expected at concentrations of 1.5 MAC or greater.

Use in rebreathing systems

Although desflurane resists degradation by soda-lime, carbon monoxide can be generated under certain conditions and may accumulate in the breathing system. The exact mechanism of CO production by desflurane is uncertain. It has been proposed that the initial reaction is the base-catalysed abstraction of a proton from the difluoromethylethyl group of desflurane, a moiety not present in sevoflurane or halothane. This reaction occurs in clinical practice when desflurane is in contact with 'dried-out' soda lime or baralyme. The amount of CO produced depends on the quantity of dry absorbent with which desflurane makes contact, the water content of the absorbent and the fresh gas flow. The percentage of water needed to prevent CO production is approximately 4.8% for soda-lime and 9.7% for Baralyme. Although high fresh gas flows generate more CO than low flows (because of the greater quantity of desflurane passing over dry absorbent) the net effect of high flows is probably beneficial by purging the system and preventing CO accumulation. The clinical signs of CO poisoning are veiled by anaesthesia. Carbon dioxide absorbents free from strong alkali do not generate carbon monoxide.

Central nervous system
Desflurane reduces cerebral metabolic rate for oxygen ($CMRO_2$) to a similar extent as isoflurane. Cerebral vascular resistance is reduced and is accompanied by an increase in cerebral blood flow (0.5–2.0 MAC). It suppresses EEG activity and there is no evidence of epileptiform activity. Somatosensory evoked potentials are preserved at clinical concentrations.

Metabolism and toxicity
The potential for desflurane to cause renal or hepatic toxicity is small given its minimal biotransformation. Prolonged exposure does not cause an increase in plasma inorganic fluoride concentrations.

Neuromuscular
Desflurane has a marked depressant effect at the neuromuscular junction. At clinical concentrations it tends to reduce the train-of-four (TOF) ratio—possibly a prejunctional effect. It prolongs neuromuscular blockade by both non-depolarising and depolarising relaxants and may trigger malignant hyperpyrexia in susceptible patients.

Enflurane

```
       F         F    Cl
       |         |    |
  H—C—O—C—C—F
       |         |    |
       F         F    H
```

Enflurane is a fluorinated methyl ethyl ether and is a structural isomer of isoflurane (Figure 3.2). It was synthesised in 1963 and introduced into clinical practice in 1966 at a time when concern was growing about the hepatotoxicity of halothane. Its main advantage over halothane was its resistance to biotransformation (2.5% compared to some 20%). For that reason it was widely used as an alternative to halothane, particularly for multiple administration.

Physical characteristics (Table 3.2)
It is a clear, colourless liquid with a characteristic ether-like odour. It does not undergo degradation by soda-lime and being stable in light, does not require a preservative. It is non-flammable at all clinical concentrations in oxygen/nitrous oxide mixtures. Like all modern volatile agents it is highly potent and should only be administered by means of an accurately calibrated, agent-specific, temperature-compensated vaporiser. The main physical properties of enflurane are shown in Table 3.2. It is relatively insoluble in blood (blood/gas solubility, 1.8) and this facilitates rapid induction and recovery. Its MAC value in adults in 100% oxygen is 1.63 making it about half as potent as halothane (0.8). In 70% nitrous oxide the MAC is 0.6. Anaesthesia can generally be induced with inspired concentrations of 3–5%.

Cardiovascular system
Enflurane produces a dose-related decrease in systemic arterial blood pressure secondary to reductions in cardiac output and systemic vascular resistance. There is evidence that cardiac output is partially maintained by a compensatory increase in heart rate. This effect seems dependent on a degree of hypercarbia and does not occur during controlled ventilation. Enflurane and halothane depress myocardial contractility to a similar extent and less than isoflurane. Enflurane does not sensitise the heart to the effects of catecholamines to any significant extent and adrenaline (epinephrine) may be given subcutaneously for control of bleeding.

Respiratory system
At high concentrations enflurane is more irritant than halothane. Coughing, breath-holding and laryngospasm are common at induction if the inspired concentration is increased too rapidly. Enflurane is a potent respiratory depressant and apnoea may occur at inspired

concentrations of 3.5% or more. In this respect, it is a more pronounced depressant than isoflurane or halothane. Minute and tidal volumes decrease and although respiratory rate is preserved initially this is insufficient to prevent hypercarbia. Enflurane acts centrally on the respiratory centre but also has a marked 'relaxant-like' effect on respiratory muscles. It has a marked bronchodilating effect similar to that of halothane.

Central nervous system

A characteristic of enflurane is its ability to induce seizure complexes in the electroencephalogram. Episodes of paroxysmal activity and burst suppression are well documented and are most marked during deep anaesthesia in the presence of hypocarbia. The effect can be terminated by reducing the inspired enflurane concentration and permitting a return to normocarbia. There is no evidence of any ill-effects as a consequence. Although patients with epilepsy are not thought to be at increased risk of seizures during or after enflurane anaesthesia, it is prudent to use an alternative agent, especially in children. Enflurane abolishes cerebral autoregulation at a concentration of 1 MAC during normocarbia resulting in an increase in cerebral blood flow and a rise in intracranial pressure. These effects are exaggerated by hypercarbia.

Metabolism and toxicity

Enflurane is metabolised by the cytochrome P-450 series, specifically P-450 2E1, but the agent is much less extensively metabolised than halothane (see above). Metabolites include trifluoroacetic acid (TFA) and inorganic fluoride ion. A small number of cases of 'enflurane hepatitis' have been reported but the overall incidence of liver damage following enflurane anaesthesia is estimated to be 1 in 800 000. Clinical studies have failed to detect any significant effects of enflurane on liver function even when given repeatedly.

In normal clinical use the peak plasma fluoride concentration rarely exceeds 25 $\mu mol \cdot L^{-1}$ and is well within the threshold for renal toxicity. Significant renal impairment is unlikely in patients with normal renal function. Prolonged enflurane anaesthesia may result in vasopressin-resistant type of renal failure with fluoride concentrations of around 30 $\mu mol \cdot L^{-1}$. In contrast to methoxyflurane peak fluoride concentrations occur early (3–4 h) after enflurane and diminish rapidly after discontinuing the agent.

Skeletal muscle

Enflurane potentiates the effects of non-depolarising muscle relaxants.

Uterus

Enflurane causes a dose-related relaxation of uterine smooth muscle. At low inspired concentrations during Caesarean section, it prevents maternal awareness without an increase in blood loss or undesirable effects on the baby.

Halothane

```
     F   H
     |   |
F —  C — C — Br
     |   |
     F   Cl
```

Halothane was introduced into clinical practice in 1956. It was not the first fluorinated anaesthetic—fluoroxene (Fluoromar) holds that distinction—but it was the first to achieve widespread acceptability. Halothane is a fluorinated alkane: 1-bromo, 1-chloro –2,2,2-trifluoroethane (Figure 3.2). It has a characteristic odour, similar to chloroform, and requires a stabiliser, thymol (0.01%), to prevent degradation by light. Halothane has a blood/gas partition coefficient of 2.4 (Table 3.2) but its lack of irritant qualities makes possible the use of relatively high inspired concentrations (2–4%). For that reason, inhalation induction is characteristically smooth and rapid. Compared to sevoflurane, and possibly isoflurane, recovery from halothane anaesthesia is delayed.

The MAC of halothane is 1.08 in infants but this declines to 0.64 in old age. In the presence of nitrous oxide the value is reduced by 60%. Halothane is soluble in rubber but only to a small extent in polyethylene. It is susceptible to degradation by soda-lime but none of the breakdown products poses a threat to health.

Cardiovascular system

The most prominent effect of halothane on the circulation is a dose-related decrease in arterial blood pressure. This is due mainly to reduced myocardial contractility and ventricular slowing. Cardiac output falls due to a decrease in stroke volume and bradycardia. Systemic vascular resistance also falls but this is less pronounced than with some other agents. Although halothane reduces myocardial oxygen consumption it also reduces oxygen demand and it is suitable for patients with myocardial ischaemia.

Halothane sensitises the myocardium to the effects of catecholamines. When high inspired concentrations are used there may be a shift of pacemaker and nodal rhythm may develop. Ventricular extrasystoles may also occur especially when there are increased circulating catecholamines (exogenous or endogenous). The use of atropine to correct changes in rate or rhythm may induce dangerous tachyarrhythmias or even ventricular fibrillation. Few halothane-induced arrhythmias persist once inspired concentrations have been reduced and normocarbia established. Arrhythmias during halothane anaesthesia are almost always associated with hypercarbia and are much less frequent during controlled ventilation.

Outpatient dental surgery in children during halothane anaesthesia is associated with a high incidence of arrhythmias. This is most likely due to breath-holding during induction (hypercarbia; hypoxia) accompanied by high levels of circulating catecholamines brought about by anxiety and 'light' anaesthesia. Sevoflurane and isoflurane are less arrhythmogenic than halothane. Full monitoring and resuscitation facilities must be available whenever general anaesthesia is administered.

Respiratory system

Halothane is non-irritant and can be inhaled at high concentrations to produce rapid, smooth induction of anaesthesia. It obtunds the protective pharyngeal and laryngeal reflexes. At deeper planes, tracheal intubation may be performed. Halothane has a pronounced bronchodilating action and this may be an advantage in patients with chronic obstructive airways disease. Both tachypnoea and slowing of respiration may be observed at deeper planes of anaesthesia.

Liver

Halothane-related hepatitis was first reported in 1958 just two years after the drug's introduction. During subsequent years it became clear from the volume of reports that there was a very small excess risk of liver failure after halothane anaesthesia, particularly when the drug was administered more than once over a short time period. The medicolegal implications of this were profound and did much to promote the search for a safer alternative agent.

It is now known that there are two types of halothane-related hepatotoxicity. The first occurs fairly commonly (perhaps as often as 1 in 3 patients) and takes the form of a minor disturbance of liver enzymes. Repeat exposure is not a requirement and the clinical significance of the biochemical changes is uncertain. The second form is rare (1 in 35 000 halothane anaesthetics) and results in a severe fulminant hepatitis with a high mortality. Previous exposure to halothane is usual and there may be a history of postoperative pyrexia or jaundice. Other risk factors have been suggested: female gender, obesity, multiple anaesthetics and genetic predisposition. Although the interval between administrations was highlighted as a risk factor by the Committee on Safety of Medicines, which recommended a 3 month interval, there is no 'safe' period between administrations and several years may have elapsed since previous exposure to the agent. The first signs of fulminant injury may be delayed for up to a month after halothane anaesthesia and pyrexia, rash or joint pains may precede jaundice. Laboratory evidence of immune involvement may include eosinophilia and circulating immune complexes or autoantibodies. Reports of liver damage after halothane in children are rare and the overall incidence has been estimated at 1 in 82 000 halothane anaesthetics.

Although both metabolic and immune factors may be involved in the aetiology of severe hepatitis after halothane the aetiology of postanaesthetic/postsurgical hepatitis is far from clear. A recent study revealed that paediatric anaesthesiologists had high titres of serum autoantibodies which react with specific hepatic proteins. Since the vast majority of these individuals have not developed hepatitis the pathological role of autoantibodies in volatile anaesthetic-induced hepatitis remains questionable (Njoku and co-workers 2002).

Central nervous system

Halothane has no significant epileptogenic properties. It is a cerebral vasodilator and increases cerebral blood flow. Autoregulation is impaired and halothane appears to raise intracranial pressure to a greater extent than isoflurane. Cerebral oxygen consumption is reduced and oxygen supply to the brain exceeds demand under stable circulatory conditions. The tendency of halothane to overperfuse the brain makes it a poor choice for most neurosurgical procedures.

GASES

Nitrous oxide (N_2O)

Nitrous oxide (N_2O) was first prepared by Priestly in 1772. Its anaesthetic properties were described by Sir Humphrey Davy in 1800 and it was first used in clinical practice by Colton and Wells in 1844.

Physical characteristics

Nitrous oxide occurs naturally and is a colourless slightly sweet-smelling non-irritant gas with the molecular weight of 44 (Table 3.3). Its boiling point is –89°C and it is compressible to a colourless liquid. The gas is stable in the presence of soda-lime and whilst it will support combustion of other agents it is neither flammable nor explosive itself.

Manufacture and storage

Nitrous oxide is manufactured by heating ammonium nitrate and is subsequently purified using water, caustic permanganate and acid scrubbers. The gas is stored under pressure in metal cylinders. The critical temperature is 36.5°C. Below that temperature some of the contents of a full cylinder will be in liquid form, the exact proportion and pressure being dependent on the ambient temperature. At 20°C, 80% of the contents of a full cylinder will be in the liquid phase at a pressure of 5170 kPa. Latent heat is required for the vaporisation of liquid nitrous oxide and this is obtained from the metal casing of the cylinder which rapidly cools and may cause freezing of the water vapour in the surrounding air. Any water present as an impurity in the gas will form ice at the reducing valve, thereby decreasing the flow rate. From this it should be clear that a pressure gauge is a poor guide to the total cylinder content of nitrous oxide whilst any of the gas is in the liquid phase.

Entonox is a 50% mixture of nitrous oxide and oxygen which remains gaseous under pressure unless the ambient temperature falls below –5.5°C. In these circumstances the contents may separate into liquid nitrous oxide and gaseous oxygen. In such a situation there is a risk that at the start high percentage concentrations of oxygen could be delivered followed by almost pure nitrous oxide.

A number of impurities are created during the manufacture of nitrous oxide. These include ammonia, nitric oxide, nitrogen, nitrogen dioxide, carbon monoxide, and water vapour. Contamination with nitrogen dioxide may result in laryngospasm, pulmonary oedema and cyanosis. Contamination with carbon monoxide may lead to high levels of carboxyhaemoglobin and marked reductions in the oxygen-carrying capacity of the blood.

Absorption and excretion

Nitrous oxide is rapidly absorbed from the alveoli. Due to its low blood/gas solubility equilibrium is rapidly established between the alveoli and the blood, and across the blood–brain barrier (Figure 3.1). The vast majority of the gas is exhaled unchanged although a small amount may defuse through the skin or be excreted in the urine.

Cardiovascular system

Nitrous oxide has both a direct depressant and sympthomimetic effect on the myocardium. In healthy patients these tend to counterbalance each other, the resultant effect being minimal cardiovascular depression. In patients with cardiovascular disease or who are taking conconcurrent medication with, e.g. β blockers, its depressant effect may be more obvious. Nitrous oxide supplementation of high-dose opioid-based anaesthesia may result in a reduction in cardiac output and heart rate although the mechanism of this is unclear. Nitrous oxide may have a venoconstrictor effect resulting in increased pulmonary vascular resistance, particularly in the presence of pulmonary hypertension. In common with all anaesthetic agents it has a depressant effect on baroreceptor reflexes.

Respiratory system

Nitrous oxide decreases tidal volume and increases the rate of breathing and minute ventilation. Although arterial carbon dioxide partial pressures tend not to be affected the normal ventilatory responses to carbon dioxide and to hypoxia are depressed. Alveolar collapse in structured lung segments may be more rapid in the presence of nitrous oxide than with oxygen due to its greater solubility. Similarly, it depresses mucous flow and chemotaxis. In theory these factors predispose to postoperative respiratory complications.

Diffusion hypoxia describes the rapid movement of nitrous oxide from the blood into the alveoli in the early recovery phase. It is usual to circumvent this problem by administering 100% oxygen for a few minutes at the end of anaesthesia.

Central nervous system

Nitrous oxide is a weak anaesthetic with a minimum alveoli concentration (MAC) value of 104%. Surgical anaesthesia is impossible with this agent alone without inducing hypoxia. At twice the normal atmospheric pressure 50% nitrous oxide in oxygen is sufficient for surgical anaesthesia. It is widely used as a supplementary agent to reduce the concentration of volatile agents (for secondary gas effect see above). It has a powerful analgesic effect when used in sub-anaesthetic doses (up to 50% in oxygen). It is now thought to exert its analgesic action by antagonising the *N*-methyl-D-aspartate (NMDA) receptor.

Closed cavities

Nitrous oxide is approximately 34 times more soluble in blood than nitrogen. It will diffuse into, and from, air-containing cavities more rapidly than nitrogen. Thus, during nitrous oxide anaesthesia, air- or gas-filled cavities will tend to expand with the risk of rupture and pneumothorax, e.g. lung cyst, bullae. Similarly, chronic inflammation in the middle ear may result in blockage of the Eustachian tube. In these circumstances, nitrous oxide may induce barotrauma and pain.

A similar phenomenon can be observed in the cuffs and balloons of tracheal tubes, flotation catheters, etc. Increases in cuff pressure may be sufficient to cause mucosal ischaemia with subsequent damage to the tracheal mucosa. In the case of pulmonary flotation catheters, there is a risk of cuff rupture followed by gas embolism and infarction. A number of factors affect the rate of volume and pressure change—time, permeability, elasticity, initial volume and pressure, nitrous oxide concentration, temperature.

Gastrointestinal tract

Nitrous oxide is associated with postoperative nausea and vomiting. This probably involves both central and peripheral mechanisms, the latter is the result of distension of the gut due to rapid movement of nitrous oxide into the lumen. It is possible that better operating conditions are achieved when nitrous oxide is avoided.

Toxicity

Nitrous oxide causes near-complete inactivation of methylcobalamin (vitamin B_{12}) after a few hours exposure. In normal circumstances, monovalent cobalamin is essential for the synthesis of methionine and tetrahydrofolate, and ultimately through a series of reactions, for the conversion of deoxyuridine to deoxythymidine. Deoxythymidine is essential for the synthesis of DNA (deoxyribonucleic acid). In the presence of nitrous oxide, monovalent cobalamin is irreversibly oxidised to a bivalent form which cannot participate in this series of reactions. Perhaps surprisingly, the only proven consequences of this oxidation in man are in the bone marrow in the short term and the nervous system in the long term.

Reversible megaloblastic changes can be detected in the bone marrow after 12–24 hours exposure. Peripheral granulocytopaenia occurs after about 3 days exposure and irreversible agranulocytosis after 5 days. Although the administration of folinic acid can protect the majority of patients, nitrous oxide should never be given for more than 24 hours. Recovery of normal function is slow and repeat administrations of nitrous oxide within a few days may also result in megaloblastic changes.

Nitrous oxide toxicity may affect staff as well as patients. The risk to staff is greatest in areas where there are absent or inefficient scavenging systems, e.g. hospital delivery suites, computerised tomographic(CT) scanning rooms. There is evidence of non-compliance with national occupational exposure standards (OES) in the UK. Despite extensive investigation there is no evidence linking low-level occupational exposure with an increased incidence of spontaneous abortion. Although nitrous oxide does not appear to be fetotoxic in humans, it is prudent to avoid lengthy exposures in the first trimester of pregnancy, given its proven effects on DNA synthesis.

Xenon

Xenon (*xenos*: Greek—'alien') was discovered, in 1898, by Ramsay and Travers but it was almost 50 years before its anaesthetic properties were identified. It was first administered to human volunteers in 1951 by Cullen and Gross. The main disadvantages of xenon were immediately apparent—its high cost and low potency aggravated by dilution in the breathing circuit due to nitrogen washout.

Environmental considerations have prompted renewed interest in xenon as a substitute for the 'greenhouse' gas—nitrous oxide. Despite some useful features, it is doubtful if xenon anaesthesia could be justified on the basis of cost-benefit. The gas may have a place as a 'niche' anaesthetic for high-risk patients or as a sedative for intensive care patients who are haemodynamically unstable.

Physical structure

Xenon is an odourless, colourless, non-explosive gas present in the atmospheres of both Earth and Mars in concentrations of approximately 0.08 ppm. Its density is approximately three times and its viscosity twice that of nitrous oxide. Like other 'noble' gases, such as helium and argon, its outer electron shell contains the maximum number of electrons (8) making the molecule highly stable chemically. Despite this, its anaesthetic activity indicates that xenon binds to cell proteins and cell membrane constituents.

Xenon has a large number of isotopes, many of which are naturally occurring. The only isotope of medical importance is ^{133}Xe which is used in the measurement of regional cerebral blood flow and in lung function testing.

Physical characteristics

These are shown in Table 3.3. Xenon (MAC 70%) has a potency of about twice that of nitrous oxide (MAC 104%). Thus, it can be given in anaesthetic concentrations in oxygen with less risk of hypoxia. It is highly insoluble in all body tissues with a blood/gas partition coefficient of 0.14 (nitrous oxide, 0.47; sevoflurane, 0.65; desflurane, 0.42).

Cardiovascular system

The initial report in 1951 indicated that arterial pressure and heart rate remained within normal limits during 50% xenon in oxygen anaesthesia. Some workers noted a slight tendency to bradycardia with 75% xenon. No ECG abnormalities were observed. During surgery there is now ample evidence that xenon tends to suppress unwanted haemodynamic responses.

Cerebral haemodynamics

Computerised tomography (CT) images can be enhanced by inhaled xenon and ^{133}Xe has been widely used to measure regional cerebral blood flow. Several studies have shown increases in cerebral blood flow during xenon inhalation in both volunteers and patients with head injury. Xenon anaesthesia is probably unsuitable in the presence of intracranial disease. Xenon-enhanced CT scanning is said to be safe, provided the lungs are hyperventilated to prevent an increase in intracranial pressure.

Respiratory system

Xenon/oxygen mixtures being non-irritant and odourless are pleasant to breathe. There is a tendency to slowing of the respiratory rate and an increase in tidal volume but the mechanism by which this occurs is unknown. Xenon has a negligible effect on gas exchange and P_{O_2}, P_{CO_2} and peak airway pressures are unaffected. Despite being denser and more viscous than nitrous oxide, xenon/oxygen mixtures are not more difficult to breathe. Expiratory resistance increases when breathing 70/30 xenon/oxygen compared to 70/30 nitrous oxide/oxygen.

Recovery characteristics

Rapidity of recovery has been one of the most consistent and compelling features of anaesthesia with xenon. After 2 hours of xenon anaesthesia recovery is two to three times as fast as recovery from equi-MAC mixtures of N_2O/sevoflurane and N_2O/isoflurane. Marked emetic effects after both nitrous oxide and xenon were reported in a volunteer study, but this was conducted under highly artificial conditions.

Analgesic action

Xenon has been reported to have a more pronounced analgesic effect than nitrous oxide. In volunteers subjected to a variety of pain modalities at equi-MAC concentrations of xenon and nitrous oxide, xenon had a slightly more potent analgesic action. This was not thought to be of clinical relevance.

Metabolism and elimination and toxicity

It is highly unlikely that xenon participates in biochemical reactions although it has been shown to have an inhibitory action at NMDA receptors. It has also been reported by Petzelt in 1999 to inhibit Ca^{2+} regulated transitions in the cell cycle of human endothelial cells. Elimination of xenon is almost entirely through the lungs. Unlike nitrous oxide, xenon does not appear to have any adverse effects on the bone marrow, and there is no evidence of teratogenicity or fetotoxicity.

Administration

Because of cost, xenon must be given using low flow rebreathing systems. It is possible to produce leak-proof breathing systems for experimental purposes, but difficult to achieve in clinical practice. Systems are now available which are near to leak-proof. Xenon diffuses freely through (silicone) rubber. A second difficulty is the dilution of xenon in the circuit due to nitrogen washout from the patient. The system must be flushed out during the initial period and recharged with a xenon/oxygen mixture.

Measuring xenon

When rebreathing systems are used for the delivery of xenon, its concentration within the system needs to be closely monitored. Infrared gas analysers cannot detect xenon, since it is a single atom, and as it is chemically inert its physical properties must be utilised. Mass spectrometry is the most accurate method but it is expensive and it is impractical for clinical use. A calibrated katharometer combined with a galvanic oxygen sensor is a satisfactory alternative which provides a reasonably accurate measure (±1%).

Mechanism of action

Unlike most general anaesthetics, xenon does not enhance the activity of the inhibitory $GABA_A$ receptors. Instead, it appears to have a marked inhibitory effect on excitatory NMDA receptors, and in that regard resembles the intravenous anaesthetic ketamine, some of whose pharmacological properties it shares (analgesia, minimal cardiovascular depression). Nitrous oxide is also thought to act, at least partly at NMDA receptors and this may account for its pharmacological similarity to xenon.

Manufacture and cost

Xenon is produced by the fractional distillation of air, mostly in oxygen separation plants with a daily oxygen production of over 1000 tonnes. It has been estimated that the lowest hourly cost achievable with near conventional anaesthetic equipment and techniques is £160–£180 for a 70/30 xenon/oxygen mixture.

Radiological uses

Xenon has been used to measure cerebral blood flow and to map regional blood flow in the brain. Two forms are used: a stable radio-dense molecule for xenon-enhanced CT scanning; a radioisotope, ^{133}Xe, whose clearance can be measured using gamma scintillography. Xenon can be injected into the carotid artery or intravenously, or given by inhalation. In a laser-induced hyperpolarised state, it may have a role as a contrast medium in magnetic resonance imaging.

Nitric oxide

Nitric oxide (NO) is a colourless, highly reactive, toxic gas which liquefies at –151.8°C. Although it is the most stable of the oxides of nitrogen it reacts rapidly with oxygen to form the highly reactive nitrogen dioxide (NO_2). The gas is highly lipid-soluble and being a small molecule diffuses rapidly across biological membranes.

Physical characteristics

These are listed in Table 3.3.

Medical applications

Nitric oxide is now known to be identical to the endothelium-derived relaxing factor described by Furchgott and Zawadzki in 1980. It is a key signalling messenger in several body systems, particularly the CVS and CNS. Nitric oxide is formed by NO synthase (NOS) enzymes, which catalyse the oxidation of L-arginine to form NO and citrulline.

The medical uses of NO are to reverse hypoxic pulmonary vasoconstriction in a variety of conditions. These include the adult respiratory distress syndrome (ARDS), pulmonary hypertension in adults, and persistent pulmonary hypertension in the newborn. There is little evidence to support the use of inhaled NO in the majority of patients with ARDS. NO may give rise to methaemoglobinaemia in infants, lung damage from reactive metabolites, nitrogen dioxide toxicity, and damage to the surfactant layer. Despite this, the evidence to date indicates that the toxicity of inhaled NO in patients is low. Guidelines and recommendations for the use of inhaled NO in adult intensive care units are available.

The use of NO in persistent pulmonary hypertension of the newborn appears to be beneficial in improving gas exchange and decreasing pulmonary resistance. NO has also been used in the treatment of chronic pulmonary hypertension and in the management of heart and lung transplantation. The results in individual cases are encouraging but large studies are required for validation.

Administration and monitoring

Medical grade NO is 99% pure and in Europe it is available for clinical use in a mixture with nitrogen at a concentration of 1000 ppm. The UK cylinder is colour coded light grey/green with a darker green shoulder and a grey stripe. In the US it is available as a mixture in either nitrogen or helium at 100 ppm or 800 ppm. The most important safety consideration from both the patient's and the carer's perspective is the oxidation of NO to NO_2. At concentrations of 20 ppm or below, environmental contamination with either NO or NO_2 is extremely low even in the absence of scavenging. Delivery systems are designed to minimise the risk to patients.

The dosage of NO is generally between 10 ppm and 80 ppm but lower doses down to 1–10 ppm are advocated by some. There is considerable interindividual variation in response but no evidence of tachyphylaxis. NO is administered only to patients with full haemodynamic and other monitoring in place. Methaemoglobin concentrations should be monitored especially when high concentrations are given to the newborn (<2% as a proportion of the total haemoglobin).

FURTHER READING

Nickalls RWD, Mapleson WW. Age-related iso-MAC charts for isoflurane, seroflurane and desflurane in man. *British Journal of Anaesthesia* 2003;91:170–4

Njoku DB, Greenberg RS, Bourdi M, et al. Autoantibodies associated with volatile anesthetic hepatitis found in the sera of a large cohort of pediatric anesthesiologists. *Anesth Analg* 2002;94: 239–40.

4

Intravenous anaesthetic agents

TJ McMurray

Introduction • The ideal intravenous anaesthetic agent • Mechanism(s) of intravenous anaesthesia • Pharmacokinetics and metabolism • Rapidly acting intravenous anaesthetics • Non-barbiturate intravenous anaesthetics • Slower-acting intravenous anaesthetics • Other drugs

INTRODUCTION

The concept of intravenous anaesthesia in the modern era was born in 1932 with the first published report by Wesse and Scharpff, of hexobarbitone, the first rapidly acting intravenous agent. However, it was thiopentone that was to dominate the field of intravenous anaesthesia until the 1980s. Thiopentone was introduced into clinical practice independently by Waters and Lundy in 1934.

The subsequent development of rapid and short-acting hypnotic, analgesic, and muscle relaxant drugs has permitted the development of total intravenous anaesthesia (TIVA) during which anaesthesia is maintained solely by intravenous drugs. Intravenous induction agents are classified in Table 4.1 according to their speed of onset and chemical group.

THE IDEAL INTRAVENOUS ANAESTHETIC AGENT

For many years, thiopentone was the 'gold standard' against which other intravenous induction agents were measured. This is probably no longer the case, and propofol could now be said to occupy this position in the developed world. Although the 'ideal' intravenous agent does not yet exist, the concept is useful when comparing agents. To date, no agent can claim all the ideal properties listed in Table 4.2 and the anaesthetist must choose those agents which are most appropriate for an individual patient undergoing a specific operation.

Table 4.1 Classification of intravenous anaesthetics
Rapidly acting agents
Barbiturates
Thiobarbiturates: thiopentone, thiamylal
Methohexitone
Imidazole compounds: etomidate
Sterically hindered alkyl phenols: propofol
Steroids: eltanolone, Althesin™, minaxolone (none currently available)
Eugenols: propanidid (not currently available)
Slower acting agents
Ketamine
Benzodiazepines: midazolam, flunitrazepam, diazepam

Table 4.2 Physical and pharmacological properties of the ideal intravenous anaesthetic agent

Physical	Drug compatibility and stability in solution
	Water-soluble: avoids the use of solubilising agents
	No pain on injection, no venous or tissue damage following extravasation
Pharmacokinetics	High lipid solubility, a high proportion of unbound, unionised drug to facilitate rapid onset of action
	Steep dose–response curve to facilitate titration and minimise accumulation
	Recovery dependent on rapid metabolism to inactive compounds
Pharmacodynamics	Rapid onset of action without excitatory activity
	Analgesic at sub-anaesthetic concentrations
	Lack of organ toxicity. This includes absence of cardiorespiratory depression, hepatotoxicity and immunosuppression
	No stimulus for porphyria, malignant hyperpyrexia
	Low potential for histamine release and hypersensitivity reactions
	Absence of postoperative nausea, emesis, psychomimetic reactions and hangover

MECHANISM(S) OF INTRAVENOUS ANAESTHESIA

We are at the beginning of understanding the mechanism(s) by which the diverse range of molecules with anaesthetic actions bring about their effects. The hypothesis of Meyer and Overton, that anaesthetics disrupt the lipid cell bilayer has been set aside in favour of the concept that they produce their effects through modulation of ligand-gated ion channels. There are a number of reasons for this shift. First, several compounds have membrane destabilising effects without having any anaesthetic actions. Second, many anaesthetics exist as enantiomers and show marked enantioselectivity in their anaesthetic potency. Third, the effects of anaesthetic agents on certain receptors have been demonstrated at clinically relevant drug concentrations.

The $GABA_A$ receptor is now believed to be the major target site for anaesthetic action. The $GABA_A$ receptors exist as a family of subtypes with their pharmacology determined by their composition. $GABA_A$ receptors are pentameric and comprise of two α, two β (or θ), and one γ (or ε) subunits, which assemble to form a chloride-sensitive pore. When the receptor is activated, transmembrane chloride conductance increases, resulting in hyperpolarisation of the postsynaptic cell membrane and functional inhibition of the postsynaptic neurone.

Sedative intravenous anaesthetic drugs interact with different components of the $GABA_A$ receptor. Benzodiazepines bind to specific sites on the $GABA_A$ receptor complex and increase the efficiency of the coupling between the GABA receptor and the chloride ion channel. This modulation of the $GABA_A$ receptor is limited, explaining the ceiling effect of benzodiazepines on central nervous system (CNS) function.

At clinically relevant concentrations, intravenous anaesthetics, with the exception of ketamine, produce their effects through potentiation of the inhibitory $GABA_A$ receptor system. The intravenous anaesthetic agents decrease the rate of dissociation of GABA from its receptor thereby prolonging its effect on Cl^- conductance. Furthermore at higher concentrations many intravenous anaesthetics exhibit GABAergic activity (Figure 4.1a). In contrast, ketamine is an inhibitor at the excitatory, glutamatergic *N*-methyl-D-aspartate (NMDA)

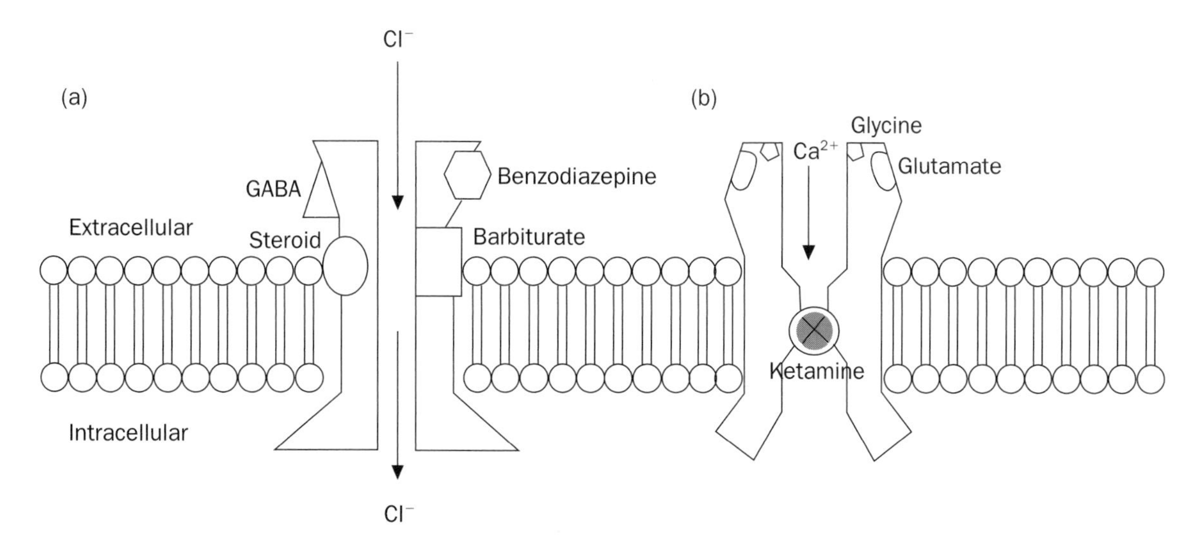

Figure 4.1 *A model depicting the different sites at which GABA, glutamate, and some intravenous (IV) anaesthetics may act. (a) The $GABA_A$ receptor. Sedative IV anaesthetic drugs interact with different components of the $GABA_A$ receptor. Benzodiazepines bind to specific receptor sites that are part of the $GABA_A$ receptor complex and increase the efficiency of the coupling between the GABA receptor and the chloride ion channel. Intravenous anaesthetic agents decrease the rate of dissociation of GABA from the receptor and the effect on Cl^- conductance requires the presence of GABA. (b) The NMDA receptor. Ketamine is an inhibitor at the excitatory, glutamatergic* N-methyl-D-aspartate *(NMDA) receptor. It is believed that ketamine acts at a site other than the primary ligand (glutamate) binding site, and that it 'sits' in the open ion channel, blocking the influx of Ca^{2+} and thus depressing excitatory transmission.*

receptor. It is believed that ketamine acts at a site other than the primary ligand (glutamate) binding site, and that it 'sits' in the open ion channel, blocking the influx of Ca^{2+} and thus depressing excitatory transmission. Recent studies have also shown that ketamine (and volatile agents) are potent inhibitors at neuronal nicotinic acetylcholine (nnACh) receptors and this may explain their analgesic effects at sub-anaesthetic concentrations (Figure 4.1b).

PHARMACOKINETICS AND METABOLISM

When an anaesthetic drug is administered as an intravenous bolus, there is a rapid increase in plasma concentration, followed by rapid distribution and redistribution of the drug throughout the body. The redistribution of intravenous (IV) anaesthetics from the richly perfused brain to other less richly supplied organs is shown in Figure 4.2. Initially, a large proportion of the drug is distributed to well-perfused viscera (brain, liver, kidneys). Although muscle has a relatively good blood supply and large mass, distribution to it is slower because of its low lipid content. Despite their high lipid solubility, IV anaesthetic drugs distribute slowly to adipose tissue because of its poor blood supply.

The rapid onset of the CNS effects of most IV anaesthetics can be explained by their high lipid solubility and the relatively high proportion of cardiac output (20%) perfusing the brain. If cerebral blood flow is significantly reduced as a consequence of decreased cardiac output, the anaesthetic effect will be delayed although the effect may be greater due to higher plasma drug concentrations.

Other factors regulating rate of transfer into the brain include:

Speed of injection The initial pharmacological effects, including CNS effects, are related to the

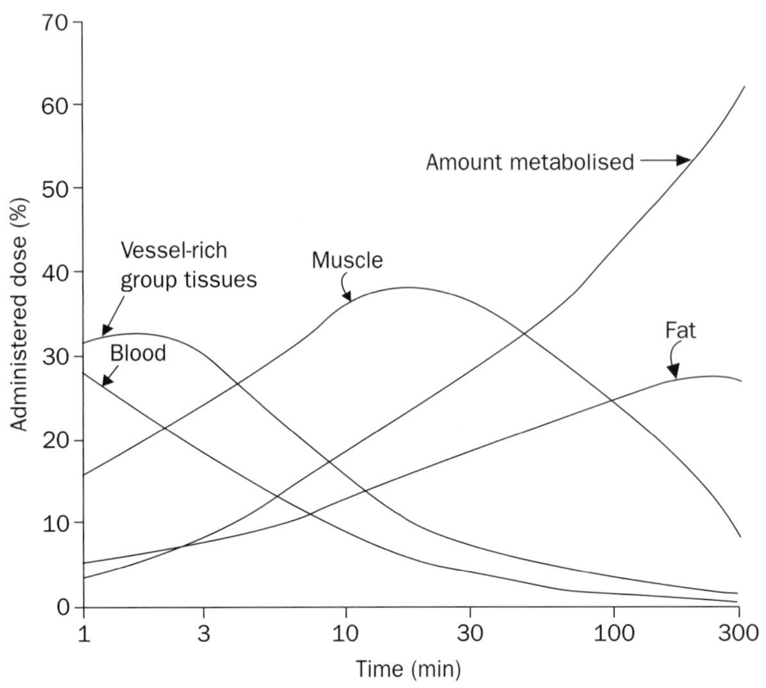

Figure 4.2 *Tissue distribution of thiopentone following intravenous injection. (Data from Saidman LJ and Eger EI.* Anesthesiology *1966;27: 118–26.)*

concentration and activity of the drug in the central compartment. Rapid IV injection results in high initial drug concentrations and increases the speed of onset of unconsciousness but will also increase the magnitude of cardiorespiratory side effects.

Extracellular pH and pKa of the drug Although lipid solubility facilitates diffusion of IV anaesthetics across cellular membranes, only the non-ionised form is able to cross these membranes. The ratio of the non-ionised to ionised fraction depends on the pKa of the drug and the pH of the body fluids (see Chapter 2).

Protein binding Protein binding determines the amount of free drug available for diffusion into the brain and most anaesthetic agents have a high protein binding characteristic (>90%). When several drugs compete for the same binding sites or when plasma proteins are reduced, due to a pre-existing disease (hepatic failure), a higher proportion of the drug will be available for diffusion and will produce an exaggerated effect. Hyperventilation, which alters blood pH, will also decrease protein binding and enhance the anaesthetic effect.

Metabolism and elimination of intravenous anaesthetics

The metabolism and elimination of IV anaesthetics starts after administration as soon as the drug reaches the liver, lungs, or other sites of removal. The primary mechanism for terminating the central effects of IV anaesthetics administered for induction is through redistribution, along concentration gradients, from the well-perfused brain to larger, relatively less well-perfused sites (muscle, fat). Most IV anaesthetic agents are eliminated by hepatic metabolism followed by renal excretion of more water-soluble metabolites. Some metabolites have pharmacological activity and can contribute to prolonged drug effects (norketamine, 1-OH midazolam). Rapid metabolism may play some part in the termination of the central action of agents, such as remifentanil. However, because of the large volumes of distribution of IV anaesthetic drugs and their high protein binding, complete elimination takes many hours or even days. A small proportion of drug may be excreted unchanged in the urine.

Marked inter-patient variability exists in the pharmacokinetics of intravenous anaesthetics. Factors that can influence drug disposition include the degree of protein binding, the efficiency of the hepatic and renal clearance systems, physiological changes with ageing, disease states, site of operation, body temperature, and drug interactions (premedicants, volatile anaesthetics).

Hypersensitivity reactions

The term *hypersensitivity* is used to cover a type of adverse reaction to a drug that resembles the effect of histamine release. Hypersensitivity reactions to IV agents and/or their solubilising agents can be severe or even life-threatening as the intravenous route bypasses many of the normal protective barriers against the entrance of foreign molecules into the body. With the possible exception of etomidate, all IV induction agents have been known to cause some histamine release and thiopentone administration has been shown to be associated with a threefold rise in circulating histamine concentrations. Estimates for life-threatening reactions are between 1:450,000 for etomidate to 1:1000 for drugs solubilised in Cremophor EL (Table 4.3). The high frequency of allergic reactions to the Cremophor EL-containing formulations led to the early withdrawal of several intravenous anaesthetics (Althesin™, propanidid, propofol EL).

Barbiturates may precipitate episodes of acute intermittent porphyria (AIP) and their use is contraindicated in patients who are predisposed to this condition. Some animal models indicate that ketamine, etomidate, and the benzodiazepines may be porphyrinogenic and propofol is considered to be the intravenous anaesthetic of choice in AIP-prone patients.

RAPIDLY ACTING INTRAVENOUS ANAESTHETICS

Barbiturates

Barbituric acid has no hypnotic action, but substitution of the side chains by organic radicals produces compounds with the ability to depress consciousness (Figure 4.3). Substitution of a sulphur atom at position 2 results in a rapidly acting drug while the presence of a methyl group at position 1 results in a more rapid onset of action but also a high incidence of dose-related excitatory phenomena. Barbiturate intravenous anaesthetics share many common pharmacological properties. Thiopentone will consequently be used as a representative agent for this group.

The most commonly used barbiturates are thiopentone [5-ethyl-5-(1-methylbutyl)-2-thiobarbituric acid], methohexitone [1-methyl-5-allyl-5-(1-methyl-2-pentynyl) barbituric acid], and thiamylal [5-allyl-5-(1-methylbutyl)-2-thiobarbituric acid]. Thiamylal is slightly more

Table 4.3 Incidence of life-threatening hypersensitivity reactions to intravenous anaesthetic agents

Agent	*Incidence*
Etomidate	1:100 000–1:450 000
Propofol (emulsion)	1:80 000–1:100 000
Thiopentone	1:14 000–1:20 000
Methohexitone	1:1600–1:7000
Drugs formulated with Cremophor EL (Althesin™, propanidid, propofol EL)	1:400 – 1:1100

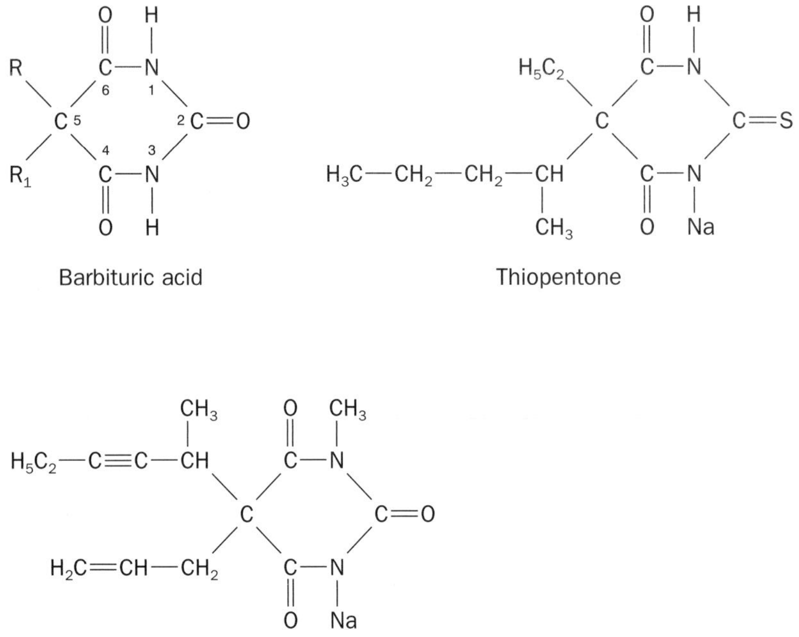

Barbituric acid

Thiopentone

Methohexitone

***Figure 4.3** Structural formulae of common barbiturate anaesthetics.*

potent than thiopentone but has very similar pharmacological properties. Although the L isomers of thiopentone and thiamylal are twice as potent as the *d*-isomers, the commercial preparations are racemic mixtures. Because methohexitone has two asymmetric carbon atoms, it has four stereoisomers. The β-L isomer is much more potent than the α-L isomer, but produces excessive excitatory reactions. Consequently, methohexitone is marketed as the racemic mixture of the two α isomers.

All three barbiturates are available as sodium salts that are soluble in water or isotonic saline.

Thiopentone sodium

Thiopentone sodium (Figure 4.3) is available as a yellow powder, stored in nitrogen to prevent atmospheric degradation, and mixed with 5% anhydrous sodium carbonate. The sodium carbonate prevents precipitation of the insoluble free acid and results in a solution with a pH of 10.5–11.0. The oil/water partition coefficient is 4.7 and the pKa 7.6. Although thiobarbiturate solutions are stable, if refrigerated, for up to two weeks, they should not be stored for longer than 24 hours as the solutions do not contain any antibacterial preservative.

Pharmacokinetics

When injected intravenously, thiopentone, which has high lipid solubility and is 61% unionised at physiological pH, rapidly diffuses into the CNS. However, between 75% and 85% is bound to plasma proteins, mainly albumin, and only the free unbound drug is available for pharmacological effect. Recovery of consciousness occurs at a higher blood concentration if a large dose is given or the drug is injected rapidly. While this has not been fully explained, it has been suggested that acute tolerance or altered redistribution may play a role.

Thiopentone is metabolised in the liver to hydroxythiopentone and the carboxylic acid metabolite, both of which are more water-soluble and almost devoid of CNS activity. The low clearance of thiopentone (3.4 $mL{\cdot}kg^{-1}{\cdot}min^{-1}$) contributes to a relatively long elimination half-life of about 12 hours (Table 4.4). The effect of the slow elimination is that residual (hangover) effects of a single dose persist for many hours and repeated small doses or infusions will lead to cumulation and more prolonged effects. During prolonged continuous infusion the elimination of thiopentone may change from a first order to a zero order process, with production of a long-acting metabolite, pentobarbitone.

Dose and administration

Thiopentone is administered as a 2.5% solution, the usual intravenous induction dose being 3–5 $mg \cdot kg^{-1}$ in adults and 5–6 $mg \cdot kg^{-1}$ in children. The dose necessary to induce anaesthesia is reduced by premedication, during early pregnancy and in critically ill patients. Patients over 70 years of age require a 30–40% lower dose because of a decrease in the volume of distribution, lower plasma proteins, and a slower redistribution of the drug from vessel-rich tissues. However, the above doses are merely guidelines, and the calculated dose should be administered over 10–20 seconds and the drug titrated to clinical effect, i.e. loss of eyelash reflex.

Induction of anaesthesia is usually smooth and pleasant and patients may comment upon a garlic-like taste before unconsciousness supervenes. No other drug should be mixed with thiopentone as precipitation, especially with muscle relaxants, may occur.

Pharmacodynamics

Central nervous system

Thiopentone rapidly crosses the blood–brain barrier causing cortical depression. Loss of consciousness normally occurs within 30 seconds, although this may be delayed in patients with a low cardiac output. A smooth, pleasant induction unaccompanied by excitatory phenomenon is characteristic of thiopentone. Thiopentone is not an analgesic and surgical anaesthesia is difficult to achieve without the use of large doses that will predispose to significant cardiorespiratory depression (Table 4.5). Following a single induction dose, consciousness is usually regained after 5–10 minutes.

The influence of IV anaesthetic agents on cerebral blood flow (CBF), metabolism ($CMRO_2$), and intracranial pressure (ICP) is of crucial importance during neuroanaesthesia. Thiopentone causes a decrease in $CMRO_2$ and CBF, thereby lowering ICP. At low concentrations it produces a predominance of high-frequency waveforms (15–30 Hz) in the electroencephalogram (EEG), along with a progressive decrease in frequency and increase in amplitude as the concentration is increased. At high concentrations a burst suppression pattern develops with an increase in isoelectric periods. The maximum reduction in $CMRO_2$ (55%) occurs when the EEG becomes isoelectric (burst

Table 4.4 Pharmacokinetic values for currently available intravenous anaesthetic agents

Agent	*Distribution half-life (min)*	*Protein binding (%)*	*Distribution volume at steady state ($L \cdot kg^{-1}$)*	*Clearance ($mL \cdot kg^{-1} \cdot min^{-1}$)*	*Terminal elimination half-life (h)*
Thiopentone	2–4	85	2.5	3.4	12
Methohexitone	5–6	85	2.2	11	4
Propofol	2–4	98	2–10	20–30	24+
Ketamine	11–16	12	2.5–3.5	12–17	2–4
Etomidate	2–4	75	2.5–4.5	18–25	2.9–5.3

Table 4.5 Main properties of intravenous anaesthetic agents

	Thiopentone	*Methohexitone*	*Propofol*	*Ketamine*	*Etomidate*
Physical characteristics					
Water-soluble	✓	✓	–	✓	a
Stable in solution	–	–	✓	✓	✓
Pain on IV injection	–	✓	✓✓	–	✓✓
Non-irritant on subcutaneous injection	–	✓–	✓	✓	–
Painful on arterial injection	✓	✓	–	–	–
No sequelae from arterial injection	–	✓–	–	–	–
Low incidence of venous thrombosis	✓	✓	✓	✓	–
Pharmacodynamic characteristics					
Rapid onset	✓	✓	✓	–	✓
Cumulation	✓✓	✓	–	✓✓	–
Excitatory effects	–	✓✓	✓	✓	✓✓✓
Respiratory complications	–	✓	✓	–	–
Hypotension	✓	✓	✓✓	–	–
Tachycardia	✓	✓✓	–	✓✓	–
Analgesic	–	–	–	✓✓	–
Emergence delirium	–	–	–	✓✓	✓
Anti-emetic	–	–	✓	–	–
Safe in porphyria	–	–	✓	?	–

✓, property is present or moderate effect; ✓✓, marked effect; ✓✓✓, severe effect.
[a] Water-soluble but not available as aqueous solution.

suppression), usually at a plasma concentration of 30–50 $\mu g \cdot mL^{-1}$. As the decrease in systemic blood pressure is usually less than the reduction in ICP, thiopentone improves cerebral perfusion and compliance leading to its use for 'neuroprotection' during neurosurgery, following acute head injury, and protection against incomplete ischaemia during cardiopulmonary bypass.

Thiopentone is a very potent anticonvulsant and continuous infusions have been used to control refractory status epilepticus.

Eye

Intraocular pressure is reduced by 40%. The pupil first dilates and then constricts, although the light reflex is maintained until surgical anaesthesia is achieved. The corneal, conjunctival, eyelash and eyelid reflexes are abolished.

Cardiovascular system

Thiopentone, given as a bolus, causes a reduction in arterial blood pressure, direct myocardial depression, vasodilatation (including venodilatation), and an increase in heart rate. In common with other intravenous anaesthetic agents, these effects are due to both a direct action on the heart and peripheral vasculature, and indirect effects through depression of the neuroregulatory mechanisms within the CNS. These cardiovascular responses are exaggerated in patients with pre-existing cardiovascular disease, especially in those with a fixed cardiac output. In the presence of hypovolaemia thiopentone should be administered very slowly and in small doses.

Respiratory system

Thiopentone has a potent dose-dependent, depressant effect on both respiratory rate and depth and depresses the sensitivity of the respiratory centre to carbon dioxide. A short period of apnoea is common, frequently preceded by a few deep breaths. Respiratory depression is influenced by premedication and is more pronounced in the presence of opioids and in patients with chronic obstructive pulmonary disease.

Cough and hiccup are uncommon during the administration of thiopentone but laryngeal sensitivity may be increased and secretions/ blood/foreign bodies in the airway may precipitate laryngospasm. There is an increase in bronchial tone although frank bronchospasm is uncommon.

Other effects

Injections of thiopentone rarely cause pain on injection or evidence of venous irritation and the incidence of venous thrombosis is very low at 3–4%.

In conventional doses, thiopentone has no effect on hepatic, renal or adrenocortical function.

Adverse effects

Local necrosis may occur following perivenous leakage of thiopentone. As median nerve damage has been reported following extravasation in the antecubital fossa, this site is not recommended for administration of thiopentone. If significant extravasation occurs then hyaluronidase should be infiltrated into the affected area to facilitate reabsorption.

Intra-arterial injection of thiopentone is a serious complication as crystals of the thiobarbiturate can form in the arterioles and capillaries, causing intense pain, vasoconstriction, thrombosis, and even tissue necrosis. Accidental intra-arterial injections should be treated promptly with intra-arterial administration of a vasodilator (papaverine 20 mg) and lignocaine (lidocaine) (*Note*: leave the needle/cannula in the artery), as well as a regional anaesthesia-induced sympathectomy (stellate ganglion block, brachial plexus block) and anticoagulation with intravenous heparin. The risk of ischaemic damage is much higher with a 5% solution and the use of this concentration is not recommended.

Allergic reactions

Thiopentone administration is associated with a threefold increase in circulating histamine concentrations. Hypersensitivity reactions range from cutaneous rashes to severe or fatal anaphylactic reactions. The incidence of life-threatening reactions is 1:14 000–1:20 000.

Indications

Thiopentone is used for:

- Induction of anaesthesia.
- Maintenance of anaesthesia. Suitable only for short procedures because cumulation occurs with repeated doses.
- Treatment of refractory status epilepticus.
- Reduction in intracranial pressure (ICP).

Absolute contraindications

- Thiopentone is contraindicated in the presence of porphyria where it may lead to circulatory collapse, alimentary crises, cutaneous rashes and lower motor neurone paralysis.
- Thiopentone should not be used if there is any doubt about the ability to maintain the airway.
- Previous hypersensitivity reaction to a barbiturate.

Use with caution in:

- *Cardiovascular disease*. The hypotensive effects of thiopentone are exaggerated in patients with myocardial dysfunction, fixed cardiac output (valvular stenosis, constrictive pericarditis), and in the hypovolaemic patient. However, if used with caution, it is probably no more hazardous than other intravenous agents.

- *Severe hepatic or renal dysfunction.* Reduced plasma proteins result in higher free, unbound thiopentone.
- *Muscle disease.* Respiratory depression is exaggerated in patients with myasthenia gravis or dystrophia myotonica.
- *Reduced metabolic rate.* Patients with myx-oedema are very sensitive to thiopentone.
- *Obstetrics.* While an adequate dose of thiopentone is required to ensure adequate anaesthesia, the barbiturate rapidly crosses the placenta. Cardiorespiratory depression in the fetus may occur if the induction–delivery interval is short.
- *Outpatient anaesthesia.* Early recovery is slow and more fluctuant in comparison with other agents. The advent of newer agents, such as propofol, with much more rapid and clear-headed recovery significantly, has reduced the role of thiopentone in outpatient anaesthesia.
- *Adrenocortical insufficiency.*
- *Asthma.*
- *Extremes of age.*

Methohexitone sodium

Methohexitone (Figure 4.3) is a water-soluble, methylated barbiturate with a pKa of 7.9. It is commercially available as a white powder, combined with 5% anhydrous sodium carbonate. The resultant 1% solution has a pH of 11.1 and although stable, when refrigerated for 6 weeks, should be discarded after 24 hours, as it does not contain an antibacterial preservative.

Pharmacokinetics

The uptake, redistribution and protein binding of methohexitone are somewhat similar to that of thiopentone. Although methohexitone is less lipid soluble than thiopentone, a greater proportion (75%) is non-ionised at body pH and therefore available for pharmacological effect. Hepatic clearance (11 $mL{\cdot}kg^{-1}{\cdot}min^{-1}$) is higher for methohexitone than for thiopentone and the elimination half-life considerably shorter (~4 hours). While cumulation is less likely to occur with repeated doses, prolongation of anaesthetic effect has been demonstrated when methohexitone was infused for longer than 60 minutes.

Dose and administration

As methohexitone is approximately 2.7 times more potent than thiopentone, a dose of 1.5 $mg{\cdot}kg^{-1}$ is equivalent to 4 $mg{\cdot}kg^{-1}$ of thiopentone in adults. As with thiopentone, the induction dose should be reduced in the elderly, in American Society of Anesthesiologists (ASA) grade III or IV patients, and in early pregnancy.

Pharmacodynamics

Central nervous system

Onset of anaesthesia is as rapid though not as smooth as after thiopentone administration, but recovery is more rapid with methohexitone and occurs within 2–5 minutes through redistribution. Drowsiness persists for much longer as the drug is slowly metabolised in the liver. While methohexitone has been reported to cause occasional EEG seizure-like activity in epileptics the drug also possesses anticonvulsant properties.

Cardiovascular system

The cardiovascular effects of methohexitone are similar to those of thiopentone except for a more marked tachycardia and less hypotension.

Respiratory system

Respiratory depression and duration of apnoea are of a lesser magnitude with methohexitone than with thiopentone.

Adverse effects

The most notable differences from thiopentone consist of a high incidence of spontaneous muscle movements, tremor and hypertonus (20% compared with 4% for thiopentone). The incidence is directly related to the dose and rate of administration and is increased by drugs, such as hyoscine and droperidol, and decreased by opioid premedication. Respiratory complications, such as cough and hiccups, are frequent (26%) and are reduced by atropine and hyoscine but unaffected by other premedicants.

Pain on injection is more common (8–20%) than with thiopentone, especially if a small vein is used for administration but can be reduced by flushing the vein with lidocaine (lignocaine) prior to methohexitone administration.

Epileptiform EEG activity has been described in epileptic subjects. Tissue damage after perivenous extravasation is uncommon. Intra-arterial injection of 1% methohexitone may cause gangrene but the risk is much less than that with 2.5% thiopentone. Allergic reactions occur but are uncommon.

Indications

- Induction of anaesthesia, especially where rapid recovery is desired.
- Anaesthetic agent to supplement electroconvulsive therapy.
- Outpatient and dental anaesthesia.

Absolute contraindications

- These are the same as for thiopentone.

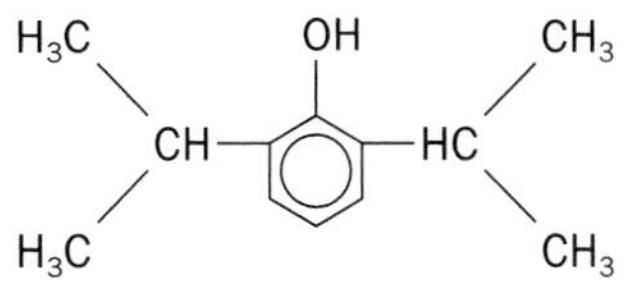

Propofol

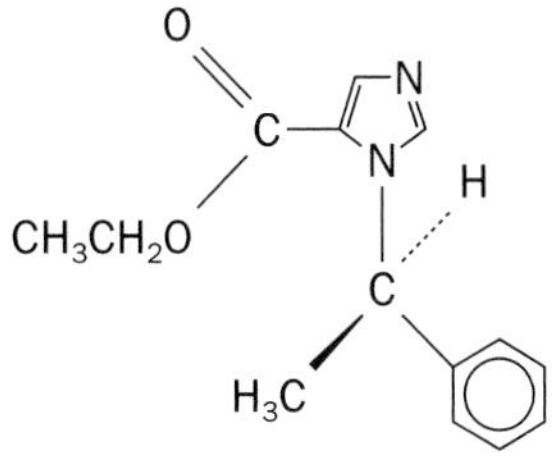

Etomidate

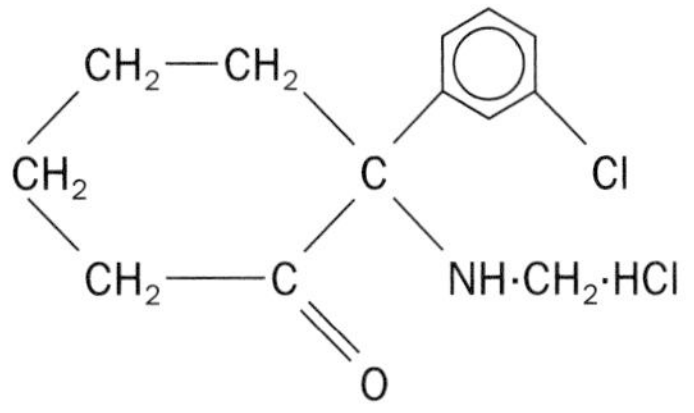

Ketamine

Figure 4.4 *Structural formulae of propofol, etomidate, and ketamine.*

NON-BARBITURATE INTRAVENOUS ANAESTHETICS

Propofol

Propofol (2,6-diisopropylphenol), an alkylphenol compound (Figure 4.4) is virtually insoluble in aqueous solution. The initial Cremophor EL formulation was withdrawn from clinical testing because of a high incidence of anaphylactic reactions. Propofol is now constituted as a 1% emulsion containing 10% soya bean oil, 1.2% egg phosphatide and 2.25% glycerol. More recently, a 2% solution and a specially tagged 50 mL prefilled syringe for target-controlled infusions (TCI) have become available. The pH is 6–8.5 and the pKa is 11.

The fat emulsion used to solubilise propofol is similar to Intralipid, used for parenteral nutrition. Its disadvantages include: (1) being an excellent culture medium if bacterially contaminated: and (2) presenting the patient with a high lipid load if infused over a prolonged period. While the emulsion is non-irritant, pain on injection occurs in 32–67% of patients when the propofol emulsion is injected into small hand veins. This can be minimised by injection into large veins, by administration of 1% lidocaine (lignocaine) (before or mixed with propofol), or a potent opioid analgesic. Diluting the solvent with additional solvent (Intralipid) or changing the lipid carrier also reduces pain on injection. A new propofol formulation with sodium metabisulphite (instead of disodium edetate) as an antimicrobial has also been recently shown to be associated with less injection pain.

Pharmacokinetics

Propofol is 98% bound to plasma proteins and, being highly lipophilic is rapidly distributed to vessel-rich tissues. Clearance from the plasma is generally accepted to follow a tri-exponential pattern giving a distribution half-life of between 2–4 min, an intermediate (or first) elimination half-life of about 60–75 min and a long terminal elimination half-life which may extend beyond 24 h. The prolonged terminal half-life reflects the return of propofol from a poorly perfused peripheral compartment into the central compartment. After a single dose, clinical recovery is rapid (2–5 min) and clear-headed. Recovery is also relatively rapid after prolonged infusions, due to a very large volume of distribution (600–1000 L). The context-sensitive half-time is less than 40 min after an 8 h infusion (context-sensitive half-time is the time taken for the concentration of a drug in the central compartment to decline by 50%, related to the context of duration of infusion). Clearance from the plasma (20–30 $mL \cdot kg^{-1} \cdot min^{-1}$) is more rapid than with other intravenous agents. Indeed, the clearance of propofol is greater than hepatic blood flow, indicating an extrahepatic site of metabolism. Propofol is rapidly metabolised (less than 20% of a bolus dose remains unchanged after 30 min) to inactive, water-soluble sulphate and glucuronide compounds that are largely excreted in the urine. While prior administration of fentanyl reduces clearance by approximately 30%, few changes in propofol kinetics have been reported in patients with renal or hepatic dysfunction.

Dose and administration

The induction dose in healthy, unpremedicated adults is 1.5–2.5 $mg \cdot kg^{-1}$, with plasma propofol concentrations of 2–6 $\mu g \cdot mL^{-1}$ producing unconsciousness depending on premedicant used, the patient's age, physical status, and the surgical stimulation. Awakening typically occurs at plasma concentrations of 1–1.5 $\mu g \cdot mL^{-1}$. An infusion rate of 100–200 $\mu g \cdot kg^{-1} \cdot min^{-1}$ is recommended when propofol is also used for maintenance hypnosis. In common with the barbiturates, children require higher induction (3–3.5 $mg \cdot kg^{-1}$) and maintenance doses of propofol, due to their larger central volume of distribution and higher rate of clearance. In premedicated patients, the elderly and those in poor health lower induction (1–1.5 $mg \cdot kg^{-1}$) and maintenance doses are recommended. While propofol infusions may be used intra-operatively in children, propofol is not licensed in the UK for sedation in the intensive care unit (ICU) in children younger than 14 years.

Pharmacodynamics

Central nervous system

Unconsciousness is usually achieved 20–40 seconds after an induction dose. Transfer to the CNS is slower than with thiopentone and there is a delay in disappearance of the eyelid reflex, normally used as a sign of unconsciousness after administration of other intravenous anaesthetics. Overdosing of propofol may occur if this sign is used; loss of verbal contact is a more reliable end-point. Recovery is more rapid and 'clear-headed' than with equivalent doses of any other intravenous anaesthetic and occurs after 2–5 minutes, again through redistribution.

Propofol reduces $CMRO_2$ and CBF, as well as ICP. Although cerebral autoregulation is not affected by propofol, when large doses are used the reduction in systemic blood pressure can lead to an unacceptable reduction in cerebral perfusion pressure. The combination of a reduction in $CMRO_2$ and possible free radical scavenging characteristics has led some to suggest that propofol may have neuroprotective properties. Although propofol has been reported to cause convulsions in patients with epilepsy the drug, paradoxically, has anticonvulsant properties.

The use of propofol is associated with a feeling of well-being during early recovery and nausea and vomiting is less common in the postoperative period than with some other intravenous agents. Sub-anaesthetic doses of propofol have been used to treat early postoperative nausea and emesis.

Cardiovascular system

In healthy patients, propofol produces a greater reduction in systemic blood pressure than equivalent doses of barbiturates. This hypotension is a consequence of both direct and indirect effects, namely, direct myocardial depression, direct veno- and vaso-dilatation, suppression of the vasomotor centre within the medulla, and a resetting of the baroreceptors to accept a lower systemic pressure. The alteration of the baroreceptor reflex may explain the minimum change in heart rate seen with propofol. There are case reports of propofol-induced bradycardia and it is recommended that a vagolytic drug should be immediately available in situations where bradycardia is a likely adverse event.

The reduction in blood pressure is dose-dependent and an appreciation of the kinetics of transfer into the brain (see above) would suggest that the drug be given slowly. In premedicated patients, the elderly, and those in poor health, lower induction (1–1.5 $mg \cdot kg^{-1}$) and maintenance doses are recommended to avoid significant hypotension.

Respiratory system

Propofol produces dose-related depression of respiration with apnoea occurring more commonly (25–35%) and being of longer duration than with equipotent doses of barbiturates. Propofol has no effect on bronchial muscle tone and suppresses laryngeal reflexes, making it the induction agent of choice to facilitate the insertion of laryngeal mask airway. A maintenance infusion of propofol decreases tidal volume and increases respiratory rate. While the ventilatory response to carbon dioxide is significantly depressed by propofol, the response to hypoxic pulmonary vasoconstriction is not inhibited.

As with other agents, prior administration of opioids leads to more marked ventilatory depression.

Other effects

Propofol has no significant effect on uterine tone but crosses the placenta easily, giving rise to neonatal depression. The drug is therefore not recommended for use in obstetric anaesthesia.

Hepatic blood flow is decreased in line with the reduction in systemic arterial blood pressure but liver function tests are not deranged following prolonged infusions (up to 24 hours). The transient decrease in renal function is of a lesser magnitude than that seen with thiopentone.

Propofol is not a trigger for porphyria or malignant hyperthermia

Adverse effects

- *Profound hypotension* (dose-dependent), especially in the elderly, the hypovolaemic, and those with pre-existing cardiovascular disease.
- *Excitatory phenomena.* More common than with thiopentone but less than with methohexitone.
- *Pain on injection* (see above).
- *Allergic reactions.* Skin rashes have been reported. Life-threatening reactions are no more common than with thiopentone.

Indications

- *Induction of anaesthesia.* Propofol is the preferred intravenous anaesthetic where a rapid induction with a rapid clear-headed recovery is desired (as in day surgery). The rapid redistribution of this drug may lead to sub-hypnotic plasma concentrations and great care must be taken to ensure adequate anaesthesia in the early operative phase.
- *Sedation* during surgery under regional or local anaesthesia but the airway and ventilation must be observed carefully.
- *Total intravenous anaesthesia (TIVA)*: as propofol shows minimal cumulation with repeated administration or following infusion, it is the hypnotic agent of choice for TIVA.
- *Sedation in ICU*: propofol has been used successfully and widely for sedation of adults in intensive care. The level of sedation is easily controlled and if the duration of infusion does not exceed 5–7 days, recovery is usually not unduly delayed.

Absolute contraindications

- Airway obstruction.
- Known sensitivity to propofol or the emulsion constituents (care with egg allergy).
- Sedation in children, < 14 years, in ICU.

Precautions

Similar to those listed for thiopentone but it is essential to use an aseptic technique (the solution is an excellent culture medium for bacterial contamination). Avoid the use of microbiological filters.

Etomidate

Etomidate (Figure 4.4) is a carboxylated imidazole-containing intravenous anaesthetic [R-1-ethyl-1-(α-methylbenzyl)-imidazole-5-carboxylate] that was introduced in 1972. Although it is soluble in water it is formulated as a 0.2% solution in 35% propylene glycol (pH 6.9) for greater stability. More recently, a new formulation has become available, using lipofundin rather than propylene glycol as the solvent. Only the *d* isomer of etomidate possesses appreciable anaesthetic activity.

Pharmacokinetics

Etomidate undergoes an intramolecular re-arrangement at body pH, analogous to midazolam, resulting in a closed-ring structure with enhanced lipid solubility. It is approximately 75% protein-bound, has a fast distribution half-life of 2–4 min, high hepatic clearance of 18–25 $mL \cdot kg^{-1} \cdot min^{-1}$, and an elimination half-life of 2.9–5.3 hours. The drug is metabolised mainly in the liver by ester hydrolysis to inactive water-soluble metabolites, about 75% being excreted in this form and only 2% excreted unchanged in urine. The clearance of etomidate is markedly reduced by the presence of a steady-state concentration of fentanyl.

Recovery occurs through redistribution but is dose-dependent and remains very short (2–5 min) even after intermittent injections and infusions of the drug.

Dose and administration

The standard induction dose of etomidate is 0.2–0.4 $mg \cdot kg^{-1}$ and a target plasma concentration of 300–500 $\mu g \cdot mL^{-1}$ is required to maintain hypnosis.

Pharmacodynamics

Central nervous system

Onset of unconsciousness is rapid but it is associated with a high incidence of excitatory effects, comparable to methohexitone, but these can be reduced by prior administration of an opioid.

Analogous to the barbiturates, etomidate decreases $CMRO_2$, CBF and ICP but the haemodynamic stability of the drug will maintain CPP. Its well-known inhibition of adrenocortical function limits its clinical usefulness for long-term control of elevated ICP. While etomidate can produce convulsion-like EEG potentials in the absence of apparent convulsions, it has been used to terminate status epilepticus.

Cardiovascular system

Etomidate, when administered as the sole agent, produces little effect on cardiovascular function. It produces a slight reduction in systemic pressure and an increase in heart rate. Myocardial oxygen consumption is not significantly affected by etomidate. The drug does not release histamine and can be safely used in the presence of cardiorespiratory disease.

Respiratory system

Equipotent doses of etomidate and methohexitone produce a similar shift in the carbon dioxide–response curve but at any given carbon dioxide tension ventilation is greater after etomidate than after the barbiturate.

Adverse effects

- *Inhibition of adrenocortical synthetic function.* Etomidate inhibits the activity of 11-β-hydroxylase, an enzyme necessary for the synthesis of cortisol, aldosterone, 17-hydroxyprogesterone, and corticosterone. Even after a single dose, adrenal suppression persists for 5–8 hours. Although the clinical significance of short-term suppression of cortisol synthesis is unknown, maintenance infusions for anaesthesia cannot be recommended.
- *Excitatory phenomena.* Involuntary movement occurs in up to 40% of unpremedicated patients and coughing and hiccup in 10%.
- *Pain on injection.* The 35% propylene glycol solvent is a significant contributor to the high incidence of pain on injection (80% with small veins, 10% with large veins) that can be further reduced by the prior administration of 1% lidocaine (lignocaine).

Injection pain is less with the new formulation containing lipofundin as the solvent rather than propylene glycol.

- *Nausea and vomiting*. The incidence of nausea and vomiting is 30%, considerably greater than that with the barbiturates or propofol.
- *Venous thrombosis* is more common than with other agents. As with pain on injection, the incidence is less when lipofundin is used as the solvent.
- *Emergence phenomena*. The incidence of restlessness and delirium is greater than that seen with the barbiturates or propofol.

Indications

There are now few indications for etomidate, although many anaesthetists still use the drug for induction in patients with compromised cardiovascular function.

Absolute contraindications

- Airway obstruction
- Porphyria
- Adrenal insufficiency
- Long-term infusions.

Precautions

These are similar to those listed for thiopentone. Although in some ways ideal for outpatient anaesthesia its usefulness is undermined by the high incidence of side effects. It has been superseded by propofol in this context.

SLOWER-ACTING INTRAVENOUS ANAESTHETICS

Ketamine

Ketamine [2-(*o*-chlorophenyl)-2-(methylamino)-cyclohexanone hydrochloride] is a phenycyclidine derivative (Figure 4.4) that was introduced in 1965. It is a water-soluble compound, with a pKa of 7.5 and is available in 1%, 5% and 10% solutions. The ketamine molecule contains a chiral centre producing two optical isomers. The anaesthetic and analgesia potency of S (+)-ketamine is three times that of the R (–) enantiomer and twice that of the racemic mixture. The therapeutic index of S (+)-ketamine is 2.5 times that of both the racemic mixture and the R (–) enantiomer. The shorter duration of action and return of cognitive function is related to the faster biotransformation (20%) of S (+)-ketamine. Although the incidence of dreaming is similar with both the S (+) and racemic mixtures, patient acceptability is higher with S (+)-ketamine. Until recently, the only commercially available solution was the racemic mixture of the two isomers and the preservative is benzethonium chloride. However, the S (+) isomer is now clinically available in several European countries.

Pharmacokinetics

Ketamine has high lipid solubility but is only 12% protein-bound. The distribution half-life is approximately 10 minutes, with an elimination half-life of 2–4 hours and recovery is due to both redistribution and metabolism. Ketamine is extensively metabolised in the liver by demethylation and hydroxylation and its primary metabolite, norketamine, has 30–50% the potency of ketamine. Approximately 80% of the metabolites of both ketamine and norketamine are excreted as water-soluble glucuronides via the kidneys with only 2.5% being excreted unchanged. Sub-anaesthetic concentrations of ketamine have been shown to be analgesic, probably through inhibition at neuronal nicotinic acetylcholine (nnACh) receptors. This, and the presence of an active metabolite, and with a contribution from redistribution explain the prolonged recovery from ketamine.

Dose and administration

Induction of anaesthesia by the intravenous route is usually achieved by a dose of 2 $mg{\cdot}kg^{-1}$. Although it is most commonly administered intravenously, oral, intranasal and intramuscular routes (6–10 $mg{\cdot}kg^{-1}$) have been used in paediatric practice.

Pharmacodynamics

Central nervous system

Loss of consciousness is slow after intravenous ketamine and may take 1–2 minutes, compared to the 15–30 seconds with the barbiturates and propofol. It is also difficult to obtain a clear end-point of unconsciousness, as the eyes may remain open with a fixed gaze. The eyelash and corneal reflexes remain unimpaired and there is usually increased muscle tone with some involuntary movements. Ketamine produces a dissociative anaesthetic state characterised by profound analgesia and amnesia. The duration of ketamine-induced anaesthesia is 10–20 minutes following a single dose but full orientation may take up to 90 minutes. Emergence times are even longer following repeated injections or continuous infusions.

Emergence delirium with restlessness, disorientation and unpleasant dreams or hallucinations may occur for up 24 hours following ketamine administration. Their incidence is reduced by psychological preparation of the patient, avoidance of verbal and tactile stimulation during the recovery period, or by concomitant administration of opioids, benzodiazepines, propofol or physostigmine. However, unpleasant dreams may persist.

Ketamine has been traditionally contraindicated in patients with increased ICP or reduced cerebral compliance because it increases $CMRO_2$, CBF and ICP. These deleterious effects can be antagonised by the concomitant administration of propofol, or thiopentone, and benzodiazepines. Furthermore, ketamine is an antagonist at the NMDA receptor. Nevertheless, ketamine can adversely affect neurological outcome in the presence of brain ischaemia.

The EEG changes associated with ketamine anaesthesia are quite unlike those seen with other intravenous anaesthetics and consist of fast β activity mixed with high-voltage δ waves. While ketamine-induced myoclonic and seizure-like activity has been seen in normal (non-epileptic) patients, ketamine appears to possess anticonvulsant properties.

Cardiovascular system

Although ketamine produces direct myocardial depression, it has significant indirect cardiovascular effects through sympathomimetic effects and stimulation of the vasomotor centre. The heart rate and systolic blood pressure increase by 30% and occasionally up to 100%. Owing to the increased cardiac work and myocardial consumption, ketamine adversely affects the balance between myocardial oxygen supply and demand. Consequently, it is not recommended for use as the sole agent in adults with severe cardiovascular disease. However, the same haemodynamic effects, particularly the raised systemic vascular resistance, make the agent particularly suitable for children with cyanotic heart disease.

Respiratory system

Respiratory depression is minimal and transient after conventional doses of ketamine but opioid premedication may lead to transitory apnoea. Ketamine is a bronchodilator and antagonises the bronchoconstrictor action of histamine, making it useful in asthmatics and for treating status asthmaticus. Coughing and hiccuping are more common than with thiopentone. The ability of ketamine to increase oral secretions can lead to laryngospasm during 'light' anaesthesia and the use of a 'drying agent' before anaesthesia has been advocated.

Laryngeal reflexes are not markedly impaired but it is a mistake to think that they remain intact. Radiopaque dye has been aspirated by supine patients given ketamine $2\ mg{\cdot}kg^{-1}$.

Other effects

Intraocular pressure is slightly increased by ketamine. Uterine tone and intrauterine pressure are increased in both the non-pregnant and pregnant uterus, effects that may be harmful in abruptio placentae and cord prolapse. Ketamine rapidly crosses the placenta and equilibrates in fetal plasma.

Transient rashes have been reported in 20% of patients although life-threatening reactions are rare.

Indications

- *High-risk patient.* In shocked states, but hypovolaemia should be corrected.
- *Anaesthesia for minor or repeated procedures* (cardiac catheterisation, burns dressing) in children.

- *Hostile environments.* Accident scenes and casualties of war.
- *Developing countries.* Ketamine is inexpensive, can be used as a sole agent for major surgery and its use does not require sophisticated additional equipment.

Absolute contraindications

- Airway obstruction.
- Raised intracranial pressure.

Precautions

These concern cardiovascular disease, particularly in patients with hypertension or ischaemic heart disease.

The main pharmacodynamic properties of commonly used agents are shown in Table 4.5.

OTHER DRUGS

Benzodiazepines and opioids have been used to induce and maintain anaesthesia. However, large doses are required resulting in prolonged recovery and their use has been restricted to specific specialist areas, e.g. cardiac anaesthesia. The pharmacology of these drugs is discussed elsewhere.

FURTHER READING

Aitkenhead AR, Rowbotham DJ, Smith G. *Text book of anaesthesia* (4th edn). Churchill Livingstone: London, 2001.

Barash PG, Cullen BF, Stoelting RK. *Clinical Anesthesia* (4th edn). Lippincott, Williams & Wilkins: Philadelphia, 2001.

Thompson SA, Wafford K. Mechanism of action of general anaesthetics—new information from molecular pharmacology. *Curr Opin Pharmacol*, 2001; 1:78–83.

5

Local anaesthetics

JP Howe and JPH Fee

Introduction • Chemical structure • Mechanism of action • Pharmacokinetics • Metabolism • Toxicity • Placental transfer • Individual drugs

INTRODUCTION

Local anaesthetics are used to inhibit the transmission of impulses in sensory and mixed nerves. The drugs are categorised as either amino esters or amino amides but both groups of drugs have an identical mode of action. Local anaesthetics comprise a large group of drugs but only a few are of *use* clinically. These are the esters: cocaine, amethocaine, benzocaine, chloroprocaine and procaine; the amides: lidocaine (lignocaine), bupivacaine, levobupivacaine ropivacaine and prilocaine. The ester drugs are associated with hypersensitivity reactions and their use is mostly confined to topical application in ENT and ophthalmic anaesthesia. There are other agents capable of depressing conduction in peripheral nerves but these are unsuitable for use in clinical anaesthesia, e.g. phenytoin, propranolol, class I anti-arrhythmic drugs such as flecanide and antihistamines such as chlorphenaramine.

Local anaesthetics can be applied topically, deposited around peripheral nerves, or infiltrated into tissues. Central neural blockade can be produced by injection into the subarachnoid or epidural spaces. Less common uses are for intravenous regional anaesthesia and attenuation of cardiovascular responses to tracheal intubation. The membrane-stabilising effect of local anaesthetics has been utilised in the treatment of myocardial arrhythmias.

CHEMICAL STRUCTURE

All typical local anaesthetics contain an aromatic amine 'head' joined to an amino group by an intermediate chain or link (Figure 5.1).

These drugs are of similar structure and size (mol. wt. 220–329) and are simultaneously lipophilic and hydrophilic—properties which are essential to their mode of action. With the exception of cocaine, all local anaesthetics in clinical use are synthetic compounds.

Aromatic 'head'

The aromatic portion consists of a benzene ring which confers lipid solubility on the molecule. In the case of the ester agents the lipophilic aromatic head is a derivative of benzoic acid. In contrast, the aromatic head in the amide agents is a derivative of aniline or xylidine (Figure 5.2).

Linkage

The intermediate link is made up of a chain of one to three carbon atoms in either ester

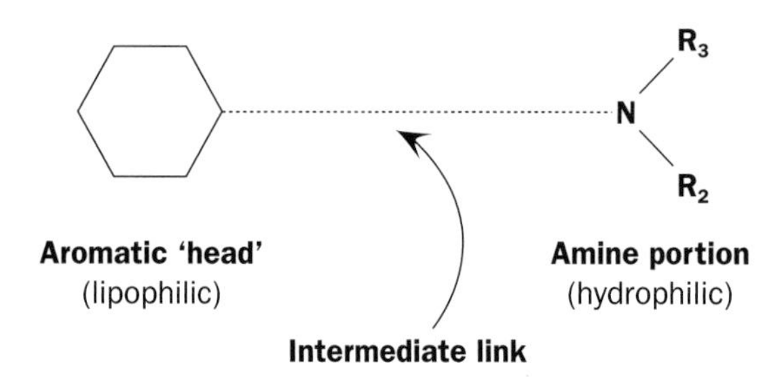

Figure 5.1 *The chemical structure of a local anaesthetic drug.*

(–COO–) or amide (–NHCO–) configuration (6–9 nm in length) (Figure 5.3).

The nature of the configuration is the basis upon which local anaesthetics are classified. Ester local anaesthetics are characteristically unstable compounds that are broken down in the plasma by plasma cholinesterases. In contrast, the amide agents are very stable compounds that require extensive hepatic biotransformation. The more complex the linkage, the greater the tendency for toxicity.

Terminal amine

The hydrophilic component of the molecule consists of a tertiary amine in all cases except for prilocaine which contains a secondary amine group (Figure 5.4). This confers water-soluble properties on the molecule.

Structure–activity relationships

The coexistence of lipid and water solubility in the same molecule is essential for the action of a local anaesthetic drug. Lipophilicity permits the migration of drug across the *phospholipid* membrane of the nerve cell; hydrophilicity is essential for the ionisation of the drug within the nerve. It follows that lipid and water solubility are the external and internal facilitators of local anaesthetic action in the nerve cell. Both within and without the nerve cell the unionised and ionised forms coexist in dynamic equilibrium. Outside the nerve, the active species is the unionised tertiary amine form. Conversely, inside the cell the ionised form predominates. The lower intracellular pH induces a shift in the equilibrium in favour of ionisation (Figure 5.5).

MECHANISM OF ACTION

The interior of a neurone is electronegative with respect to its exterior and in a typical human nerve is of the order of –80 mV. This transmembrane potential is due to the unequal distribution of anions and cations on either side of the cell membrane. The difference in potential is due to a number of factors of which the most important are: (1) the tendency of ions to migrate towards electrical stability; and (2) the tendency of substances to move in the direction of a concentration gradient. These processes are sometimes referred to as the electrochemical properties of the ions. It is the summation of these processes that helps determine the difference in potential across the cell membrane. This is the resting membrane potential (RMP). The evolution of the RMP begins with the large, complex intracellular organic molecules, which cannot migrate across the membrane of a normal healthy cell. These are negatively charged anions and require a high concentration of cations within the cell, mostly in the form of K^+, in order to achieve electrical stability. Outside the cell a similar process operates but in this

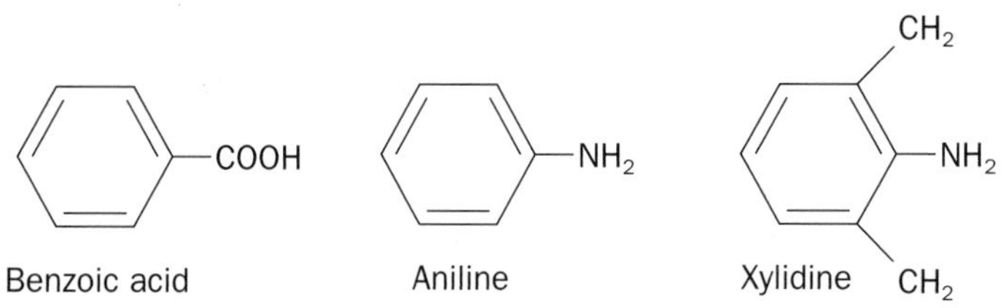

COOH
Benzoic acid
NH_2
Aniline
CH_2
NH_2
CH_2
Xylidine

Figure 5.2 *Structural formulae for benzoic acid, aniline and xylidine.*

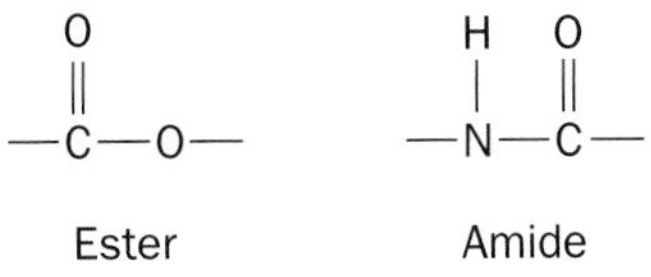

$-C(=O)-O-$ Ester

$-N(H)-C(=O)-$ Amide

Figure 5.3 *Intermediate linkages.*

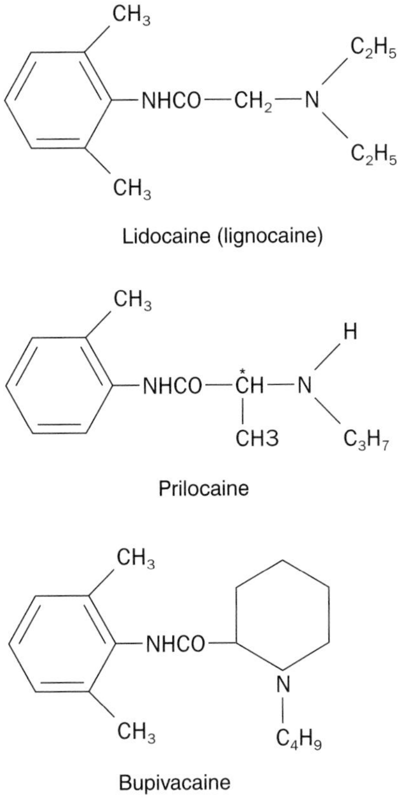

CH_3, NHCO—CH_2—N, C_2H_5, C_2H_5, CH_3

Lidocaine (lignocaine)

CH_3, NHCO—$\overset{*}{C}H$—N, H, CH3, C_3H_7

Prilocaine

CH_3, NHCO, N, CH_3, C_4H_9

Bupivacaine

Figure 5.4 *Structural formulae showing tertiary (lidocaine (lignocaine), bupivacaine) and secondary (prilocaine) amines. * Asymmetrical carbon atom.*

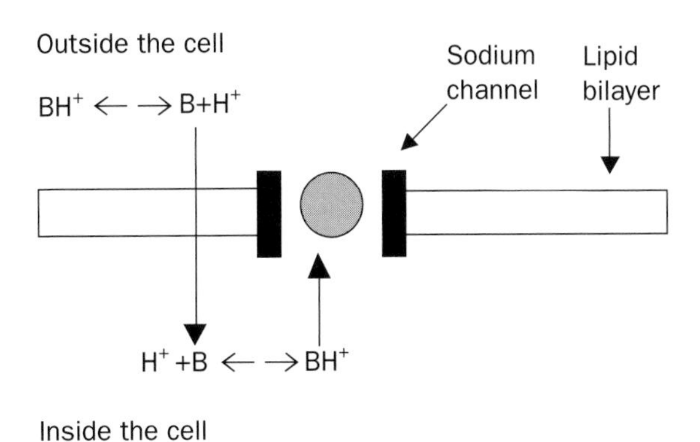

Figure 5.5 *Ionisation equilibrium inside and outside the neuronal membrane.*

instance the anion is Cl^- and the cation is Na^+. Consequently, the concentration of K^+ is much greater inside the cell than out and the reverse is true of Na^+. The maintenance of this ionic disequilibrium across the cell wall is attributable to a number of factors. First, the cell membrane is much more permeable to K^+ ions than to Na^+ ions by a factor of approximately 100 and second, the neuronal membrane contains Na^+/K^+ ATPase, the Na^+/K^+ 'pump'. This is an energy-dependent process that transfers Na^+ *from* the intracellular cytoplasm to the extracellular fluid in exchange for K^+ ions against the existing concentration gradients.

When the RMP becomes less negative the cell undergoes depolarisation and when the RMP becomes more negative the cell undergoes hyperpolarisation. When the RMP increases from –80 mV to a critical value of –55 mV (the threshold potential) an action potential ensues. If an individual spike potential fails to reach the threshold value then an action potential is not generated. This is an all-or-none phenomenon.

The development of an action potential depends on a particular property of the axonal membrane, namely the ability to undergo a rapid increase in Na^+ conductance resulting in massive influx of Na^+ ions into the cell via ion specific channels. These channels are voltage-sensitive and sequentially gated. Voltage dependence implies that the conductance of the Na^+ channel increases markedly when the transmembrane potential in its immediate vicinity becomes more positive. The resulting influx of Na^+ further elevates the membrane potential and this in turn has a similar effect on adjacent Na^+ channels. A wave of depolarisation spreads down the axon as more Na^+ channels are recruited. This process has been likened to the progression of a burning fuse where the heat of combustion of the fuse causes the next segment to ignite. The process becomes self-propagating; as the ignition spreads distally the proximal segment behind cools and becomes inactive.

The concept of sequential gating describes the capacity of the Na^+ channel to facilitate or hinder the movement of Na^+ ions into and out of the neurone at the time of depolarisation and repolarisation. During resting conditions, i.e. in the absence of a neural stimulus, the ion channel is closed to the passage of Na^+ ions by a gating mechanism within the channel which is responsible for maintaining the normal RMP of –80 mV. The gating mechanism consists of a specific channel protein that undergoes a configurational change in such a way as to facilitate or hinder Na^+ ion transfer.

In the absence of a stimulus the channel is described as resting. An approaching action potential causes a small rise in the membrane potential resulting in a rapid increase in the conductance of the Na^+ channel, facilitating a large influx of Na^+ ions into the cell. At this point the channel is said to be in the open state. Depolarisation begins during this phase of the process and lasts less than a millisecond. When the depolarising potential reaches a critical value of somewhere in the region of +40 mV the inward migration of Na^+ ions is terminated. The channel now switches to the inactive state and remains so until full repolarisation has taken place. These changes are summarised in Figure 5.6.

A channel for K^+ ions functions in a similar voltage-sensitive, gated manner. Typically, a depolarising current induces a slow opening of the K^+ channels delaying maximal K^+ ion conductance until after closure of the Na^+ channel. An efflux of K^+ ions from the cell occurs due to the marked concentration gradient and renders the interior of the axon more electronegative, ultimately leading to hyperpolarisation. During the inactivation phase of the sequence, the neurone is said to be refractory and cannot generate an action potential. During the hyperpolarisation phase it is relatively refractory and can only generate an action potential in response to a supramaximal stimulus.

Local anaesthetics bind to a single, specific site on the channel protein and act as non-depolarising Na^+ channel blockers. This inhibits the usual conformational change in the channel protein that facilitates inward transfer of Na^+ ions during depolarisation. The channel proteins contain multiple anionic fragments and since the local anaesthetic must be in the cationic form to be effective the binding process is probably electrostatic in origin. According to the modulated receptor hypothesis, local anaesthetics preferentially bind to the channel in the open and inactive states when access is relatively uninhibited (Figure 5.6). It is unclear whether or not the affinity for the binding site is fixed or variable. The modulated receptor theory proposes that the affinity varies as the channel undergoes conformational change during depolarisation and repolarisation. An alternative is the guarded receptor hypothesis that suggests that the binding affinity is constant but that access of local anaesthetic to the channel is facilitated or hindered by the same conformational changes.

Local anaesthetics slow the rate of rise of the action potential and reduce its height. They also slow impulse conduction and lengthen the refractory period (Figure 5.7). They may elevate the threshold potential but do not affect the RMP. As more and more Na^+ channels are blocked by local anaesthetic the value of each successive spike potential gradually decreases to the point where it fails to achieve the value of the threshold potential (Figure 5.7). At this point nerve conduction ceases.

Some local anaesthetics, such as benzocaine, are totally insoluble in water and cannot ionise. Consequently, there is no cation and therefore no Na^+ channel block from within the cell. It is suggested that agents, such as benzocaine, which are very lipid-soluble, exert their effect in the phospholipid bilayer of the axon. This is the basis of the membrane expansion theory of local anaesthetic action. It is also possible that they diffuse laterally form the bilayer into the Na^+ channel without ever accessing the axoplasm and in effect produce another variety of Na^+ channel block.

Repetitive depolarisation of a nerve recruits more Na^+ channels and maintains them in the open state for a longer period than normal.

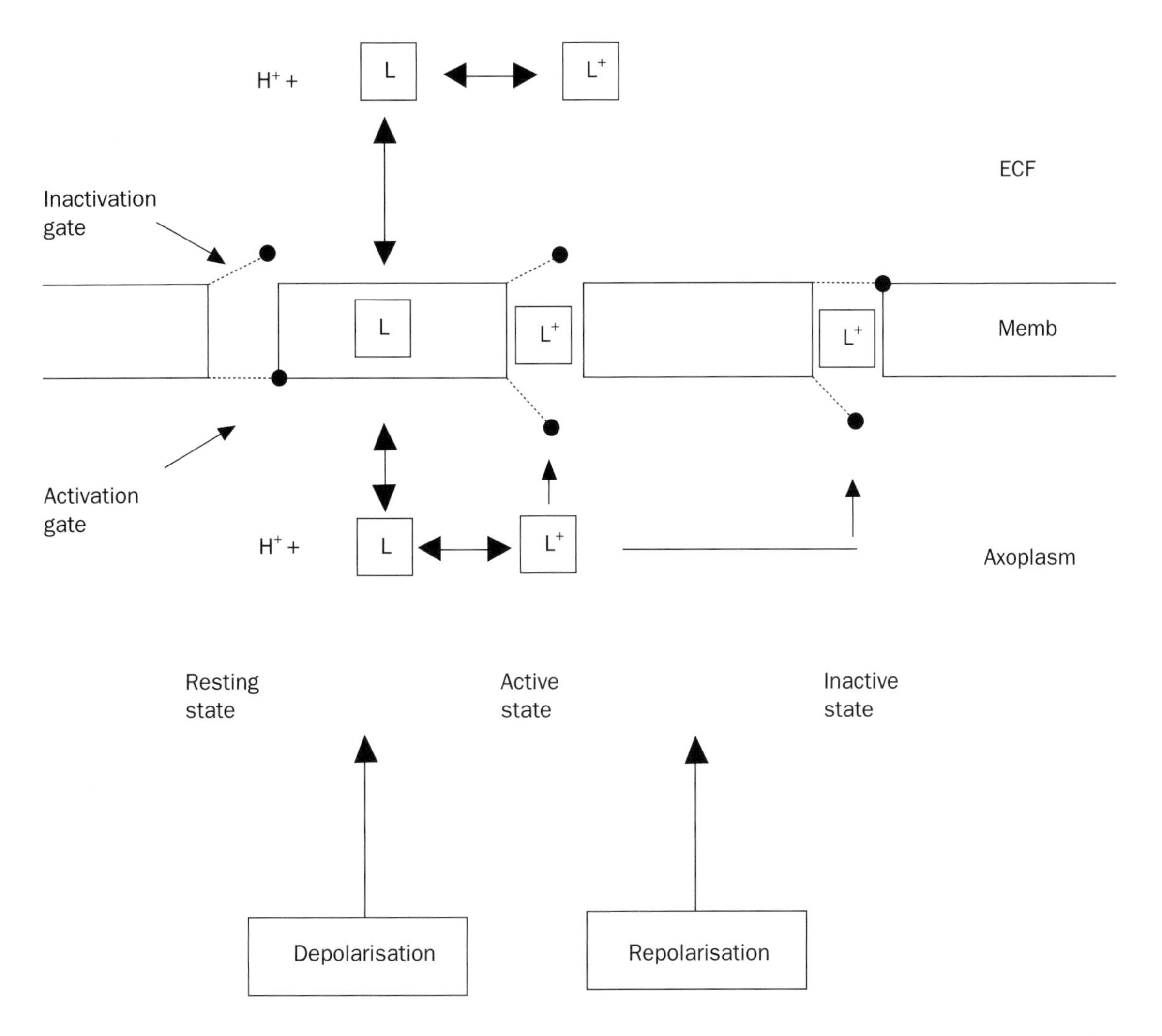

Figure 5.6 *Sodium channel blockade by local anaesthetic drug, mechanism of action. L, local anaesthetic free base; L^+, ionised local anaesthetic; ECF, extracellular fluid; Memb, axonal cell membrane.*

Drug uptake by the channel will therefore be facilitated. If a nerve is artificially depolarised in this manner by a small electric current in the presence of a local anaesthetic the onset of the block is more rapid than usual and the block is more dense compared to the unstimulated state. This phenomenon is known as *frequency dependent block* or *biphasic block* and is explained by the fact that stimulated axons have a relatively large number of Na^+ channels in the open and inactive states.

Nerves differ in their sensitivity to local anaesthetics. When lidocaine (lignocaine) is applied to a mixed peripheral nerve the onset of the block is in the order, vasodilatation (B fibres), loss of pain and temperature (C and Aδ fibres), muscle spindle reflex (Aγ fibres), motor and pressure (Aβ fibres) and large motor and proprioception (Aα fibres). This phenomenon is called *differential block*. There are other minor variations in this ranking order among the local anaesthetics. The basis of differential block is thought to be the result of variability in the sensitivity of different nerves to the same agent.

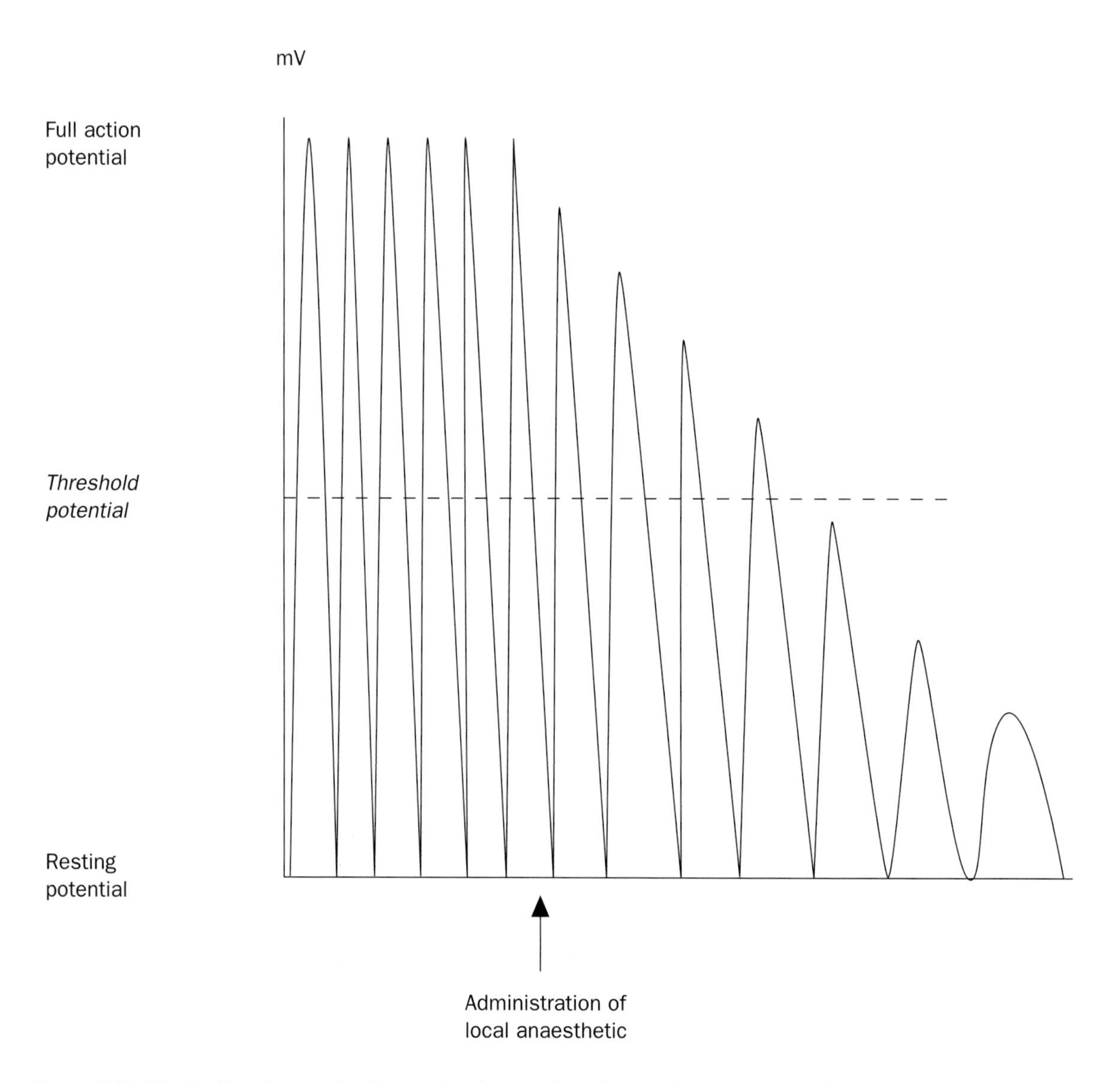

Figure 5.7 *Effect of local anaesthetics on the propagation of an action potential. A full action potential occurs when a spike potential reaches the level of the threshold potential. Local anaesthetics decrease the rate of rise and the frequency of spike potentials. When the value of the spike potential falls below the threshold potential neural transmission ceases.*

The variability can be accounted for largely by the diffusion barriers of the different fibre types and by Na^+ channel density. For example, the presence of a Schwann cell and myelin sheath poses a considerable barrier to the diffusion of local anaesthetic to the interior of the cell. There is *in vitro* evidence to indicate that all desheathed nerves require a similar minimum concentration of local anaesthetic to induce block irrespective of fibre type. A consequence of the physical architecture of a mixed nerve is that access of the drug to the outer fibres is easier than access to fibres at the core. It is for this reason that the onset of proximal analgesia of the limb precedes distal analgesia with a brachial plexus block.

PHARMACOKINETICS (Table 5.1)

The standard pharmacokinetic approach to the understanding of drug uptake, disposition and elimination cannot easily be applied to local anaesthetic drugs. Uniquely, this group of drugs have fulfilled their function before they reach the vascular compartment. In contrast, all other anaesthetic drugs (intravenous induction agents, opiates, inhalation agents, muscle relaxants) are distributed from the vascular compartment to their sites of action. In other words, the presence of such a drug in the vascular compartment represents the first phase of the kinetic process. In the case of a local anaesthetic the appearance of drug in the vascular compartment represents an intermediate phase in the kinetic process.

Tissue kinetics

Factors that affect drug dispersal at the site of injection are *bulk flow* and *diffusion*.

Bulk flow

This is the physical mass movement of a drug about the site of its administration. Its importance in the production of neural blockade is not known. It is likely that bulk flow is facilitated in areas where tissue barriers, such as aponeuroses, sheathes, and multiple tissue planes, are minimal.

Physical barriers

The most important obstacles to drug migration across the axon are the Schwann cell and the myelin sheath. The structure of a mixed peripheral nerve means that access of a local anaesthetic to the core fibres is delayed relative to the outer fibres. This explains the differences in onset times between proximal and distal dermatomes.

Diffusion

This is the capacity of a drug to pass across cell membranes. It is a function of the molecular weight of the drug, its lipid solubility, the concentration gradient, and the properties of the cell wall. Low molecular weight and high lipid solubility are characteristic features of all local anaesthetic drugs.

Tissue binding

A further property which is of central importance in diffusion is the tissue-binding capacity (or affinity) of a drug. Drugs that are highly lipid-soluble and protein-bound, such as bupivacaine and ropivacaine, are extensively bound to tissue. This limits the rate at which they are transferred from their intracellular sites of action to the vascular compartment. When tissue affinity is great the local anaesthetic effect is prolonged.

Tissue acidosis

Ambient pH in the extracellular fluid (ECF) is approximately 7.4 but the value varies and this determines the proportions of ionised and unionised local anaesthetic drug. A decrease in ambient pH will increase the amount of ionised drug and reduce the unionised fraction available for transfer across the cell membrane. A common example of this is when infection or inflammation reduces the ambient pH. In the case of lidocaine (lignocaine), a fall in tissue pH from 7.4 to 7.0 will halve the amount of unionised drug. This has obvious implications for efficacy. Similar effects occur following repeated administrations of acidified local anaesthetic solutions.

Alkalinisation and carbonation

Alkalinisation of local anaesthetic solution with sodium bicarbonate ($NaHCO_3$) increases the pH of the solution to a value near its pKa. This results in an increased proportion of unionised drug available for neural penetration and thereby reduces the onset time. Carbonation is a term used to describe the acidification of a local anaesthetic solution with carbon dioxide. Following injection, the carbon dioxide diffuses into the axoplasm causing a decrease in the pH. This results in a higher proportion of ionised drug within the cell. In theory this should enhance the Na^+ channel block but in practice the results are disappointing.

Table 5.1 Pharmacokinetic characteristics of local anaesthetic agents

	Lidocaine (lignocaine)	*Prilocaine*	*Bupivacaine*	*Ropivacaine*	*Levobupivacaine*
pKa	7.7	7.7	8.1	8.1	8.1
Protein binding (%)	65	55	95	94	95
$t_{1/2}$ (h)	1.6	1.6	3.5	2	3.3
Metabolism	Intermediate Liver (monoethyl glycine xylidide to xylidide)	Faster than lidocaine Liver (hydrolysis to *o*-toluidine)	Slow Liver *N*-desbutyl bupivacaine	Slow Liver	Slow Liver (3-hydroxylevobupivacaine)
Chemistry	Amide	Amide	Amide	Amide	Amide
Relative potency	1	1	4	3	4
Onset	Fast	Fast	Slow	Slow	Slow
Topical	Yes	Yes	No	No	No

METABOLISM

Ester and amide local anaesthetics differ in the manner, site and rate of metabolism. There is little relation between the elimination of local anaesthetics and their duration of action. Amethocaine has a prolonged action due to its high affinity for nerve tissue despite being rapidly removed from plasma. Bupivacaine can be detected in the plasma many hours after its effects have worn off due to continuing absorption from the site of injection. The renal excretion of unchanged local anaesthetics is minimal.

Esters

Most of the ester-linked local anaesthetics are rapidly hydrolysed by *plasma cholinesterases* and *liver esterases*. Because the cerebrospinal fluid contains little or no esterase, intrathecal administration of these drugs produces a prolonged effect, which persists until the agent is absorbed into the bloodstream.

Amides

These are generally metabolised in the hepatic endoplasmic reticulum, the initial reaction being *N*-dealkylation, with subsequent hydrolysis. An exception to this is prilocaine, where the initial step is hydrolysis, forming *o*-toluidine. This is further metabolised to 4- and 6-hydroxytoluidine. The latter is believed to be responsible for the methaemoglobinaemia which may follow high doses. The amide-linked local anaesthetics are extensively protein-bound (between 55% and 95%) particularly to α_1-acid glycoprotein.

TOXICITY

This may be the result of systemic toxicity, hypersensitivity, drug interactions and agent-specific effects. Serious toxicity is almost always the result of overdosage or inadvertent intravascular injection. The maximum recommended doses are shown in Table 5.2.

Systemic toxicity

Local anaesthetic toxicity is directly related to the amount of free drug in the plasma and is influenced by the drug, the dose and the site of injection. Mild and short-lived CNS toxicity is common when doses close to the maximum recommended are employed. The brain and heart are the organs most affected by overdosage and the rate of rise of the plasma concentration would appear to be as important as the peak concentration. The symptoms correlate best with the arterial rather than the venous concentrations. There is no good evidence that the maximum dose should be calculated on the basis of body weight.

Table 5.2 Maximum recommended doses of commonly used local anaesthetic agents

Agent	*Plain (mg)*	*With adrenaline (epinephrine) (mg)*
Lidocaine (lignocaine)	300	500
Prilocaine	400	600[a]
Bupivacaine	150	150
Levobupivacaine	150	400
Ropivacaine	225	800

[a] With felypressin as vasoconstrictor.

Central nervous system

The earliest signs of CNS toxicity are circumoral and tongue numbness, tinnitus, tremor, and dizziness. These appear at plasma lidocaine (lignocaine) concentrations of about 5 $\mu g \cdot mL^{-1}$. The value for prilocaine is similar to lidocaine but bupivacaine toxicity appears at about half those of lidocaine. Further progression is evidenced by drowsiness, visual disturbances, or muscle twitching (plasma lidocaine of 5–10 $\mu g \cdot mL^{-1}$). Over 10 $\mu g \cdot mL^{-1}$ grand mal convulsions, coma and respiratory arrest are likely. Serious CNS toxicity is indicative of imminent and potentially fatal cardiac toxicity since lidocaine is associated with direct cardiac depression at plasma concentrations in excess of 20 $\mu g \cdot mL^{-1}$.

The rate of progression of the symptoms and signs of local anaesthetic toxicity may be shortened or absent. The time course may be accelerated by intravascular injection or when large doses are inadvertently injected into the subdural space.

Cardiovascular system

Local anaesthetics directly depress myocardial conduction and contractility in a dose-dependent manner. They bind to and inactivate myocardial sodium channels, reducing the velocity of the cardiac action potential and prolonging the QRS interval. As plasma concentrations approach toxic values sodium channels become progressively inactivated until there is a generalised reduction in automaticity (cardiac slowing) with negative inotropy. Slow increases to near- or above-toxic levels are better tolerated than rapid rises seen following intravascular injection.

The heart is more resistant to the toxic effects of local anaesthetics than the brain. The ratio of the plasma drug concentration which will induce cardiovascular collapse relative to CNS toxicity is different for each agent and is a crude measure of the safety margin of individual drugs. Lidocaine (lignocaine) has a ratio of 7:1 compared to 4:1 for bupivacaine. The differences in toxicity are due, at least in part, to the different tissue affinities of local anaesthetics, specifically their affinity for myocardial sodium channels. Lidocaine is believed to bind to the channel in its open and inactive state whereas bupivacaine binds to the channel in the inactive state only. Dissociation is greatest in the closed and resting states for both agents but is approximately 10 times slower for bupivacaine than for lidocaine. Prolonged binding of bupivacaine to the sodium channel is thought to be the basis for its 'selective' cardiotoxicity. This may also explain the difficulty in performing successful resuscitation from ventricular fibrillation.

The sodium channel binding properties of racemic bupivacaine are stereospecific. The binding affinity of *laevo*- bupivacaine is less than *dextro*—hence the reduced cardiotoxic potential of the *laevo* form of the drug.

Drug interactions and other factors

Hypoxia, hypercarbia, and acidosis make toxic reactions more likely. Pregnancy may exacerbate bupivacaine toxicity by a combination of reduced drug binding and progesterone sensitisation of the myocardium. Concurrent medication with cardioactive drugs, such as calcium channel blockers, digoxin, and β-adrenoceptor blocking drugs, may all increase the likelihood of unwanted cardiac side effects with local anaesthetics. Both enzyme induction, e.g. barbiturates, phenytoin, alcohol, and inhibition, e.g. cimetidine, may decrease or increase the plasma clearance of local anaesthetic drugs. Local anaesthetics reduce the minimum alveolar concentration (MAC) values of volatile anaesthetics.

Local tissue toxicity

Local anaesthetics are rarely associated with localised nerve damage. There have been a number of reports of prolonged motor and sensory deficits after large doses of chloroprocaine. This is believed to be related to the antioxidant sodium bisulphite. Radiculopathy has been reported following the subarachnoid administration of lidocaine (lignocaine) 5%.

Allergic reactions

Only rarely are individuals hypersensitive to local anaesthetics, manifest as urticarial skin reactions, asthma, or fatal anaphylaxis. More commonly, side effects of systemic toxicity are mistaken as being allergic in nature. These reactions appear to be more common with the ester group of local anaesthetics. This is the main reason why esters are rarely used nowadays, with the possible exceptions of the topical use of cocaine in otolaryngological surgery where its vasoconstricting properties are an advantage, and amethocaine as a surface anaesthetic in ophthalmic surgery.

Prolongation of action by vasoconstrictors

The duration of action of a local anaesthetic is proportional to the time that the drug remains bound to the sodium channels. Measures that prolong contact time will prolong the duration of the local anaesthetic effect. Cocaine has a vasoconstricting effect on blood vessels and prevents its own absorption. Many local anaesthetics are prepared with adrenaline (epinephrine) in order to achieve this effect. Concentrations are usually of the order of 1:200 000 or more dilute than this. Care should be exercised when using adrenaline-containing solutions in the presence of halothane as it is known to sensitise the myocardium to the effects of catecholamines.

PLACENTAL TRANSFER

The majority of drugs cross the placenta by diffusion, the rate depending on placental blood flow, the concentration gradient, and the properties of the drugs concerned. The most crucial of these are lipid solubility and molecular weight. Amide local anaesthetics have low molecular weights and high lipid solubility so that transfer is almost completely flow-dependent and is achieved in a single circulation. Only unbound drug can cross the placenta so the amount transferred is dictated by the extent of maternal and fetal protein binding. Binding of local anaesthetic to α_1-acid glycoprotein is greater in the mother than the fetus so distribution (of unbound drug) across the placenta will favour movement outwards into the maternal circulation. Drugs that are highly protein-bound have lower maternal to fetal ratios than agents which have low protein binding. For these reasons, extensive protein binding reduces the risk of toxicity in the fetus. The fetal:maternal ratios are 0.3 for bupivacaine, levobupivacaine, and ropivacaine; 0.6 for lidocaine (lignocaine); and 1.0 for prilocaine.

In contrast, fetal acidosis promotes ionisation of local anaesthetic in the fetal circulation resulting in ion trapping in the fetus, and thereby increasing the risk of toxicity.

Of all the local anaesthetics available, levobupivacaine and ropivacaine have the most favourable pharmacological characteristics for use in obstetrics. They have the lowest potential for cardiotoxicity and, unlike lidocaine and prilocaine, there is little risk of cumulation when they are administered by epidural infusion at effective doses. Elimination of all amides is prolonged in the neonate, exceeding 20 h in the case of bupivacaine.

INDIVIDUAL DRUGS

Bupivacaine

Bupivacaine is an amide compound with a duration of nerve blocking effect of around 3 hours. It is about four times more potent than lidocaine (lignocaine) and has an intermediate-to-slow onset of action. Bupivacaine is prepared as the hydrochloride salt in aqueous solutions in concentrations of 0.25%, 0.50%, and 0.75%. The incidence of motor block increases with increasing concentration. High doses of bupivacaine are associated with cardiac toxicity. Particular care must be exercised to avoid inadvertent overdosage or when the drug is administered to patients taking concurrent cardioactive medication.

Indications

Bupivacaine is used for most types of regional, spinal and epidural block. It is not suitable for intravenous regional anaesthesia and the 0.75% solution is not recommended in obstetrics because of the risks of overdosage. The safe single dose is 150 mg and the maximum daily dose is 400 mg. The addition of adrenaline (epinephrine) has only a marginal effect on these recommendations. The maximum recommended doses are shown in Table 5.2 but dosages should be reduced in the elderly and in debilitated patients. The drug is not recommended for children under the age of 12 years.

Pharmacokinetics

Bupivacaine is about 95% bound to plasma proteins (Table 5.1). The reported elimination half-life ranges from 1.5 hours to 5.5 hours in adults and about 8 hours in neonates. It is metabolised in the liver and is excreted in the urine principally as metabolites with only 5–6% as unchanged drug. High potency and long duration of effect mean that bupivacaine is suitable for repeat administration or epidural infusion as the risk of cumulation is low. Epidural infusions containing opioid additives, such as fentanyl and alfentanil, are effective for controlling postoperative pain with only a small risk of overdosage or toxicity.

Bupivacaine is distributed into breast milk in small quantities. It crosses the placenta but the ratio of fetal-to-maternal concentrations is low.

Lidocaine (lignocaine)

This is an amide local anaesthetic and is widely used on account of its rapid onset, medium duration of effect, and low toxicity. It is less highly protein-bound than the longer-acting amides (Table 5.1) but it has a useful duration of effect and is the most versatile of all local anaesthetics. It is of intermediate potency and has less toxic potential than bupivacaine. It is available in aqueous solution as the hydrochloride salt in concentrations of 0.5–2.0% with and without adrenaline (epinephrine). Topical preparations are also available as gels or aerosols in 2–4% concentrations.

Indications

Lidocaine is used for all forms of infiltration anaesthesia, in addition to peripheral, regional, spinal and epidural block. Unlike bupivacaine, it is suitable for use in intravenous regional anaesthesia. Duration of anaesthesia is about 1 hour but this can be prolonged to 2 hours by the addition of adrenaline. The maximum doses are shown in Table 5.2.

Lidocaine is also a class Ib anti-arrhythmic drug and is used to treat ventricular arrhythmias. Administered by intravenous infusion it has also been found to have a useful role in the management of acute pain and chronic pain syndromes.

Prilocaine

This amide drug has a similar pharmacodynamic and kinetic profile to lidocaine (lignocaine) (Table 5.1) and is equipotent with it. It has a rapid onset of action but a longer duration of effect. Its main advantages over lidocaine are its lower toxic potential, due to rapid clearance from the circulation, and its very large volume of distribution (twice that of lidocaine). Doses in excess of those recommended cause methaemoglobinaemia which can be reversed with methylene blue (1 $mg{\cdot}kg^{-1}$ given intravenously). Injectable preparations are available in 0.5–2.0% concentrations with, and without felypressin as a vasopressor. The addition of felypressin is thought to double the duration of effect and this combination is widely used in dentistry.

Indications

Prilocaine is suitable for most types of local anaesthetic block but is not suitable for epidural use in obstetrics because of the need for repeat administration. Its main uses are for infiltration anaesthesia and intravenous regional anaesthesia where its low toxicity makes it the drug of choice.

Levobupivacaine

This amide local anaesthetic is the S enantiomer of bupivacaine and is available in concentrations 2.5 mg·mL^{-1}, 5.0 mg·mL^{-1} and 7.5 mg·mL^{-1} as the hydrochloride in aqueous solution. It is claimed to have less cardiotoxic potential than racemic bupivacaine but it is not suitable for regional intravenous anaesthesia. Adverse reactions to levobupivacaine are similar to those seen with bupivacaine and other amide local anaesthetics. The pharmacokinetic properties of racemic bupivacaine, S (–)-bupivacaine, and R (+)-bupivacaine appear to be near identical at normal doses (Table 5.1). It is not known if levobupivacaine is excreted in human breast milk.

Indications

For continuous epidural analgesia, levobupivacaine may be administered in combination with fentanyl or clonidine. Levobupivacaine has been approved in European Union states for ilio-inguinal and ilio-hypogastric nerve blockade in children. (See also bupivacaine, above.)

Ropivacaine

Ropivacaine is an amide anaesthetic prepared as the pure S enantiomer of the racemic drug. Adverse cardiac effects appear to be stereoselective for the R (–) enantiomer and so the intrinsic cardiotoxic potential of the drug may be reduced. Unlike other amide local anaesthetics it has a slight vasoconstricting effect.

Pharmacokinetics

The lipid solubility of ropivacaine is less than that of bupivacaine and this may slow the penetration of the myelin sheaths of motor nerve fibres. The plasma protein binding of ropivacaine is somewhat less than that of bupivacaine and this may account for the slightly shorter duration of its nerve blocking effect. It has a lower volume of distribution, greater clearance, and shorter elimination half-life than bupivacaine. Ropivacaine undergoes hepatic biotransformation and renal clearance of the intact drug accounts for a minor proportion of total clearance. Peak plasma concentrations of ropivacaine following epidural or peripheral nerve block may rise twice as high as those of bupivacaine, possibly due to its decreased lipid solubility and volume of distribution.

Indications

When used for spinal anaesthesia, 0.75% ropivacaine produces less intense sensory and motor block than 0.5% bupivacaine. It is suitable for regional, spinal and epidural block but not for regional intravenous anaesthesia. The addition of adrenaline (epinephrine) does not prolong the duration of anaesthesia in brachial plexus or epidural block. Ropivacaine is indistinguishable from bupivacaine when used in obstetric anaesthesia. Its direct myocardial toxicity is somewhat less than that of bupivacaine.

EMLA cream

EMLA cream (lidocaine (lignocaine) 2.5% and prilocaine 2.5%) is an emulsion in which the oil phase is a eutectic mixture of lidocaine and prilocaine in a ratio of 1:1 by weight. It is available in 5 g and 30 g tubes. It is also available as an anaesthetic disc. This consists of a single-dose unit of EMLA contained within an occlusive dressing. The disc contains 1 g EMLA emulsion, the active contact surface being approximately 10 cm^2. The surface area of the entire anaesthetic disc is approximately 40 cm^2. EMLA (1 g) contains lidocaine 25 mg, prilocaine 25 mg with thickening agents, water, $NaHCO_3$, etc., at a pH of about 9.

Mechanism of action

EMLA applied to intact skin provides dermal analgesia by the release of lidocaine and prilocaine from the cream into the epidermal and dermal layers of the skin. There is cumulation of lidocaine and prilocaine in the vicinity of dermal pain receptors and nerve endings. The quality and duration of dermal analgesia depends primarily on the duration of application. EMLA should be applied 1–2 hours before the planned intervention, e.g. venepuncture, split skin harvesting.

Amethocaine

This is a potent ester anaesthetic with a rapid onset of action (about 10 min) and an intermediate duration of action (60–90 min). The maximum recommended dose is 40 mg. Its properties are similar to the other ester drugs in this group and its main use has been as a spinal anaesthetic. It is widely used as a surface anaesthetic in the eye. In general, the disadvantages of this drug—toxicity and hypersensitivity—outweigh its advantages except as a topical agent.

Chloroprocaine

2-Chloroprocaine is a member of the ester group of local anaesthetics. The drug has a rapid onset time (6–12 min) but it is rapidly hydrolysed in the plasma and has a short duration of action (60 min). Its rapid clearance accounts for its low toxicity although in the past it was associated with prolonged motor and sensory block, possibly due to the sodium metabisulphite preservative. More recently, a higher than expected incidence of back pain has been reported following epidural administration and it has been suggested that this is caused by the preservative, EDTA. Maximum recommended doses are 800 mg and 1000 mg, without and with adrenaline (epinephrine).

6

Neuromuscular blocking and reversal agents

Rajinder K Mirakhur

Introduction • Neuromuscular transmission • Depolarising neuromuscular blocking agents • Non-depolarising neuromuscular blocking agents • Other neuromuscular blocking agents • Antagonists of neuromuscular blocking agents

INTRODUCTION

Neuromuscular blocking agents were introduced into clinical practice in 1942 when the first use of curare in clinical practice was reported. Since then, these agents have been used regularly and have facilitated many types of surgery. While the earlier drugs had many side effects, greater understanding of physiology and pharmacology has helped in the introduction of newer, safer, and more predictable neuromuscular blocking agents. One of the great advantages of the use of neuromuscular blocking agents is avoiding the need for deep anaesthesia with its attendant side effects.

NEUROMUSCULAR TRANSMISSION

The process of neuromuscular transmission includes the synthesis and storage of acetylcholine (ACh), its release and passage across the synaptic cleft, the interaction with nicotinic ACh receptor, and the process of actual muscle contraction.

Acetycholine is synthesised from choline and acetylcoenzyme A in the cholinergic nerve terminals. The transmitter is present throughout the cholinergic neurones and exists within the axon terminals in vesicles. About 1% of the vesicles are the readily 'releasable' store that maintains transmitter release but more than 80% is in motor nerve endings in the 'releasable' store, which is released in response to a nerve impulse. The remainder of ACh is in the so-called 'stationary' store. The release of ACh may be spontaneous or in response to nerve impulses. Spontaneous release of ACh results in the production of random miniature endplate potentials. It is, however, in response to a nerve impulse that we see a large release of ACh provided there is adequate calcium present in the extracellular fluid. Evoked release of ACh usually results in the production of an endplate potential due to depolarisation of the motor endplate.

ACh receptors are present in the postjunctional membrane of the endplate, in the junctional folds. The nicotinic ACh receptor at the motor endplate has five subunits, two αs, β, δ and ε. In addition, a γ subunit instead of an ε subunit may be present in the so-called extrajunctional or the fetal receptor. The five subunits are arranged as a cylinder around a central funnel-shaped pore, the ion channel. The two α subunits each carry a recognition site which binds nicotinic agonists such as ACh and antagonists such as the neuromuscular blocking agents. Whilst ACh must bind to both subunits to produce an effect, it is sufficient for neuromuscular blocking agents to bind to only one of the α subunits. The margin of safety of neuromuscular transmission is such that it is necessary to have about 75% receptor occupancy for a neuromuscular blocking agent to show its effect.

While most of the muscle relaxants exert their predominant actions at the post-junctional nicotinic receptors, many also have variable pre-junctional effects. Although pre-junctional receptors have not been demonstrated there is putative evidence for their existence. The pre-junctional mechanisms are supposed to be responsible for the development of fade in response to tetanic or train-of-four (TOF) stimulation following administration of non-depolarising neuromuscular blocking drugs.

Potency of muscle relaxants is estimated by constructing dose–response curves and calculating the ED_{50} or the ED_{95}, the doses required to produce 50% or 95% block of the adductor pollicis muscle. The sensitivities of different muscles to muscle relaxant drugs differ. In clinical practice, 2–3 × ED_{95} doses are usually administered to facilitate tracheal intubation, due to relative resistance of the laryngeal muscles to neuromuscular blocking agents. The relative potency of commonly used muscle relaxants in terms of their ED_{95} is given in Table 6.1.

Table 6.1 Relative potency (ED_{95}) of currently used neuromuscular blocking agents

Agent	*ED_{95} (mg·kg^{-1})*
Pancuronium	0.06
Vecuronium	0.04
Atracurium	0.25
Rocuronium	0.30
Cisatracurium	0.05
Mivacurium	0.08
Suxamethonium	0.30

DEPOLARISING NEUROMUSCULAR BLOCKING AGENTS

Suxamethonium is the only agent from this class of drugs in current use. Depolarising drugs are agonists at the nicotinic receptor and, like ACh, produce depolarisation at the end-plate. However, since the breakdown of suxamethonium is not as rapid as that of ACh, the receptor is held in a prolonged depolarised state which is unresponsive to further stimulation until suxamethonium has been metabolised.

Suxamethonium produces a typical depolarising block that is characterised by the appearance of fasciculations before the onset of block, absence of fade in response to tetanic and TOF stimulations, and potentiation of block by anticholinesterase drugs.

The block may change into a non-depolarising type (phase II block) after high doses (7–10 mg·kg^{-1}) of the drug have been administered. A phase II block shows the characteristics of a non-depolarising block with slow recovery.

Muscle relaxation following administration of suxamethonium is preceded by muscle fasciculations representing the ACh-like agonist activity of suxamethonium. It is also thought that fasciculations may be due to a presynaptic action through binding of the drug to the presynaptic receptors and depolarising nerve terminals.

Maximum block after suxamethonium develops in 60–90 seconds following a dose of 1 mg·kg^{-1} (about 3 × ED_{95}) with a duration of action of 5–10 minutes. This dose provides near ideal intubating conditions in 60–90 seconds. It is because of a rapid onset and a short duration of action that suxamethonium is considered as the ideal agent for facilitating tracheal intubation during rapid sequence induction.

The pharmacokinetics of suxamethonium are difficult to estimate due to its rapid metabolism. However, its half-life has been indirectly estimated at between 16 seconds and 4 minutes.

The use of suxamethonium is associated with a range of side effects (Table 6.2). Some of these, such as myalgias, are inconvenient and troublesome while others, such as anaphylaxis

Table 6.2 Side effects of suxamethonium

- Myalgia
- Increase in intraocular pressure
- Increase in intracranial pressure
- Masseter muscle spasm
- Hyperkalaemia in susceptible patients
- Cardiovascular effects
- Prolonged block
- Anaphylaxis
- Malignant hyperpyrexia

and malignant hyperthermia, are associated with a high morbidity and mortality. Muscle pains may occur in over 50% of patients receiving suxamethonium and are more common in young, fit patients and those who are mobilised early. Small doses of non-depolarising relaxants 3–4 minutes before suxamethonium administration remains the most commonly used prophylactic measure, although these do not abolish pain completely. Suxamethonium can give rise to vagally mediated bradycardia, particularly in children and after a second dose, but also hypertension and tachycardia due to an increase in circulating catecholamines. Serum potassium can increase significantly, and have adverse consequences, in patients with lesions of the spinal cord, extensive burns, skeletal muscle diseases, renal failure, and after immobility. Masseter muscle spasm may sometimes be severe enough to make intubation difficult. Suxamethonium administration has been associated with malignant hyperthermia in susceptible individuals. This condition is characterised by rapidly increasing temperature, metabolic acidosis, hypercarbia, and increase in serum potassium and is associated with considerable mortality.

Suxamethonium shows a prolonged response in patients with low plasma cholinesterase activity or in those with genetically abnormal enzyme. The enzyme activity is low in conditions, such as pregnancy, liver disease, old age, malignancy, malnutrition, and following anticholinesterase drugs. The prolongation of block in these conditions is not very long. Very prolonged block, however, is associated with the presence of silent or atypical genes in homozygous individuals. The prolongation in these individuals lasts several hours until suxamethonium is broken down and eliminated at a very slow rate.

NON-DEPOLARISING NEUROMUSCULAR BLOCKING AGENTS

Non-depolarising neuromuscular blocking drugs act by competing with ACh molecules for binding sites on the nicotinic receptor. Non-depolarising block is characterised by reduction in the twitch response, presence of fade in response to tetanic and TOF stimulations, post-tetanic facilitation, and antagonism of block by anticholinesterase agents.

Most of the currently used non-depolarising neuromuscular blocking agents are structurally either aminosteroid or benzylisoquinolinium compounds (Figures 6.1 and 6.2). They are generally classified according to the duration of their action as long, intermediate, or short acting (Table 6.3).

Tubocurarine

Tubocurarine was the first muscle relaxant used in clinical anaesthesia, although it is now rarely used and is not available in many countries. The ED_{95} of tubocurarine is approximately

Table 6.3 Classification of non-depolarising relaxants

Long acting	Tubocurarine
	Pancuronium
Intermediate acting	Atracurium
	Vecuronium
	Rocuronium
	Cisatracurium
Short acting	Mivacurium

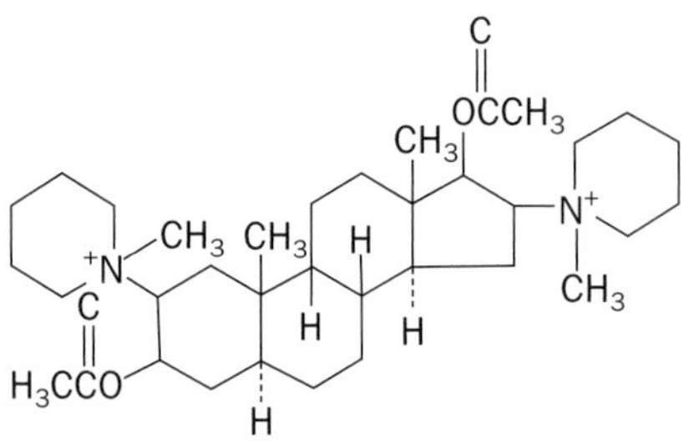

Pancuronium

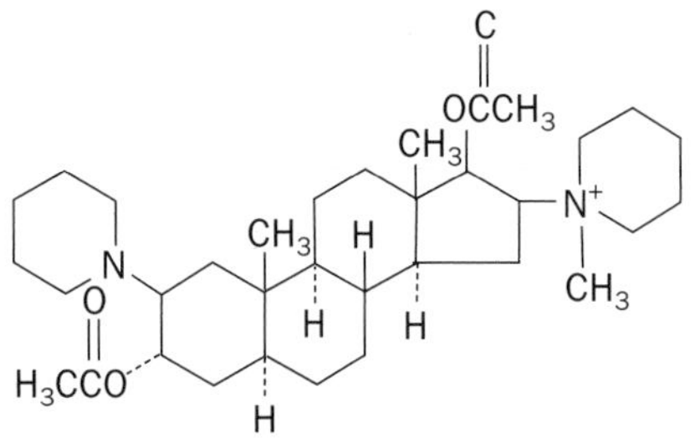

Vecuronium

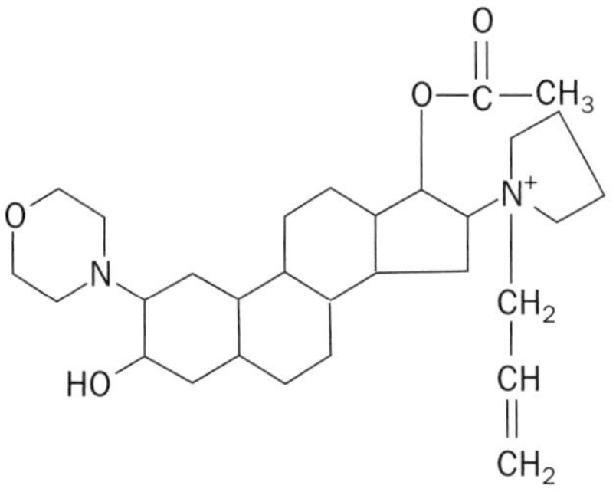

Rocuronium

__Figure 6.1__ Chemical structures of currently used aminosteroid relaxants.

0.5 mg·kg^{-1} and this is the dose commonly employed to facilitate tracheal intubation and abdominal muscle relaxation (in contrast to the frequently used dose of 2–3 × ED_{95} with other relaxants). Tubocurarine has a slow onset and a long duration of action, being over 5 minutes and up to 100 minutes, respectively. The duration of action is prolonged after successive doses.

Tubocurarine produces significant hypotension which has led to decline in its use. This is due to ganglion blocking effects, histamine liberation and possible myocardial depression. It has a long elimination half-life (Table 6.4), which is further prolonged in patients with renal disease and in old age. This agent is mainly of historical interest now.

Pancuronium

Pancuronium is a bisquaternary aminosteroid muscle relaxant with an ED_{95} of about 0.06 mg·kg^{-1}, the commonly administered doses for facilitating tracheal intubation being about 0.1 mg·kg^{-1}. It is a slow-acting agent producing maximum effect and acceptable intubating conditions in 3–4 minutes. The clinical duration (25% recovery of twitch height) with a dose of 0.06 mg·kg^{-1} is similar to that of tubocurarine, 60–90 minutes. Higher doses act more rapidly but have a longer duration of action. A progressive increase in the duration of action occurs with repeated administration.

A pancuronium block can be effectively antagonised with 40–50 μg·kg^{-1} of neostigmine provided some spontaneous recovery has taken place before the administration of the anticholinesterase agent. The recovery is slow if the block is deep. Edrophonium in doses of 0.5–1.0 mg·kg^{-1}, although acting more rapidly, is effective only if the block is relatively superficial.

Pancuronium undergoes some hepatic metabolism, producing the 3-hydroxy metabolite which has neuromuscular blocking properties. The main route of elimination is via the kidney, about half of it in an unchanged form, with a relatively low rate of clearance and a long elimination half-life (Table 6.4). Its clinical duration and elimination half-life are therefore markedly increased in patients with significant renal and hepatic disease.

Unlike tubocurarine, pancuronium does not produce ganglionic block or histamine release. For this reason it became popular soon after its introduction and became the drug of choice for use in sick patients. However, it increases the heart rate, arterial pressure, and cardiac output in clinical doses. While this may be advantageous when using high-dose opiate anaesthesia in cardiac surgery, it can be associated with arrhythmias and myocardial ischaemia. The

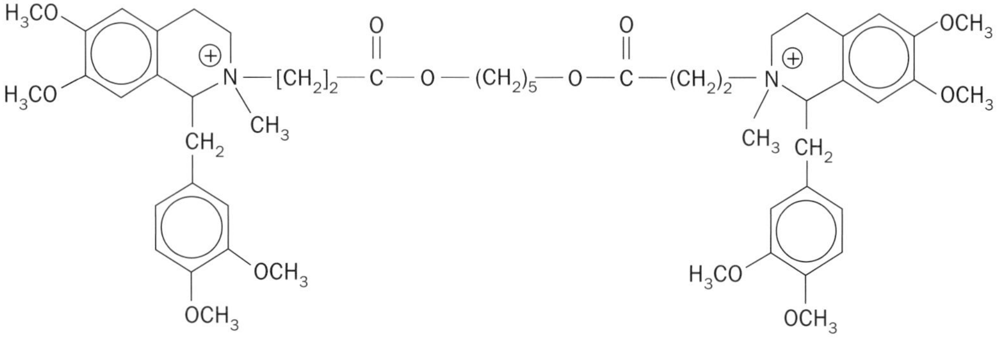

H_3CO OCH_3

H_3CO $\oplus$ N—$[CH_2]_2$—$\overset{O}{\overset{||}{C}}$—O—$(CH_2)_5$—O—$\overset{O}{\overset{||}{C}}$—$(CH_2)_2$—$N$ $\oplus$ OCH_3

CH_3 CH_2 CH_3 CH_2

OCH_3 H_3CO

OCH_3 OCH_3

Atracurium

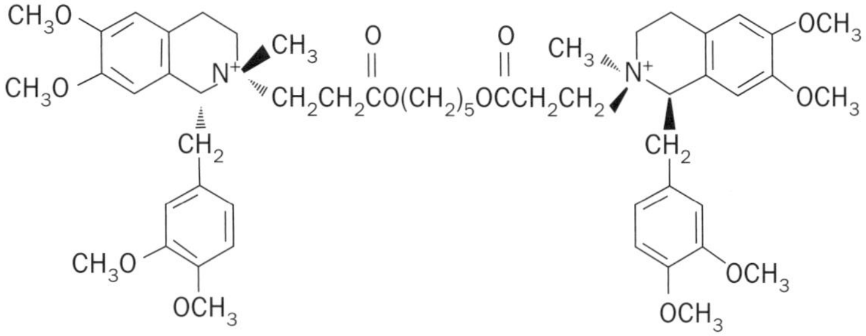

CH_3O OCH_3

CH_3O N^+ CH_3 $CH_2CH_2\overset{O}{\overset{||}{C}}O(CH_2)_5O\overset{O}{\overset{||}{C}}CH_2CH_2$ CH_3 N^+ OCH_3

CH_2 CH_2

CH_3O OCH_3

OCH_3 OCH_3

Cisatracurium

H_3CO OCH_3

H_3CO $\oplus$ N—$(CH_2)_3$—O—$\overset{O}{\overset{||}{C}}$—$(CH_2)_2$—CH=CH—$(CH_2)_2$—$\overset{O}{\overset{||}{C}}$—O—$(CH_2)_3$—$N$ $\oplus$ OCH_3

CH_2 CH_3 CH_3 CH_2

H_3CO OCH_3 H_3CO OCH_3

OCH_3 OCH_3

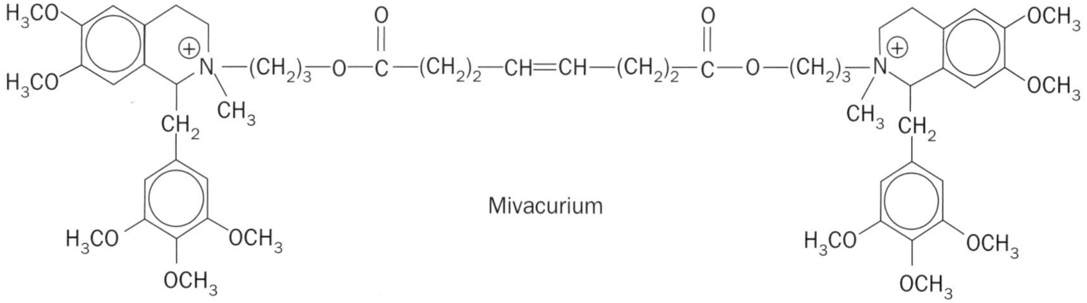

Mivacurium

Figure 6.2 *Chemical structures of benzylisoquinolinium drugs.*

Pharmacokinetic parameters for muscle relaxants

	Clearance ($mL \cdot kg^{-1} \cdot min^{-1}$)	Elimination half-life (min)
Tubocuranine	1.70	164
Pancuronium	1.50	130
Vecuronium	4.26	58
Atracurium	6.10	20.6
Rocuronium	3.70	97.2
Cisatracurium	5.09	24.8
Mivacurium		
Cis-trans isomer	95	1.53
Trans-trans isomer	70	2.32
Cis-cis isomer	5.2	50.3

mechanisms for this include increased release of catecholamines and their decreased reuptake, muscarinic receptor blockade, and possible direct myocardial effect.

Although the use of pancuronium has decreased markedly, and with good justification, it still retains some popularity in anaesthesia for cardiac surgery in conjunction with the use of high doses of opiates.

One of the problems with the use of long-acting relaxants has been the high incidence of postoperative residual curarisation which can increase the incidence of pulmonary complications.

Vecuronium

Vecuronium, a monoquaternary analogue of pancuronium, was among the first of a new generation of intermediate-acting nondepolarising muscle relaxants. A dose of 0.1–0.15 $mg \cdot kg^{-1}$ (approximately 2–3 × ED_{95}) provides acceptable intubating conditions within 90–120 seconds with a clinical duration of 25–40 minutes. The onset of action of a standard intubating dose of 0.1 $mg \cdot kg^{-1}$ is in about 3 minutes. Both the onset and duration of action are dose-related. The onset of vecuronium block is slightly faster in children and with a shorter duration of action. While the duration of action remains similar after a few repeat doses, cumulation will eventually occur due to the formation of metabolites. Both neostigmine and edrophonium, in equipotent doses, are effective antagonists of a vecuronium block although the latter is slow and somewhat ineffective if the block is deep.

Vecuronium has an elimination half-life of about one hour (Table 6.4) and is metabolised to 3-, 17-, and 3,17-hydroxy metabolites, the main route of elimination being via the liver. The metabolites have potent neuromuscular blocking action and are eliminated by the kidneys. As a result, the effects of vecuronium are prolonged in hepatic and renal disease. The metabolites may be responsible for cases of prolonged paralysis seen after long-term administration of vecuronium to patients in intensive care units. The effects of vecuronium are also prolonged in the elderly and in hypothermia due to the kinetic factors.

Vecuronium, unlike pancuronium, does not give rise to tachycardia or hypertension, even when used in large doses, as there is a wide separation between the vagal and neuromuscular blocking doses (≅ 70:1) and it has little ganglion blocking or sympathetic activity. The drug can therefore be used in larger doses (3–4 × ED_{95}) in order to achieve a faster onset of action and good intubating conditions. While it does not cause tachycardia or hypotension, its use may be associated with bradycardia when given in combination with some other drugs, e.g. opioids, or due to vagal stimulation.

Vecuronium can be given by repeated bolus administration or by a continuous infusion for maintenance of block. A general rule of thumb for administration by infusion is to use $0.1\ mg{\cdot}kg^{-1}{\cdot}h^{-1}$ following some recovery from a bolus dose of $0.1\ mg{\cdot}kg^{-1}$. The dose requirements diminish with time as peripheral storage sites become saturated. It is strongly advocated that neuromuscular block be routinely monitored during prolonged administration.

The drug is formulated as a freeze-dried preparation because the aqueous solution is unstable when stored for a prolonged period. However, the freeze-dried preparation does not need storage in a refrigerator.

Atracurium

Atracurium is a synthetic bisquaternary benzylisoquinolinium compound with a novel method of metabolism, the Hofmann elimination reaction. This reaction takes place at a pH of 7.4 and a temperature of 37°C. It is thus metabolised at body temperature and pH, and has to be stored in a refrigerator. The usual intubating dose of atracurium is $0.5–0.75\ mg{\cdot}kg^{-1}$ ($2–3 \times ED_{95}$). The onset of action with this dose is 2–3 minutes and intubating conditions are acceptable in 90–120 seconds. Spontaneous recovery occurs reliably from an atracurium neuromuscular block, such that an intubating dose of about $0.5\ mg{\cdot}kg^{-1}$ can be expected to provide surgical muscle relaxation for 25–40 minutes in the normal healthy patient. Repeated administration of atracurium leads only to a small increase in the duration of action.

About half of administered atracurium is eliminated by spontaneous degradation at physiological pH and temperature through Hofmann elimination and ester hydrolysis, the rest being cleared via other pathways, presumably by metabolism or excretion by the liver and/or the kidney. The elimination half-life is about 20 minutes (Table 6.4). Hofmann degradation of atracurium produces the tertiary compound, laudanosine, which produces central nervous system (CNS) excitation at high concentrations. Ester hydrolysis of atracurium produces monoquaternary alcohol, which also undergoes Hofmann degradation to laudanosine. However, concentrations high enough to produce CNS excitation have not been reported in humans even after prolonged administration of atracurium. The duration of action of atracurium is little changed in the elderly or in those with renal or hepatic dysfunction due to its unique mode of metabolism.

Atracurium causes minimal cardiovascular effects except those associated with some histamine release if the drug is given rapidly or in high doses. As with vecuronium, it produces little increase in heart rate; in fact, decreases in heart rate have been reported. This is once again thought to be due to the effects of other agents, such as the opiates, or as a result of vagal stimulation. The incidence of histamine release with atracurium is about one-third of that observed after tubocurarine administration.

Satisfactory neuromuscular block can be maintained with an atracurium bolus of $0.5–0.6\ mg{\cdot}kg^{-1}$ followed by an infusion at a rate of about $0.5\ mg{\cdot}kg^{-1}{\cdot}h^{-1}$. The unique metabolism of atracurium makes it suitable for use in critically ill patients with organ dysfunction, in whom it can be used for even longer periods of time as long as hypothermia is not present. The reversal of an atracurium block can be easily accomplished with anticholinesterase agents.

Rocuronium

Rocuronium is a desacetoxy analogue of vecuronium which is stable in solution and formulated as an aqueous ready-to-use solution. It was deliberately designed as a low-potency relaxant in an attempt to develop a non-depolarising agent which would have a fast onset of action, closer to that of suxamethonium. The basis for this development was the observation that potency and the speed of onset of action are inversely related. The potency of rocuronium is between one-sixth and one-eighth that of vecuronium, with an estimated ED_{95} of approximately 0.3 mg·kg^{-1}, the common intubating doses being 0.6–0.9 mg·kg^{-1}. While intubating conditions with 0.6 mg·kg^{-1} are acceptable during normal induction, a dose close to 1.0 mg·kg^{-1} is required to obtain acceptable conditions within 60–90 seconds during a rapid sequence induction.

Early animal and subsequent human studies showed the onset of action of rocuronium to be faster than that of other non-depolarising relaxants. Maximum block following an intubating dose of 0.6 mg·kg^{-1} occurs in about 2 minutes, larger doses having a more rapid onset. The duration of action of rocuronium is similar to that of vecuronium and atracurium in comparable doses and is dose-related with a clinical duration of about 30 minutes with 0.6 mg·kg^{-1}. The block can be readily antagonised by neostigmine. As with other relaxants, the duration of action is prolonged by potent inhalational agents, and in particular sevoflurane.

The block of rocuronium is reversed with neostigmine 35–50 μg·kg^{-1} provided some spontaneous recovery has taken place. The reversal may be slowed in the presence of agents like sevoflurane, however discontinuation of sevoflurane before neostigmine administration results in fairly prompt recovery.

About a third of an administered dose of rocuronium is excreted in the urine, the rest being taken up by the liver and excreted unchanged in the bile. Its elimination half-life is just under 100 minutes (Table 6.4). Unlike other aminosteroid relaxants, only very small amounts of the metabolite 17-desacetyl rocuronium have been found in plasma. The clearance of rocuronium is reduced in patients with significant renal and hepatic disease, with a possible prolongation of effect. The same mechanisms are responsible for prolongation of the block in the elderly.

Rocuronium produces only small changes in the heart rate with 0.6–0.9 mg·kg^{-1} doses, although higher doses may produce some increase in heart rate due to a lower vagal:neuromuscular blocking ratio compared to vecuronium. Like other aminosteroid agents, rocuronium causes little histamine release. However, like all drugs, there are some reports of anaphylaxis consistent with its frequency of usage.

The initial dose of rocuronium is 0.6 mg·kg^{-1} but a larger dose can be given depending upon the anticipated duration of surgery. The block can be maintained by repeated doses or by a continuous infusion (about 0.5 mg·kg^{-1}·h^{-1} for a 90% block). While the use of intermediate acting agents, such as rocuronium, may not help with the early discharge of patients undergoing relatively long cardiac surgery, it facilitates early tracheal extubation in such patients and is associated with a lower incidence of residual curarisation in these patients. With its rapid onset of action, rocuronium may be useful for facilitating tracheal intubation during rapid sequence induction of anaesthesia as an alternative to suxamethonium or where the latter is contraindicated. It is, however, important to assess the airway carefully if the use of rocuronium is contemplated in this setting.

Cisatracurium

Cisatracurium, one of the 10 stereoisomers of atracurium, has been developed in order to reduce the histamine-liberating and laudanosine-generating potential of atracurium. It also differs from atracurium in being more potent (ED_{95} of 0.05 mg·kg^{-1} compared to about 0.25 mg·kg^{-1} for atracurium), and being predominantly metabolised via the Hofmann elimination pathway. Being more potent, the drug has a slower onset of action than atracurium, taking 3–5 minutes for maximum block with a dose of 0.1 mg·kg^{-1}. For this reason it is usually advocated to use three times the ED_{95} dose (0.15 mg·kg^{-1}) for facilitating intubation with cisatracurium. The intubating conditions 2 minutes after relaxant administration are however still somewhat better with atracurium 0.5 mg·kg^{-1}.

The duration of clinical relaxation with cisatracurium is slightly longer than following equipotent doses of atracurium and ranges from about 35–65 minutes with doses of

0.1–0.15 mg·kg^{-1} and is dose-dependent. Administration of neostigmine accelerates the recovery significantly and produces effective reversal.

The major metabolic pathway for cisatracurium is Hofmann elimination, although renal and other organ clearance accounts for some elimination. The pharmacokinetics of cisatracurium are independent of dose in healthy adult patients up to doses of 0.2 mg·kg^{-1} and its elimination half-life is similar to that of atracurium (Table 6.4). In contrast to atracurium, the clearance of cisatracurium is slightly reduced and recovery slightly slower in patients with renal failure. Much less laudanosine is produced as a metabolite of cisatracurium as compared with atracurium even when the drug is given by continuous infusion over a prolonged period of time.

An important attribute of cisatracurium is its minimal cardiovascular effects resulting in no significant changes in arterial pressure or heart rate even in doses of up to 8 × ED_{95}. Cisatracurium does not in general liberate as much histamine as atracurium although individual patients may occasionally show significant increase in plasma histamine levels. Several cases of anaphylaxis have also been reported following cisatracurium administration.

Cisatracurium can either be administered by repeat dosing or by a continuous infusion (about 2 µg·kg^{-1}·min^{-1} for a 90% block) for lengthy procedures.

Mivacurium

Mivacurium is unique among non-depolarising relaxants in being hydrolysed by plasma cholinesterase and also capable of being reversed by anticholinesterase agents. Enzymatic hydrolysis, which occurs at about 80% of the rate for suxamethonium, is responsible for its short duration of action. Mivacurium is a mixture of three stereoisomers, the *cis-trans*, the *trans-trans*, and the *cis-cis*. The onset of action of 0.15–0.2 mg·kg^{-1} of mivacurium (2–3 ED_{95}) varies from 2–4 minutes with a clinical duration of about 15 minutes (approximately 2–2.5 times that of suxamethonium and one-half to one-third that of the intermediate-acting relaxants). The increase in the duration of action with increasing doses is not as marked as with other non-depolarising relaxants. It is currently the shortest-acting non-depolarising relaxant available. The intubating conditions following mivacurium are not consistently acceptable at 2 minutes after drug administration, even with doses of 0.2 mg·kg^{-1}. The quality of muscle relaxation with bolus doses can also be variable.

Although the recovery of block can be shortened by anticholinesterase administration, the effect is only minimal, perhaps due to an inherently short duration of action of the drug. Neostigmine which is a potent anticholinesterase agent, may prolong the action of mivacurium, particularly if given in the presence of deep block and edrophonium may be a better alternative. Previous administration of neostigmine prolongs the effects of subsequently administered mivacurium.

Mivacurium is a mixture of three stereoisomers, the two short-acting *cis-trans* and *trans-trans* isomers comprising about 94% of the mixture. Both have very short half-lives of about 2 minutes, while the much less potent *cis-cis* isomer has about one-tenth the neuromuscular blocking potency of the other two isomers. The *cis-cis* isomer undergoes some renal excretion as well as being broken down by plasma cholinesterase with a half-life of about 50 minutes (Table 6.4). The short-acting isomers are broken down almost entirely by plasma cholinesterase with a high rate of clearance and a short duration of action. The duration of action of mivacurium is increased when there is a reduction in plasma cholinesterase activity as in patients with marked renal and hepatic disease. The same is true for elderly patients.

Mivacurium is a potent histamine liberator even in clinically useful doses of 0.15–0.2 mg·kg^{-1}; this can result in a significant reduction in arterial pressure.

Mivacurium block is significantly prolonged in patients with inherited homozygous silent or atypical plasma cholinesterase variants; the effect of a single dose may last several hours in such patients. The prolongation of effect is only moderate in heterozygotes.

Mivacurium is a suitable agent for maintaining relaxation by infusion; in fact this is the preferred method of mivacurium administration for anything but brief procedures. The dose required to maintain approximately 90% block is 6–8 $\mu g \cdot kg^{-1} \cdot min^{-1}$.

OTHER NEUROMUSCULAR BLOCKING AGENTS

Gallamine, alcuronium and fazadinium have all been used in the past but are rarely used now; in fact only gallamine is still available in some European countries. All of these have significant side effects, particularly on the cardiovascular system. All are long acting and at least gallamine and alcuronium are almost totally dependent on the kidneys for elimination.

Doxacurium and pipecuronium are two long-acting relaxants without any significant side effects which were introduced as possible replacements for tubocurarine and pancuronium. Both are devoid of any cardiovascular effects. However, both are relatively slow acting and have a long duration of action, particularly doxacurium. Both are dependent on the kidneys for elimination with consequent prolongation of effect in renal disease. Although both agents are available in the US, their use is infrequent and these are unlikely to become available elsewhere.

Rapacuronium is a low-potency rapid- and short-acting non-depolarising agent with an aminosteroid structure which was introduced in the US as a possible replacement for suxamethonium. Although not short acting like suxamethonium, it was originally shown that its effect could be antagonised soon after its administration to give it an overall profile similar to that of suxamethonium. However, in clinical practice the duration of action was similar to that of mivacurium and early reversibility was not always attained. The drug was withdrawn due to an unacceptable frequency of bronchospasm.

ANTAGONISTS OF NEUROMUSCULAR BLOCKING AGENTS

While recovery from the effects of non-depolarising relaxants will occur spontaneously, it can take a long time and can be unpredictable. Therefore, pharmacological antagonism of neuromuscular block is commonly carried out in clinical practice by administering anticholinesterase drugs. Such agents include neostigmine, pyridostigmine, and edrophonium, neostigmine being the one used most commonly (Figure 6.3).

The main mechanism of action of anticholinesterase agents is inhibition of the enzyme acetylcholinesterase, resulting in increased concentration of acetylcholine (ACh). Acid-transferring inhibitors, neostigmine and pyridostigmine, are carbamated compounds that combine at both the anionic and the esteratic sites on the enzyme in almost the same way as ACh but with a longer dissociation half-life. Their breakdown products also have weak anticholinesterase effects. The prosthetic inhibitor, edrophonium, attaches mainly to the anionic site but dissociates more readily from the enzyme. Anticholinesterase agents may also stimulate the endplate receptors directly and/or increase the liberation of ACh (presynaptic effect); the contribution of these is, however, small. Out of the three agents, edrophonium has the greatest presynaptic effect.

Anticholinesterase drugs if administered in large doses or in the absence of muscle relaxants may produce fasciculations and even a depolarising type of block, similar to that with suxamethonium. Neostigmine prolongs the effect of suxamethonium.

Pyridostigmine is about five times less potent that neostigmine and edrophonium 10–15 times less potent, the equipotent doses for reversal being 0.05, 0.25, and 0.5–0.75 $mg \cdot kg^{-1}$ for neostigmine, pyridostigmine, and edrophonium, respectively. Edrophonium is the most rapid acting of the three with peak effect apparent in 1–2 minutes while neostigmine may take up to 10 minutes and pyridostigmine even longer. Pyridostigmine is therefore too slow for routine use. On the other

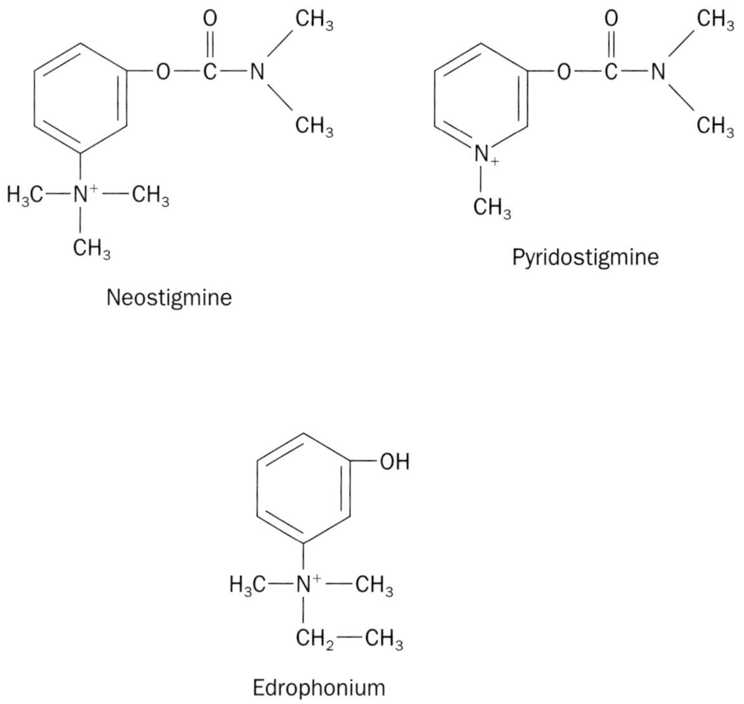

Neostigmine

Pyridostigmine

Edrophonium

***Figure 6.3** Chemical structures of anticholinesterase drugs.*

hand, while edrophonium is faster acting, it is not always effective for antagonising a relatively deep block. The duration of action of pyridostigmine is the longest but all three in the doses given above have sufficiently long durations of action for antagonising block.

About half of administered neostigmine is metabolised, the rest being renally excreted. The elimination half-life of neostigmine is about 80 minutes (Table 6.5). The clearance is markedly reduced in the presence of significant renal disease. Kinetics of pyridostigmine follow a similar pattern. The elimination half-life of edrophonium when given in a dose of 0.5–1.0 $mg{\cdot}kg^{-1}$ is similar to that of neostigmine and pyridostigmine. Elderly patients show a reduced rate of clearance for all three agents.

While the effects of anticholinesterase agents at the nicotinic receptors are desirable these agents also act at the muscarinic receptors, resulting in undesirable side effects, such as bradycardia, increased secretions, and increase in the activity of smooth muscles. Contraction of smooth muscles of the bowel, in particular, could theoretically lead to the breakdown of bowel anastomosis but in practice this is not a problem. Contraction of the bronchial smooth muscle may result in bronchospasm. It is therefore routine to administer antimuscarinic (anticholinergic) agents like atropine (20–30 $\mu g{\cdot}kg^{-1}$) or glycopyrrolate (10 $\mu g{\cdot}kg^{-1}$) in combination with drugs, such as neostigmine. Use of glycopyrrolate is associated with greater stability of the heart rates when neostigmine is used, although atropine is the preferred agent with

Table 6.5 Pharmacokinetic parameters for anticholinesterase agents

Agent	*Clearance ($mL{\cdot}kg^{-1}{\cdot}min^{-1}$)*	*Elimination half-life (min)*
Neostigmine	9.0	80
Edrophonium	9.6	110
Pyridostigmine	8.6	112

edrophonium. Glycopyrrolate may have other advantages as it does not cross the blood–brain barrier.

Some believe that administration of neostigmine may increase the incidence of postoperative emetic symptoms but critical assessment of the evidence shows this not to be the case. Neostigmine and pyridostigmine, but not edrophonium, produce marked inhibition of plasma cholinesterase activity which may prolong the effect of subsequently administered suxamethonium or mivacurium.

Edrophonium requires a lower dose of the anticholinergics as it exerts muscarinic effects of a smaller magnitude.

RECENT DEVELOPMENTS

Org 25969 which is a γ-cyclodextrin has recently been developed as a specific reversal agent for rocuronium and possibly vecuronium. This novel compound acts on the principle of chemical chelation forming complexes with the aminosteroid relaxant molecule resulting in a rapid reversal of the relaxant effect. The block is reversed even from a very deep level and without needing any anticholinergic drugs, as the mechanism of action does not involve cholinergic system. The agent is currently undergoing clinical trials and the first results appear to be very promising.

FURTHER READING

Berg H, Viby-Mogensen J, Roed J, et al. Residual neuromuscular block is a risk factor for postoperative pulmonary complications. A prospective, randomised and blinded study of postoperative pulmonary complications after atracurium, vecuronium and pancuronium. *Acta Anaesthesiol Scandinavica* 1997;41:1095–103.

Bevan DR, Donati F, Kopman AF. Reversal of neuromuscular blockade. *Anesthesiol* 1992;77:785–805.

Bowman WC, Rodger IW, Houston J, et al. Structure: action relationships among some desacetoxy analogs of pancuronium and vecuronium in the anesthetized cat. *Anesthesiol* 1988;69:57–62.

Donati F. Onset of action of relaxants. *Can J Anaesth* 1988; 35(Suppl):S52–S58.

Fuchs-Buder T, Sparr HJ, Zeigenfu BT. Thiopentone or etomidate for rapid sequence induction with rocuronium? *Br J Anaesth* 1998;80:504–6.

Ibebunjo C, Donati F. Sensitivities of different muscles to relaxant drugs. *Bailliere's Clin Anaesthesiol* 1994;8:369–94.

Mirakhur RK. Newer neuromuscular blocking drugs: An overview of their clinical pharmacology and therapeutic use. *Drugs* 1992;44:182–99.

Mirakhur RK. Antagonism of neuromuscular block. *Bailliere's Clin Anaesthesiol* 1994;8:461–81.

Mirakhur RK, McCoy EP. The new relaxants. *Curr Opin Anaesthesiol* 1994;7:365–9.

Mirakhur RK, McCarthy GJ. Basic pharmacology of reversal agents. *Anesthesiol Clin North Am* 1993;11:237–50.

Whittaker M. Plasma cholinesterase variants and the anaesthetist. *Anaesthesia* 1980;35:174–97.

Zhang M-Q. Drug-specific cyclodextrins: the future of rapid neuromuscular block reversal? *Drugs of the Future* 2003;28:347–54.

7

Opioids and NSAIDs

JG Bovill

Opioids • Individual drugs • Pure antagonists • Partial agonists • Other drugs • Non-steroidal anti-inflammatory analgesics (NSAIDs) • Individual drugs

OPIOIDS

Opioids are potent analgesics that act through G protein-coupled opioid receptors. The three classical opioid receptors are μ, δ, and κ. Three subtypes of the μ receptor have been described, μ_1, μ_2 and μ_3. The supraspinal mechanisms of analgesia produced by μ agonists are thought to involve the μ_1 receptor whereas spinal analgesia, respiratory depression, and the gastrointestinal effects are associated with the μ_2 receptor. The μ_3 receptor binds opioid alkaloids, such as morphine, but has exceedingly low affinity for the endogenous opioid peptides or non-alkaloid opioids, such as fentanyl, and is thought to be mainly involved in immune processes. There is evidence that morphine-6β-glucuronide (M6G), an active metabolite of morphine, and diamorphine act via a unique receptor site, which may be a splice variant of the μ receptor (Rossi and co-workers 1996). Subtypes of the δ and κ receptors have also been described, but their physiological functions are not known. A new receptor, the 'opioid receptor like 1' (ORL1), also referred to as an orphan receptor because the endogenous ligand was initially unknown, has been identified in several species, including humans (Darland and Grandy 1998). Its endogenous ligand is the heptadecapeptide, nociceptin, also known as orphanin FQ, since Phe (F) and Gln (Q) are the first and last amino acids of its primary sequence (Figure 7.1). Nociceptin produces a range of actions that differ from other opioids. It produces analgesia when administered intrathecally but causes hyperalgesia and reverses opioid-induced analgesia when given intracerebroventricularly.

The endogenous ligands for the opioid receptors are the enkephalins, endorphins and dynorphins, encoded by separate genes. These pentapeptides vary in their affinity for the opioid receptor, but none binds exclusively to one type. A new class of endogenous tetrapeptides, endomorphin-1 and endomorphin-2, with more than 1000-fold greater affinity for μ receptors than for δ or κ receptors, are thought to be the endogenous ligands for the μ receptor. Although the endogenous opioids are analgesic, their clinical usefulness is severely limited by rapid biodegradation by peptidases. Enkephalinase inhibitors are analgesic in animals, and mixed inhibitors of enkephalin degrading enzymes are now undergoing preclinical trials.

Activation of opioid receptors produces effects that are primarily inhibitory. Opioid-mediated inhibition of adenylyl cyclase decreases cAMP production. Opioids also close *N*-type voltage-operated calcium channels and

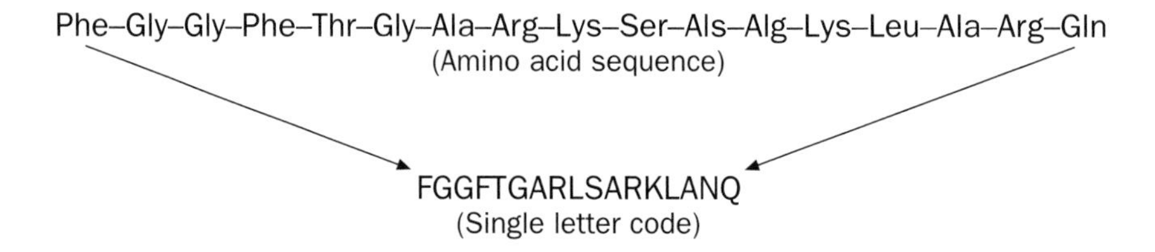

Figure 7.1 *Amino acid structure of nociceptin/Orphanin FQ.*

open calcium-dependent inwardly rectifying potassium channels (Figure 7.2). This results in hyperpolarisation and a reduction in neuronal excitability. Inhibition of calcium channels is important since intracellular Ca^{2+} levels influence the release of neurotransmitters and modulate the activity of protein kinases. In contrast to inhibitory activity, nanomolar concentrations of opioids can produce excitatory effects by activating excitatory G_s proteins.

Analgesia

Two anatomically distinct sites exist for opioid-mediated analgesia, supraspinal and spinal, and systemically administered opioids produce analgesia at both sites. Studies using mice deficient in the μ-opioid receptor have demonstrated that the μ receptor is essential for the analgesic and respiratory depressant properties of morphine (Keiffer 1999), although δ and κ agonists also mediate antinociception at spinal and supraspinal sites. In the dorsal horn the release of substance P, glutamate and other nociceptive neurotransmitters from the afferent terminals of sensory fibres is inhibited by activation of presynaptic μ, δ and κ receptors. Opioids selectively modulate 'second pain' sensation carried by slowly conducting, unmyelinated C fibres but have little effect on 'first pain' carried by small, myelinated Aδ fibres. Opioid receptors have been demonstrated on peripheral terminals of sensory nerves. Activation of these receptors seems to require an inflammatory reaction since locally applied opioids do not produce analgesia in healthy tissue. Intra-articular morphine, 1–5 mg, provides analgesia after arthroscopic surgery, without systemic side effects.

Respiratory depression

All pure μ agonist opioids produce a dose-related depression of ventilation. Pure κ agonists have little effect on respiration. The primary effect of opioids is a reduction in the sensitivity of the respiratory centre to CO_2. They also depress the medullary and peripheral chemoreceptors. Initially, respiratory rate is affected more than tidal volume, which may even increase. With increasing doses respiratory rhythmicity is disturbed resulting in the irregular, gasping breathing characteristic of opioid overdose. The hypoxic drive to ventilation is also depressed by opioids.

Muscle rigidity

Muscle rigidity, commonly associated with opioids, seems to be primarily associated with central activation of the μ receptor. Rigidity involving the thoracic and abdominal muscles can sometimes interfere with ventilation to such an extent that manual ventilation is

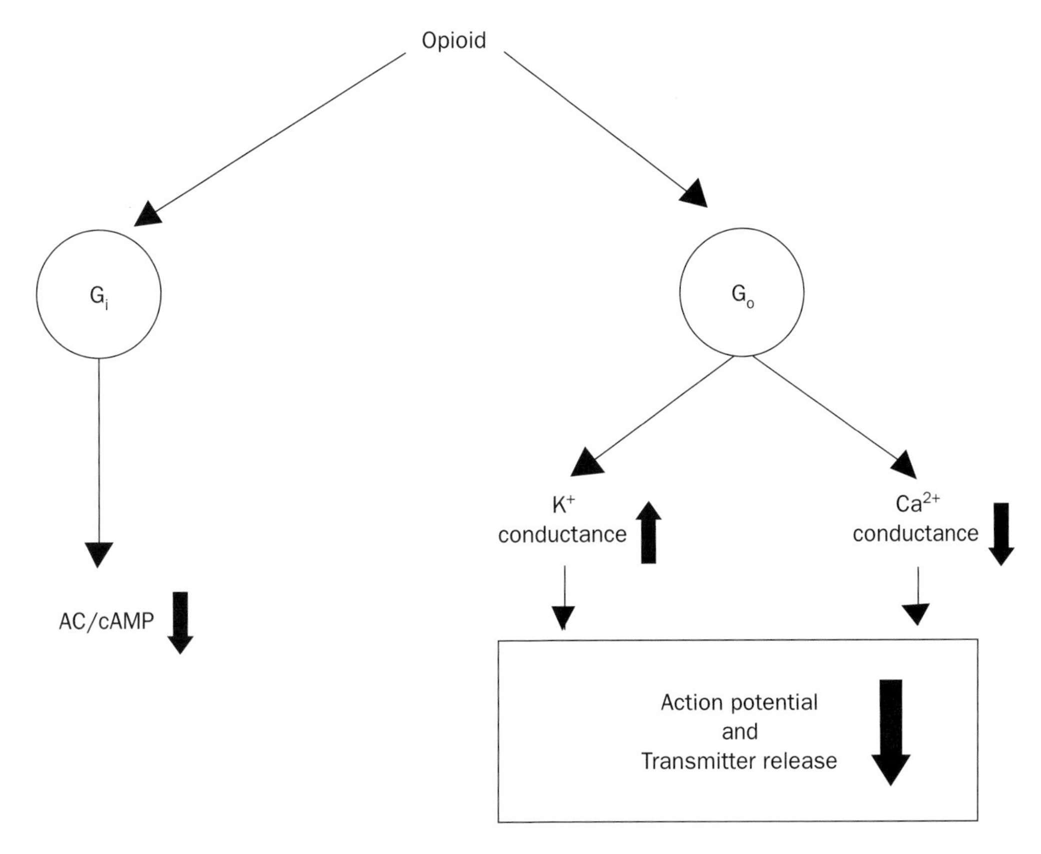

Figure 7.2 *G protein-mediated mechanisms of opioid cellular actions. Activation of the μ receptor results in inhibition of adenylyl cyclase (AC), the enzyme responsible for the formation of cAMP, via the* G_i *protein, and increased potassium conductance and decreased calcium conductance, mediated via* G_o *proteins.*

impossible without the use of a muscle relaxant. It is common when an opioid is given during induction of anaesthesia, but may manifest itself in the postoperative period. It is reversed by naloxone and muscle relaxants and attenuated by barbiturates and benzodiazepines. The mechanism of opioid-induced muscle rigidity remains unresolved, but may involve inhibition of dopamine release in the striatum. Catatonic movements of the limbs are frequently observed in patients given high doses of opioids.

Tolerance and physical dependence

Following prolonged or repeated exposure to opioids, a diminished responsiveness to their actions develops. While tolerance is often associated with chronic exposure for days or weeks, it can develop after minutes to hours. Physical dependence is a state, sometimes associated with drug tolerance, whereby adaptive changes occur as a consequence of sustained exposure to a drug, so that it becomes required for normal function. Withdrawing the drug or antagonising its action elicits a 'withdrawal syndrome', with restlessness and an intense craving for the drug, accompanied by yawning, running nose, lacrimation, perspiration, and aches and pains.

The pupils become dilated and there are associated signs of hyperactivity of the sympathetic nervous system, such as hypertension and pilomotor stimulation. The mechanism(s) underlying tolerance and dependence are poorly understood. While acute activation of $G_{i/o}$-coupled receptors leads to inhibition of adenylyl cyclase, chronic activation of such receptors produces an increase in cAMP accumulation, particularly evident upon withdrawal of the inhibitory agonist. This phenomenon, referred to as adenylyl cyclase superactivation, is believed to play an important role in opioid addiction.

Gastrointestinal tract

The gastrointestinal tract is the only system outside the central nervous system (CNS) with significant concentrations of opioid receptors. This reflects their common embryonic origins. Opioids increase intestinal tone and decrease propulsive peristalsis, resulting in delayed gastric emptying and constipation or ileus. Opioids increase common bile duct pressure and decrease bile production and flow, primarily because of spasm of the sphincter of Oddi. The tone of the bile duct itself is also increased.

Emetic effects

Nausea and vomiting are common and undesirable side effects of opioids. Opioids initiate the vomiting reflex by stimulating a specialised area of the brain located in the area postrema called the chemoreceptor trigger zone (CTZ). This in turn leads to activation of the 'vomiting centre' located in the reticular formation of the medulla close to the area postrema. Nausea and vomiting are more common in ambulatory patients, due to vestibular stimulation of the CTZ, which is sensitised by opioids. Opioids depress the vomiting centre and with increasing plasma concentrations this effect overcomes the CTZ stimulant effect.

Cardiovascular system

Most of the haemodynamic effects of opioids are related to decreased central sympathetic outflow, specific vagal effects or, in the case of morphine and pethidine, histamine release. Fentanyl and its analogues do not cause histamine release. All opioids, with the exception of pethidine, produce bradycardia by actions on the afferent fibres of the vagus and the nucleus tractus solitarius and nucleus commissuralis, which have very high densities of opioid receptors. Pethidine often produces tachycardia, possibly due to its structural similarity to atropine. In isolated heart or heart-muscle preparations, opioids produce a dose-related negative inotropic effect, but only at concentrations 100 to several thousand times those found clinically.

INDIVIDUAL DRUGS

Morphine

Morphine, the prototype μ agonist, is available as the sulphate or hydrochloride salt. Morphine sulphate contains two moles of anhydrous morphine per molecule, the hydrochloride salt only one mole per molecule. It is the amount of anhydrous morphine that is important and 10 mg of either salt contains approximately equal amounts of anhydrous morphine (~ 7.5 mg). Morphine is poorly lipid-soluble, due to the presence of two hydroxyl groups that confer polar characteristics to the molecule (Figure 7.3). Masking the hydroxyl group by acetylation or methylation, as in diamorphine (heroin) or codeine, changes the pharmacological effect. The low lipophilicity of morphine means that it cannot easily cross the blood–brain barrier. Morphine is well absorbed from the gastrointestinal tract although significant presystemic metabolism occurs. An intramuscular dose of 10–15 mg will produce maximum analgesia in about 30 min, and lasting 4 to 5 hours. With larger doses, the incidence of side effects increases out of proportion to the increase in analgesia. For severe pain, it is

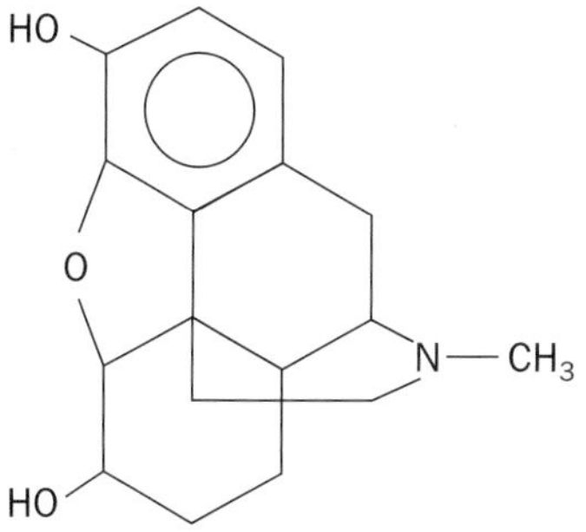

Morphine

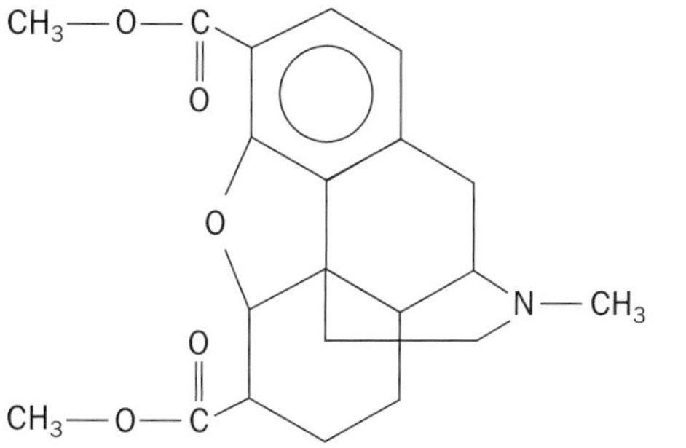

Heroin

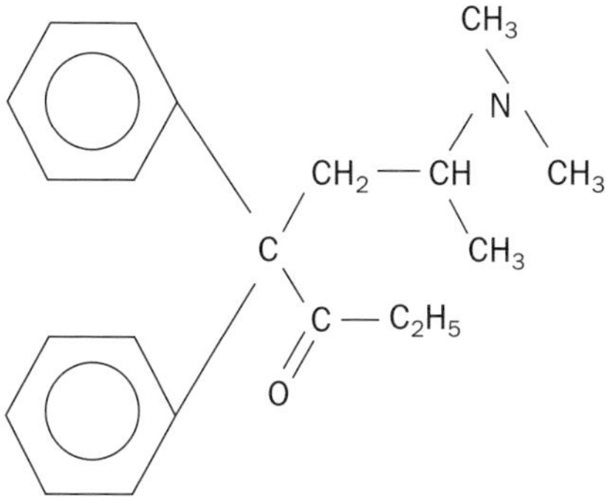

Methadone

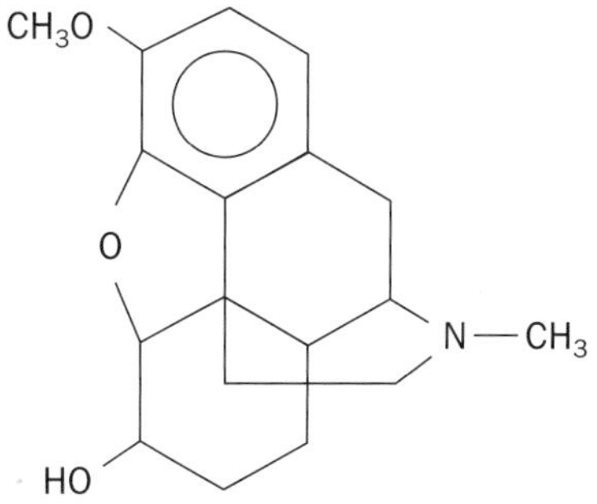

Codeine

Figure 7.3 Chemical structure of morphine and allied opioids.

preferable to titrate small doses, e.g. 1–2 mg, intravenously until adequate analgesia is achieved. The oral dose is about 50% higher than the intramuscular dose.

Central nervous system depression is the usual effect of morphine, and sedation and drowsiness are frequently observed with therapeutic doses. When given in the absence of pain morphine may sometimes produce dysphora—an unpleasant sensation of fear and anxiety. The most important stimulatory effects of morphine in man are emesis and miosis. Miosis, due to stimulation of the Edinger-Westphal nucleus of the third nerve, occurs with all opioids. The combination of pinpoint pupils, coma, and respiratory depression are classical signs of morphine overdosage. Stimulation of the solitary nuclei may also be responsible for depression of the cough reflex (antitussive effect).

Pharmacokinetics and metabolism

The pharmacokinetic parameters for morphine and other agonist opioids are given in Table 7.1. Morphine undergoes extensive hepatic biotransformation, principally by phase II conjugation to morphine-3-glucuronide (M3G), the major metabolite, 5–10% to morphine-6-glucuronide (M6G), and the remainder undergoes sulphate conjugation. Although the liver is the primary organ of conjugation, extrahepatic metabolism of morphine occurs in the kidney and possibly in the gut.

M3G has no analgesic activity but may antagonise the analgesic effects of morphine. M6G is pharmacologically active with potency higher than morphine. The plasma concentration of M6G exceeds that of the parent drug by a factor of nine within 30 minutes of intravenous (IV) administration (Figure 7.4). Despite

Table 7.1 Pharmacokinetic parameters for the opioid agonists

Agonist	*pKa*	*Unionised (%)*	*Lipid solubility*	*Protein binding (%)*	*Oral availability (%)*	*CL (L/min)*	*V_{Dss} (L)*	*$t_{\frac{1}{2}}$ (h)*
Morphine	7.90	24	1.4	35	25–50	1.20	200	1.7
Methadone	8.30	5.9	57	85	90	0.18	410	35
Pethidine	8.60	7.4	39	70	50–55	1.02	260	4–8
Diamorphine	7.63	37	280	40	–	–	–	–
Fentanyl	8.40	9.1	816	84	negligible	1.53	335	3.6
Alfentanil	6.50	88.8	128	92	–	0.24	27	1.6
Sufentanil	8.00	19.7	1757	93	negligible	0.90	123	2.8
Remifentanil	7.07	68	18	70	–	3–4	21–28	10–20 (min)

Lipid solubility is expressed as the octanol:water partition coefficient.

its polarity it crosses the blood–brain barrier and undoubtly contributes to the analgesic effect. Despite slower penetration into the brain (blood–brain equilibration half-life 3–16 h for M6G versus 2–4.5 h for morphine), it may be that 50% or more of the respiratory depression observed by 1 h following systemic administration of morphine is due to this metabolite. Patients with renal insufficiency have impaired elimination of morphine glucuronides and M6G makes a significant contribution to morphine intoxication in these patients.

In neonates, and especially in premature infants, the mechanism for glucuronide conjugation is poorly developed. Renal function is also very inefficient. The pharmacokinetics of morphine in neonates is thus markedly different from that in older children and adults. This, together with age-related differences in the development of opioid receptors, may explain their increased sensitivity to morphine.

Codeine phosphate

Codeine, one of the principal alkaloids of opium, has an analgesic efficacy much lower than other opioids, due to an extremely low affinity for opioid receptors. It is approximately one-sixth as potent as morphine. It has a low abuse potential. In contrast to other opioids, with the exception of oxycodone, codeine is relatively more effective when administered orally than parenterally. This is due to methylation at the C3 site on the phenyl ring (Figure 7.3), which may protect it from conjugating enzymes. It is used in the management of mild-to-moderate pain, often in combination with non-opioid analgesics, such as aspirin or paracetamol. It is valuable as an antitussive and for the treatment of diarrhoea. Side effects are uncommon and respiratory depression, even with large doses, is seldom a problem.

Diamorphine

Diamorphine (3,6-diacetyl morphine, heroin) is a semi-synthetic derivative of morphine. It was first synthesised in 1874 and put on the market in 1898 as a non-habit-forming alternative to morphine! It is a prodrug with no opioid activity itself. All its pharmacological activity derives from hydrolysis to monoacetylmorphine (MAM) and then to morphine in the plasma and tissues. Diamorphine also

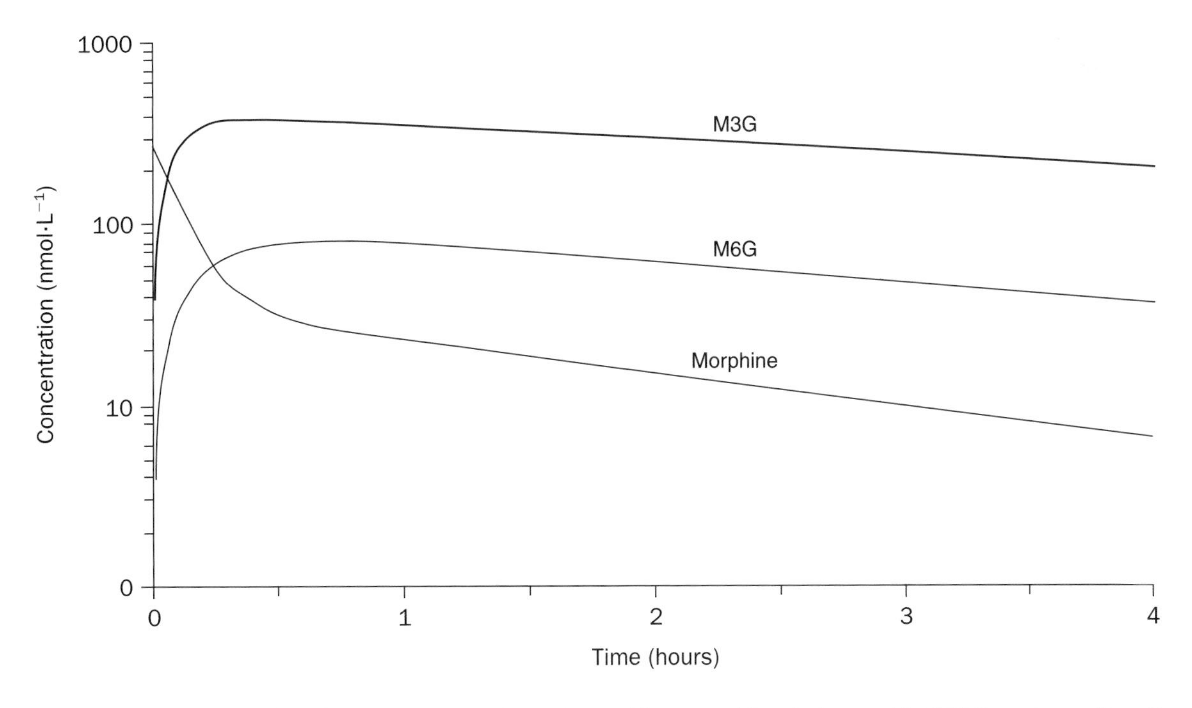

Figure 7.4 *Changes in the plasma concentrations of morphine, morphine-3-glucuronide (M3G), and morphine-6-glucuronide (M6G) following an IV bolus of morphine 10 mg.*

undergoes metabolism in the tissues, including the CNS, by esterases. Diamorphine and MAM are more lipid-soluble than morphine and may act as carriers to facilitate the entry of morphine into the CNS. It is a potent analgesic with a high potential for addiction and its manufacture and use, even for medical purposes, is illegal in the US and some other countries. Although it is claimed that diamorphine produces more sedation and less nausea and vomiting than morphine, it is likely that the incidence of side effects with equi-analgesic doses is similar to other opioids. A dose of 5 mg diamorphine is equi-potent with 10 mg morphine, but the duration of action is shorter, about 2 hours. Because diamorphine in solution rapidly undergoes deacetylation, injections should always be freshly prepared. Interest in the use of diamorphine by the epidural or intrathecal routes has recently become more evident due to its greater lipid solubility in comparison with morphine.

Methadone

Methadone is a synthetic opioid commercially available as a racemic mixture. The R(–) isomer is 50 times more potent than the S(+) -isomer. It produces less sedation and euphoria but in other respects the side effects are similar to those of morphine. Its high bioavailability after oral administration (80%) and its long half-life make it useful in the management of cancer pain. It is widely used in the treatment of withdrawal symptoms in opioid addicts. Methadone is equipotent with morphine when given orally or intramuscularly, but may be somewhat less potent when given intravenously. Although the duration of a single dose is comparable to that after morphine, with repeated doses accumulation occurs so that there needs to be either lower doses or longer intervals between doses to avoid overdosage.

The phenylpiperidines

The phenylpiperidines share a common chemical structure; a phenyl ring connected either directly (pethidine and phenoperidine) or by a nitrogen atom to a 6-membered piperidine ring (Figure 7.5). The phenyl ring confers high lipophilicity to the phenylpiperidine opioids. Clinically important phenylpiperidines include pethidine, phenoperidine, fentanyl, alfentanil, sufentanil and remifentanil. Pethidine was the first synthetic opioid. It is less potent than morphine, 75 mg pethidine being approximately equivalent to 10 mg morphine. Phenoperidine is an *N*-phenylpropyl derivative of norpethidine, a metabolite of pethidine. As a supplement during anaesthesia the usual dose is 0.5–1 mg intravenously in spontaneously breathing patients, and up to 5 mg when intermittent positive pressure ventilation (IPPV) is used. Remifentanil is a μ-receptor agonist with an analgesic potency similar to that of fentanyl, a rapid onset and a very short duration of action.

The combination of pethidine with monoamine oxidase inhibitors (MAOIs) can cause serious adverse reaction, which can present in two distinct forms. The excitatory form is characterised by sudden agitation, delirium, headache, hypo- or hypertension, rigidity, hyperpyrexia, convulsions and coma. It is thought to be caused by an increase in cerebral 5-HT concentrations because of inhibition of monoamine oxidase. This is potentiated by pethidine, which blocks neuronal uptake of 5-HT. The depressive form, which is frequently severe and fatal, consists of respiratory and cardiovascular depression and coma. It is the result of the inhibition of hepatic microsomal enzymes by the MAOI, leading to accumulation of pethidine. Phenoperidine should also be avoided in patients taking MAOI drugs but other opioids appear to be safe.

Pharmacokinetics and metabolism

The phenylpiperidines are basic compounds, with pKa values varying from 6.5 (alfentanil) to 8.4 (fentanyl). Due to its low pKa, 85% of alfentanil in blood is non-ionised resulting in rapid passage across the blood–brain barrier and a fast onset of action. Its blood–brain equilibration half-time ($t_{\frac{1}{2}}k_{e0}$) is about 1 min compared to 5–6 min for fentanyl and sufentanil. The $t_{\frac{1}{2}}k_{e0}$ of remifentanil is similar to that of alfentanil. As with many basic drugs, the phenylpiperidines are highly protein bound, particularly to α_1-acid glycoprotein (AAG).

The biotransformation of the phenylpiperidines is primarily by hepatic phase I metabolism, catalysed by cytochrome P-450 isoenzymes. The elimination of alfentanil is significantly slowed in patients treated with erythromycin, a P-450 inhibitor, with delayed recovery and prolonged postoperative respiratory depression (Bartkowski and McDonnell 1990). Apart from pethidine and phenoperidine, none of the phenylpiperidines has pharmacologically active metabolites.

Pethidine undergoes extensive hepatic metabolism by *N*-demethylation to norpethidine and hydrolysis to pethidinic acid. Phenoperidine is metabolised to pethidine, norpethidine, and pethidinic acid. Norpethidine has a long plasma half-life in normal patients (14–21 h) and even longer in those with diminished renal function. Pethidine and norpethidine can readily cross the placental barrier and accumulate in the fetus. Both compounds are weak bases and ion-trapping occurs in the fetal plasma. The elimination of pethidine in neonates is slower than in adults with half-lives prolonged up to 6 days. Only about 7% of unchanged pethidine is excreted in the urine. This amount is markedly influenced, however, by urinary pH. Acidification of the urine reduces the excretion of unchanged pethidine to less than 1% whereas with urinary alkalinisation this is increased to 20–25%. With increasing doses of pethidine, signs of CNS excitation—tremors, muscle twitching and eventually convulsions—predominate over CNS depression. Norpethidine, a major metabolite of pethidine, may be the principal mediator of those CNS excitatory effects. CNS toxicity is most likely to occur in patients with renal failure and where the oral route is used, due to the significant presystemic metabolism, which results in rapid accumulation of norpethidine. It may take

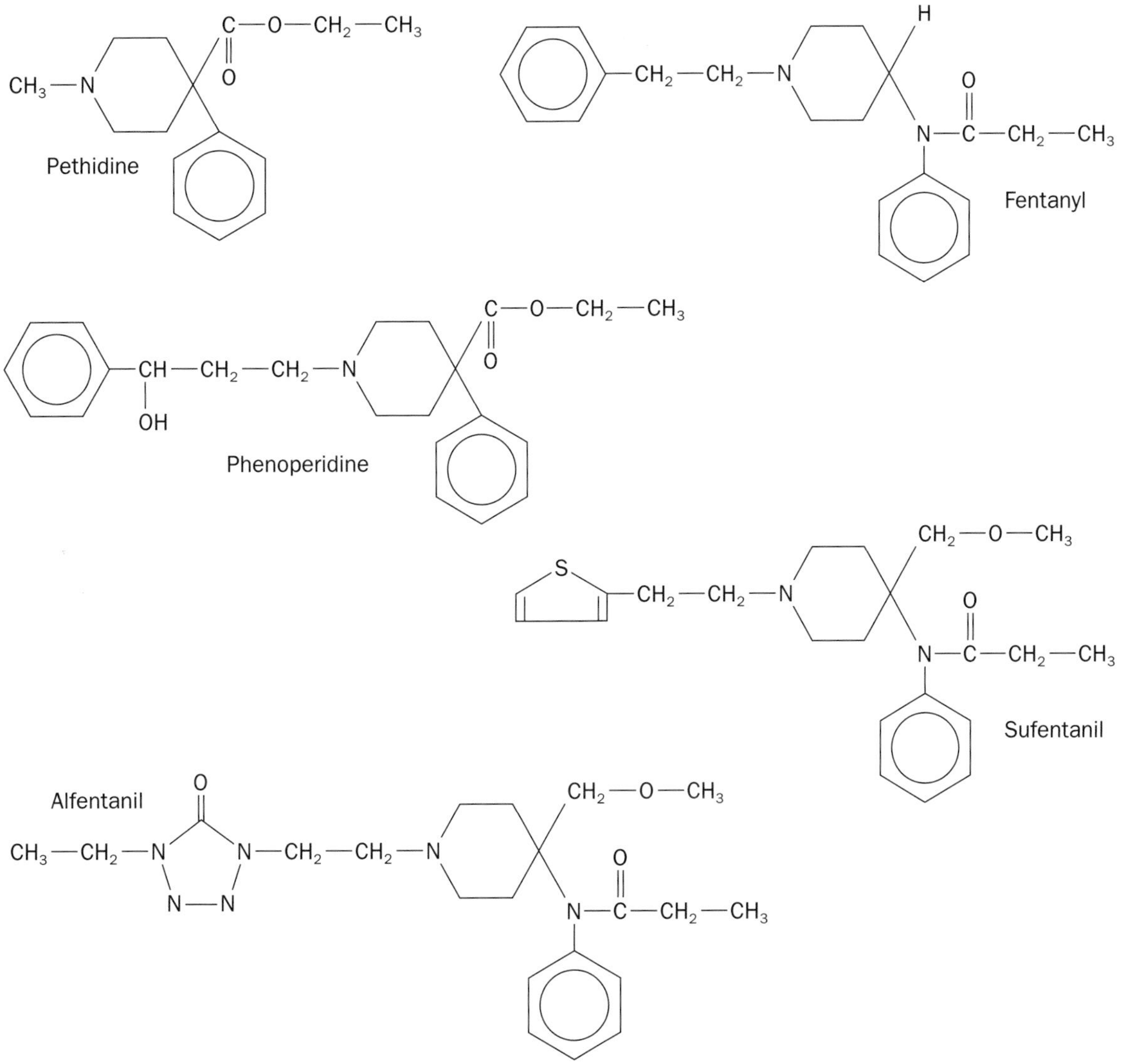

Figure 7.5 *Chemical structures of the phenylpiperidine class of opioids.*

several days for normal neurological functions to return.

Remifentanil incorporates a methyl ester group attached to the nitrogen of the piperidine ring, making it susceptible to hydrolysis by non-specific esterases in the blood and tissues, with very rapid degradation to inactive metabolites (Figure 7.6). The β-adrenoceptor antagonist esmolol is metabolised by a similar mechanism. Clearance is not affected by the presence of a cholinesterase inhibitor such as neostigmine. Remifentanil is not a good substrate for butyrylcholinesterase (pseudo-cholinesterase) so its pharmacokinetics will not be different in patients with cholinesterase deficiency.

For fentanyl and sufentanil, hepatic extraction is high and hepatic clearance is dependent on liver blood flow. Factors decreasing this will slow elimination and prolong effect. Conversely, because the liver has such a large reserve capacity of metabolising enzymes, their elimination is not significantly altered in patients with hepatic disease until liver function becomes severely compromised. In

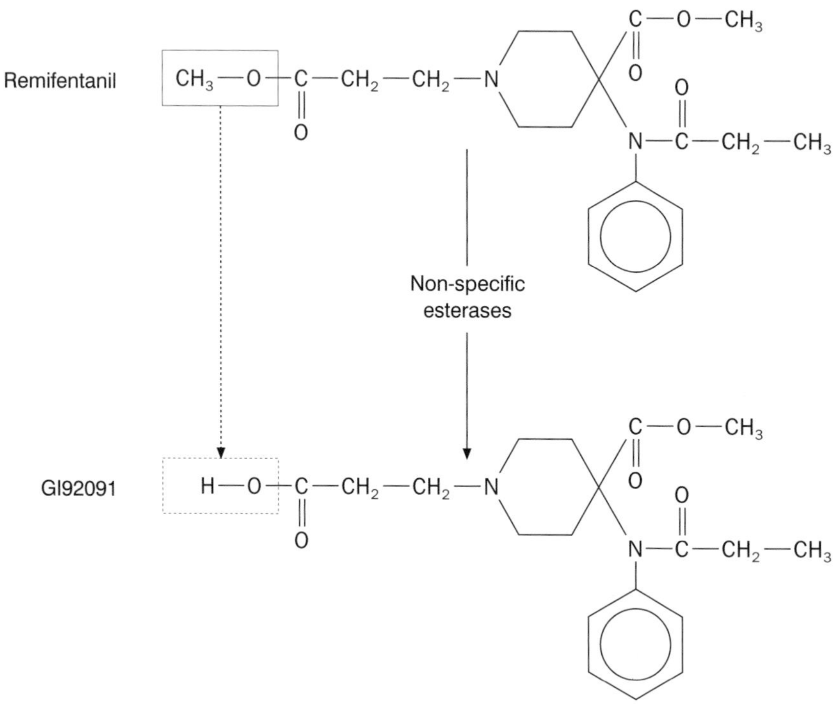

Remifentanil

Non-specific esterases

GI92091

Figure 7.6 Structure of remifentanil and its major metabolite formed by ester hydrolysis.

contrast, alfentanil has an intermediate hepatic extraction (0.3–0.5) and alfentanil clearance will be sensitive to changes in both liver blood flow and reduced enzyme capacity in patients with liver disease. Although the kidneys play a minor role in the elimination of most opioids, renal disease can influence their pharmacokinetic profile, secondary to alterations in plasma proteins and intra- and extravascular volumes. Neither the pharmacokinetics nor the pharmacodynamics of remifentanil is significantly altered in patients with liver or renal disease.

Epidural and intrathecal opioids

Epidural and intrathecal opioids are widely used for postoperative and obstetric analgesia. In contrast to local anaesthetics, spinal opioids cause minimal sympathetic efferent and motor blockade. Pethidine, which has local anaesthetic activity, can produce sensory and motor blockade. Because remifentanil is formulated with glycine as a vehicle, it should not be used epidurally or intrathecally, since glycine is neurotoxic.

After epidural injection, an opioid may transfer into the cerebrospinal fluid (CSF), into the blood or bind to epidural fat, the extent depending on their lipophilicity. After epidural administration, morphine passes slowly into the CSF. Sufentanil, which is highly lipid soluble, can be detected in the plasma within 2–5 minutes after epidural injection and part of the analgesic effect of the more lipid soluble opioids may be due to a supraspinal action amplifying the direct spinal action. Epidural fentanyl and sufentanil produce a more consistent and intense analgesia than morphine, with a faster onset. However, the duration is short but this can be overcome by giving them by continuous epidural infusions.

Side effects and complications tend to be higher with the intrathecal than the epidural route. A common side effect is pruritus, the incidence of which is higher with intrathecal than with epidural administration. It is dose-dependent, with an incidence of about 10% after epidural morphine 5 mg. The risk of severe, distressing itching is about 1%. Pruritus may be related to cephalad spread of morphine within the CSF. Prophylactic naloxone infusion at a rate of 5 $\mu g \cdot kg^{-1} \cdot h^{-1}$ will reduce the frequency of pruritus without reversing analgesia. A small, 10 mg, IV dose of propofol may be equally effective.

Rostral spread is largely responsible for emetic symptoms and respiratory depression. The incidence of respiratory depression is low (0.25–0.5%) with epidural morphine but is potentially the most serious complication and is frequently delayed until several hours after drug administration. It can be profound and long lasting. Although late-onset respiratory depression is rare with the more lipid-soluble opioids, respiratory depression within 30 min of injection can occur due to extensive uptake into the systemic circulation. The other important side effect is urinary retention with an overall incidence of about 40%. It can develop insidiously and since bladder sensation is partially or wholly lost may not be reported by the patient until gross overdistension of the bladder has occurred. Naloxone, 0.4 mg intravenously, will immediately restore normal micturition but will also reverse analgesia.

Because epidural opioids are usually ineffective in controlling pain during the final stages of labour they are commonly combined with a low concentration of a local anaesthetic, e.g. 0.125% bupivacaine. There has been speculation that epidural opioids may reactivate herpes simplex in pregnant patients. The aetiology is unclear. Herpes simplex after delivery is potentially dangerous because of the risk of herpes encephalitis in the infant. Spinal opioids should therefore be avoided in the parturient with a history of recurrent herpes simplex.

PURE ANTAGONISTS

Naloxone

Naloxone is the *N*-allyl derivative of oxymorphone (Figure 7.7). It is a competitive antagonist at μ, δ and κ receptors but is more potent at the μ receptor. When given to patients who have had an excessive perioperative dose of an opioid, naloxone will reverse not only the respiratory depression but also analgesia. A dose of 0.2–0.4 mg is effective in reversing opioid-induced respiratory depression, although it is better to titrate naloxone in increments of 0.04 mg to avoid acute reversal of analgesia. When used to reverse the effects of large doses of an opioid intense pressor responses, tachycardia, and severe pulmonary oedema may occur. The plasma half-life of naloxone (1.0–1.5 h) is considerably shorter than most opioids, and the clinical effects of a single injection last only 30–90 min. On occasions, repeated doses or a continuous intravenous infusion might be required. An infusion of 0.2–0.4 $mg \cdot h^{-1}$ will usually suffice to prevent opioid-induced respiratory depression without affecting analgesia.

Naltrexone and nalmefene

Naltrexone and nalmefene are structurally related to naloxone. Naltrexone is the *N*-cyclopropylmethyl analogue of oxymorphone while nalmefene is the *N*-allyl analogue. They have similar pharmacological properties to naloxone but with longer durations of action, with elimination half-lives in excess of 8 hours. They also have significant oral availability. They are used mainly in the management of addicts.

Peripheral opioid antagonists

Postoperative ileus occurs after all major abdominal surgery, and is exacerbated by opioids used for pain relief. Constipation is also a common side effect of chronic opioid therapy. Opioid-induced inhibition of gastrointestinal motility is caused by activation of μ opioid receptors in the gastrointestinal tract, and can be blocked by oral opioid antagonists. Unfortunately, most antagonists are absorbed and reverse the analgesic effects of opioid agonists in postoperative patients and produce withdrawal effects in patients on long-term opioid therapy. One solution is to use an antagonist that is not absorbed but can antagonise opioid binding to gut receptors. Two peripheral opioid antagonists have recently been introduced, methylnaltrexone

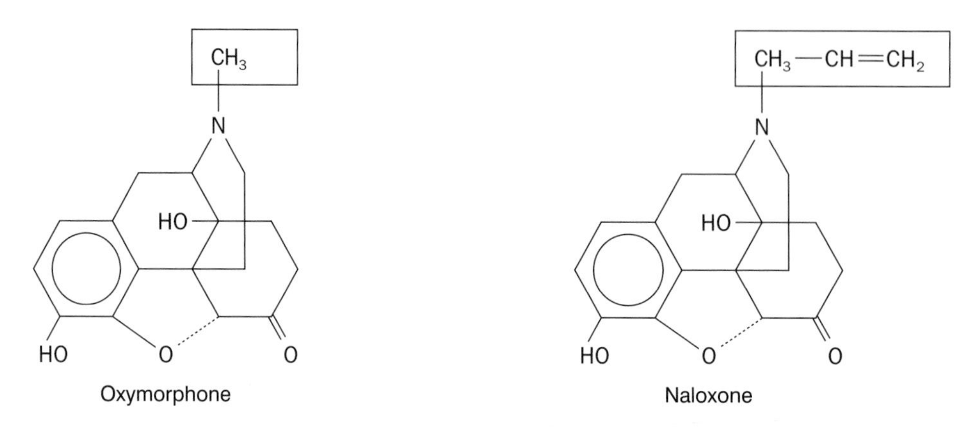

Figure 7.7 *Chemical structure of naloxone and oxymorphone. Note how the small difference in structure changes the full agonist, oxymorphone, into the antagonist, naloxone.*

and alvimopan, with activity that is restricted to peripheral receptors.

Methylnaltrexone is a quaternary derivative of the opioid antagonist, naltrexone. The addition of the methyl group forms a compound with greater polarity and lower lipid solubility, so that it is poorly absorbed, and does not cross the blood–brain barrier. Methylnaltrexone distributes selectively (> 200-fold selectivity) to peripheral receptors. In human trials it prevented morphine-induced delay in gastrointestinal transit time, while sparing centrally mediated analgesic effects.

Alvimopan is a μ-selective opioid receptor antagonist whose moderately large molecule and polarity prevent penetration of the blood–brain barrier. It has minimal systemic bioavailability (0.03%) with a short plasma half-life (10 min when given IV). Plasma concentrations of alvimopan are undetectable at the usual oral doses. Alvimopan 6 mg, administered orally before surgery and twice daily starting on the first postoperative day speeded recovery of bowel function after major abdominal surgery, without affecting postoperative analgesia by morphine. It improved bowel function in patients receiving opioid therapy for chronic pain or methadone for opioid addiction, without CNS signs of opioid withdrawal or reversal of analgesia (Kurz and Sessler 2003; Bates and co-workers 2004).

PARTIAL AGONISTS

The first drug in this class was nalorphine (*N*-allylmorphine). Nalorphine is equipotent with morphine but produced severe psychotomimetic activity, which precluded its use as an analgesic. Until the discovery of naloxone it was widely used for its antagonist properties in the treatment of opioid overdose. The dysphoric side effects of some of this class of drugs is thought to be due to binding to the non-opioid σ receptor.

Pentazocine

Pentazocine was the first member of the so-called agonist–antagonist opioids to be clinically successful. Its analgesic potency is one-third to one-fifth that of morphine. In equi-analgesic doses pentazocine causes the same degree of respiratory depression as morphine. However, as with other partial agonists, the response curves for respiratory depression and analgesia are plateau-shaped, with the plateau being reached at a dose of approximately 60 mg for the average adult. Peak blood concentrations after oral administration are reached by 1–3 h and between 15 and 45 min after intramuscular administration. The oral bioavailability is about 20%.

Pentazocine is contraindicated in the treatment of patients with acute myocardial infarction because of cardiovascular stimulation. Psychotomimetic side effects, such as hallucinations, bizarre dreams, and sensations of depersonalisation, occur in about 6–10% of patients. They are more common in elderly patients, in those who are ambulatory, and when doses above 60 mg are given. Nausea occurs in approximately 5% of patients although vomiting is less common. Other commonly reported side effects are dizziness and drowsiness. The risk of physical dependence is low.

Butorphanol tartrate

Butorphanol tartrate is a weak partial μ-receptor agonist, 3.5–5 times as potent as morphine. The incidence of psychotomimetic effects is relatively low. The recommended doses are 1–4 mg intramuscularly every 3–4 h or 0.5–2 mg intravenously. Respiratory depression produced by butorphanol 2 mg IV is similar to that of 10 mg morphine. However, there is a ceiling effect for respiratory depression, and near-maximum depression occurs after 4 mg in normal adults. In healthy volunteers, butorphanol 0.03–0.06 $mg{\cdot}kg^{-1}$ produces no significant cardiovascular changes. However, in patients with cardiac disease, progressive increases in cardiac index and pulmonary artery pressure occur, and butorphanol should be avoided in patients with recent myocardial infarction. Butorphanol is metabolised mainly in the liver to inactive metabolites. The terminal half-life is 2.5–3.5 h.

Nalbuphine hydrochloride

Nalbuphine hydrochloride is structurally related to oxymorphone and naloxone. It is approximately equipotent with morphine. Nalbuphine is metabolised in the liver to inactive metabolites. The plasma terminal half-life is approximately 5 h. The onset of analgesia is within 2–3 min of intravenous administration and 15 min after intramuscular injection, and lasts 3–6 h with an adult dose of 10 mg. With equi-analgesic doses, similar degrees of respiratory depression to that of morphine occur up to a dose of approximately 0.45 $mg{\cdot}kg^{-1}$. With higher doses a 'ceiling effect' occurs. Sedation, possibly mediated by κ-receptor activation, occasionally occurs. The incidence of psychotomimetic side effects is lower than with pentazocine. The abuse potential is low, but is can cause withdrawal symptoms in opioid-dependent subjects. It has occasionally been used to reverse opioid-induced respiratory depression.

Buprenorphine

Buprenorphine is a semi-synthetic derivative of thebaine, one of the opium alkaloids. It is approximately 30 times as potent as morphine. A dose of 0.3 mg intramuscularly has a duration of analgesic action of 6–18 h. Buprenorphine is also effective sublingually. The average bioavailability by this route is about 55%, but absorption is slow and the time to achieve peak plasma concentrations is variable, with a range of 90–360 min. The onset of action is rather slow (5–15 min) after both intramuscular and intravenous administration, possibly due to slow receptor association.

Buprenorphine binds to and dissociates from the μ receptor very slowly, which may account for its low potential for physical abuse. It also means that buprenorphine-induced respiratory depression is difficult to reverse with naloxone, even with very high doses. Doxapram may in these circumstances be useful. Drowsiness and dizziness are the most common side effects, although they rarely constitute a major problem. In comparison with other opioids, buprenorphine appears to have a very low abuse potential. Buprenorphine is almost completely metabolised in the liver by *N*-dealkylation and conjugation. The terminal half-life is approximately 5 h. The oral bioavailability is only 3–6%.

OTHER DRUGS

Meptazinol is structurally related to pethidine and has approximately similar potency. It can be given orally or by injection. Clinically it behaves as a partial μ agonist, but part of its analgesic activity is mediated via central cholinergic activation. In clinically effective analgesic doses it is almost devoid of respiratory side effects, but does cause emesis, sedation, and atropine-like side effects. **Dezocine** is a partial μ agonist with analgesic activity similar to morphine. In single doses, however, dezocine is a slightly more potent respiratory depressant than morphine, but a 'ceiling' effect occurs with increasing dose. Maximum respiratory depression occurs at about 2.3 $mg{\cdot}kg^{-1}$ intravenously.

Tramadol hydrochloride is a centrally acting analgesic that acts at opioid receptors and also modifies nociceptive transmission by inhibition of noradrenaline (norepinephrine) and serotonin. It has a low affinity for opioid receptors, 10-fold less than that of codeine. It is approximately equipotent to pethidine. It may be administered orally, rectally or intravenously. Oral tramadol is effective for the treatment of patients with cancer pain. The tolerance and dependence potential of tramadol is low, even with prolonged treatment. It can cause respiratory depression, although this is considerably less than with the classical opioid agonists. It is generally well tolerated, with dizziness, nausea, sedation, dry mouth and sweating the most common side effects. The mean oral availability of tramadol is 68%, with peak plasma concentrations achieved by 1.5–2 hours. It is extensively metabolised by the liver and the elimination half-life is about 5–6 hours. Tramadol, like pethidine and phenoperidine, should not be given to patients taking monoamine oxidase inhibitors (MAOIs).

NON-STEROIDAL ANTI-INFLAMMATORY ANALGESICS (NSAIDs)

Non-steroidal anti-inflammatory analgesics are a heterogeneous group of compounds with analgesic, anti-inflammatory and antipyretic properties. Many, e.g. phenylbutazone, have a high toxicity that restricts their use to the treatment of chronic inflammatory conditions, such as rheumatoid arthritis. Other less toxic compounds, e.g. paracetamol, diclofenac and ketorolac, are used for the treatment of postoperative pain. NSAIDs are weak organic acids (pK_a 3–5) that bind extensively to plasma albumin. An exception is paracetamol, which has a pK_a of 9.3 and negligible protein binding. Most are completely absorbed from the gastrointestinal tract and have high oral bioavailability. Because of their very high protein binding, NSAIDs can displace other drug, e.g. warfarin and phenytoin, from plasma proteins.

NSAIDs act by inhibition of cyclooxygenase (COX), the enzyme which catalyses the synthesis of prostaglandins and other endoperoxides, such as thromboxane and prostacyclin, from arachidonic acid (Figure 7.8). Prostaglandins are involved in many homeostatic processes and are important mediators of inflammation. A component of the analgesic action of NSAIDs is due to a central action by reduction of prostaglandin (PG) production within the CNS. This is the main action of paracetamol.

There are two distinct COX enzymes, COX-1 and COX-2. COX-1 is the constitutive form responsible for the production of prostaglandins involved in cellular 'housekeeping' functions, such as the regulation of vascular homeostasis. COX-2 is induced 20–80-fold by exposure to mediators of inflammation, such as cytokines and endotoxin, and is responsible for the production of prostanoids that mediate inflammation, pain and fever. It is, however, constitutively expressed in small amounts in gastric mucosa, and may be involved in renin production in the kidney.

Toxicity associated with NSAID therapy is largely due to inhibition of COX-1, whereas therapeutic benefit derives from inhibition of COX-2. Selective COX-2 inhibitors cause less gastric or renal toxicity than non-selective NSAIDs. Also, because only COX-1 is present in platelets, selective COX-2 inhibitors will have no effect on haemostasis. There is increasing evidence, however, that the physiological and

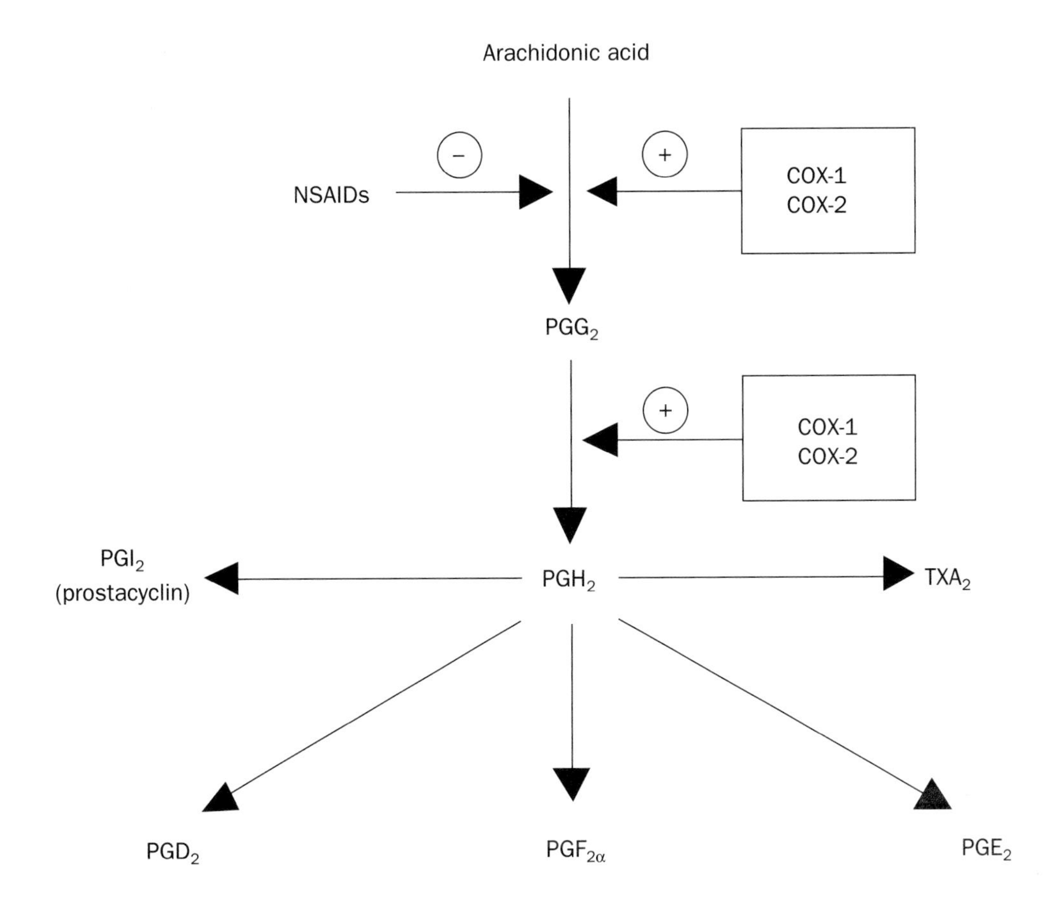

Figure 7.8 *Formation of prostaglandins (PG) from arachidonic acid.*

pathological activities of the two COX isoforms overlap to a considerable degree (Wallace 1999).

There are wide differences in the selectivity of conventional NSAIDs for the two isoforms (Table 7.2). Some, such as aspirin, indometacin and ibuprofen are more potent inhibitors of COX-1 than COX-2. Diclofenac, paracetamol and naproxen are equipotent inhibitors of both types. Several COX-2 selective drugs have been developed. Meloxicam is moderately selective for COX-2, while celecoxib, rofecoxib, etoricoxib and valdecoxib are highly COX-2 selective. These drugs are not available in a parenteral formulation. Parecoxib, a water-soluble COX-2-specific inhibitor that can be given intravenously or intramuscularly, is a prodrug that is rapidly hydrolysed to the active COX-2 inhibitor, valdecoxib. Valdecoxib has *in vitro* selectivity for COX-2 versus COX-1 90 times greater than celecoxib and 34 000 times greater than ketorolac. The COX-2 selective NSAIDs cause fewer gastrointestinal side effects and do not affect platelet function. Several studies have demonstrated that the COX-2 inhibitors, like their predecessors the non-selective NSAIDs, decrease postoperative pain and opioid requirements by 20–50%. The primary advantage of COX-2 inhibitors compared with non-selective NSAIDs for postoperative analgesia is their lack of effect on platelet function and bleeding. The renal effects of perioperative COX-2 inhibitors, particularly in populations susceptible to NSAID nephropathy (volume depletion, renal insufficiency, heart failure, diabetes) still needs to be considered when using these drugs.

Rofecoxib was withdrawn from the market worldwide in September 2004 by the pharmaceutical supplier because of a reported high

Table 7.2 Data, from various sources, on the selectivity of NSAIDs for inhibition of COX-1 versus COX-2. The ratios are based on measurements of IC_{50} values, so that the lower the ratio the greater the COX-2 selectivity

NSAID	*COX-2/COX-1 (selectivity ratio)*
COX-1 selective	
Piroxicam	250–600
Aspirin	166
Indometacin	60
Less COX-1 selective	
Paracetamol	7.5
Ibuprofen	0.6–3
Diclofenac	1.6–7.6
Naproxen	3–6
Ketorolac	1–10
COX-2 selective	
Meloxicam	0.5
Celecoxib	0.15
Rofecoxib	0.03–0.003
Etoricoxib	0.01
Valdecoxib	~0.03

incidence of adverse cardiovascular events such as myocardial infarctions and strokes in patients taking the drug.

Adverse effects

Gastrointestinal tract

A major limitation to the use of NSAIDs is gastrointestinal ulceration and bleeding, particularly in the stomach, due to suppression of protective gastric prostaglandins (PGs). NSAID-induced ulceration is often asymptomatic, the initial presentation frequently being severe haemorrhage or perforation. Conventional anti-ulcer therapy, such as antacids, histamine H_2-receptor antagonists, or proton pump inhibitors, are relatively ineffective in preventing NSAID-induced ulceration. The concomitant administration of the PGE_1 analogue, misoprostol, is more effective but is expensive and associated with an appreciable incidence of side effects, notably diarrhoea.

Renal adverse effects

Prostaglandins modulate renal blood flow and glomerular filtration rate, although they are not essential to maintaining renal function in the unstressed kidney. Renal dysfunction is uncommon in patients with normal kidneys but rarely can present as acute renal failure. In the presence of dehydration or hypovolaemia prostaglandins become essential for maintening renal perfusion, and NSAIDs will decrease renal blood flow and glomerular filtration rate. This is reversible if the drug is discontinued, but if not recognised can lead to permanent renal damage. NSAIDs can also cause acute renal insufficiency in patients with pre-existing renal disease.

While adverse renal effects have largely been attributed to inhibition of COX-1, it is now recognised that COX-2 has a physiological role in renal homeostasis. To date, there is no firm evidence for adverse renal effects in humans with the presently available COX-2 selective NSAIDs. However, the experience with these drugs is limited and caution is advised with their use in susceptible patients.

Hypersensitivity reactions

In susceptible individuals, NSAIDs may precipitate acute bronchospasm. It affects 10–20% of adults with asthma but is rare in asthmatic children. The mechanism is related to cyclooxygenase inhibition, with shunting of arachidonic acid metabolism from the prostaglandin pathway to the biosynthesis of leukotrienes with increased mucosal permeability and bronchospasm. Susceptible patients should avoid NSAIDs since the bronchospasm may be severe and has been fatal. Paracetamol in doses up to 1000 mg daily will be tolerated by most patients. True type I allergic reactions to NSAIDs, with specific IgE, are rare but anaphylоactoid reactions have occasionally been described in patients with a history of allergy or bronchial asthma.

INDIVIDUAL DRUGS

Aspirin

Aspirin (acetylsalicylic acid, Figure 7.9) is a derivative of salicyclic acid, which was first used in 1875 as an antipyretic and antirheumatic. The usual dose for mild pain is 300–600 mg orally. In the treatment of rheumatic diseases, larger doses, 5–8 g daily, are often required. Aspirin is rapidly hydrolysed in the plasma, liver and erythrocytes to salicylate, which is responsible for some, but not all, of the analgesic activity. Both aspirin and salicylate are excreted in the urine. Excretion is facilitated by alkalinisation of the urine. Metabolism is normally very rapid, but the liver enzymes responsible for metabolism are easily saturated and after multiple doses the terminal half-life may increase from the normal 2–3 h to 10 h. A soluble salt, lysine acetylsalicylic acid, with similar pharmacological properties to aspirin, has been used by parenteral administration for postoperative pain. Aspirin in low doses (80–160 mg daily) is widely used in patients with cardiovascular disease to reduce the incidence of myocardial infarction and strokes. The prophylaxis against thromboembolic disease by low-dose aspirin is due to inhibition of COX-1-generated thromboxane A_2 production. Because platelets do not form new enzymes, and COX-1 is irreversibly inhibited by aspirin, inhibition of platelet function lasts for the lifetime of a platelet (8–10 days).

Aspirin is the non-steroidal anti-inflammatory (NSAID) analgesic most commonly involved in adverse hypersensitivity reactions. With plasma concentrations over 350 $\mu g \cdot mL^{-1}$, such as occur with overdose, aspirin directly stimulates the respiratory centre, resulting in marked hyperventilation. Overdose is also associated with metabolic acidosis, particularly in infants and children, circulatory collapse and renal impairment.

Paracetamol

Paracetamol (Figure 7.9) has analgesic and antipyretic effects similar to those of aspirin, but has negligible anti-inflammatory activity. It is a weak COX inhibitor whose activity is mainly restricted to within the CNS. Paracetamol is widely used in the treatment of mild-to-moderate pain, and is incorporated as an ingredient of many proprietary compounds. The adult dose is 0.5–1 g orally. It is well absorbed from the gastrointestinal tract and does not cause gastric irritation. Indeed, side effects with paracetamol are uncommon with normal doses. Occasional haemolytic anaemia has been reported in patients with glucose-6-phosphate dehydrogenase deficiency.

Overdosage with paracetamol is extremely dangerous and potentially fatal, due to liver

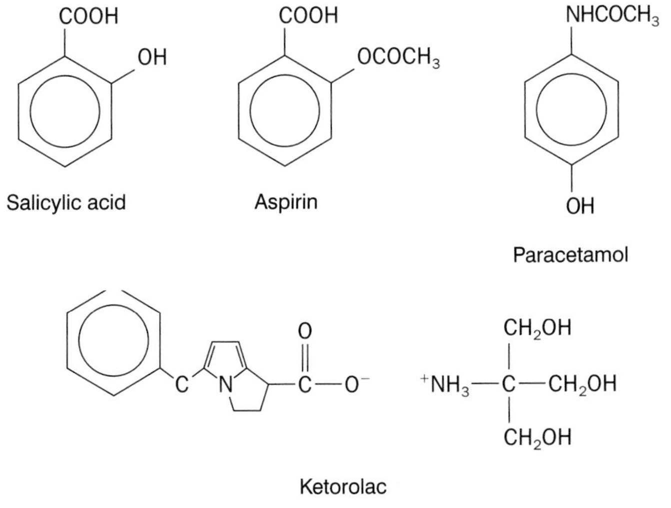

Salicylic acid

Aspirin

Paracetamol

Ketorolac

Figure 7.9 *Structures of some NSAIDs.*

damage. Renal damage also occurs. When the liver enzymes responsible for the conjugation reactions (Figure 7.10) become saturated P-450-mediated oxidation to the toxic metabolite *N*-acetyl-*p*-benzoquinone predominates. This metabolite is normally excreted as the harmless glutathione conjugate. When glutathione reserves become depleted, the metabolite accumulates and reacts with cellular proteins to cause hepatic and renal necrosis. The initial symptoms of overdose are nausea and vomiting, and signs of hepatotoxicity may be delayed for 24–48 hours. The treatment of paracetamol poisoning involves gastric lavage followed by oral activated charcoal and agents that increase glutathione formation (acetylcysteine intravenously or methionine orally). These agents are usually only effective if given within 12 hours of the ingestion of paracetamol.

Propacetamol, the soluble diethylglycidyl ester of paracetamol, is a prodrug which is completely and rapidly hydrolysed by non-specific plasma esterases to paracetamol, and is available for intravenous use. One gram IV propacetamol yields 0.5 g paracetamol. Propacetamol has similar analgesic efficacy to ketorolac for the treatment of postoperative pain (Varrassi and co-workers 1999).

Diclofenac

Diclofenac, a derivative of phenylacetic acid, is equipotent as an inhibitor of COX-1 and COX-2. In addition to prostaglandin inhibition a central analgesic action of diclofenac mediated by endogenous opioid peptides has been demonstrated. It can be administered orally, intramuscularly or intravenously, and is effective as a postoperative analgesic in a dose of 75–150 mg. The risks of adverse gastrointestinal effects is moderate and diclofenac does not appear to increase blood loss during or after surgery.

Ketorolac tromethamine (trometamol)

Ketorolac, which appears to have a greater analgesic than anti-inflammatory or antipyretic activity, is widely used to treat postoperative as well as chronic pain. The tromethamine salt possesses sufficient water solubility to allow for parenteral administration. When administered orally or intramuscularly, ketorolac is rapidly and well absorbed, with peak plasma concentrations attained between 30 min and 50 min. In doses of 10–30 mg intramuscularly it is

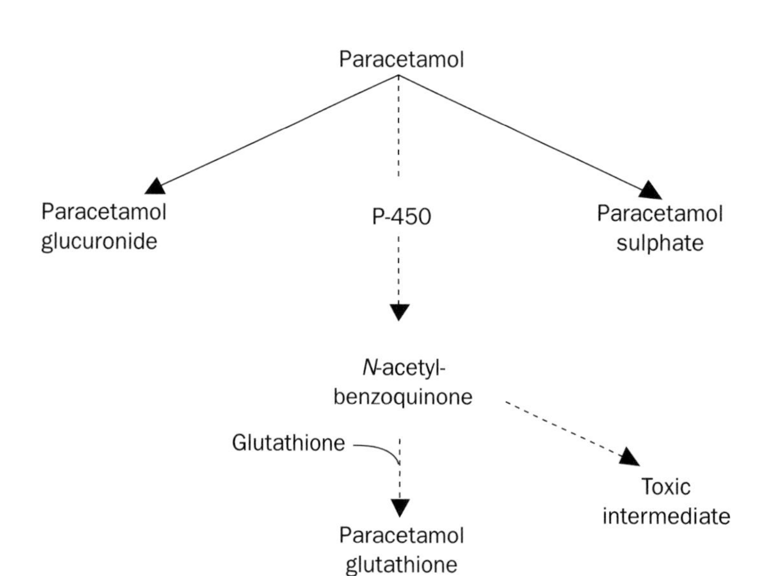

Figure 7.10 *Metabolism of paracetamol. With therapeutic doses, paracetamol is metabolised to the glucuronide and sulphate conjugates. With higher doses these pathways become saturated and metabolism proceeds via the P-450-mediated route, with the formation of the toxic metabolite benzoquinone. This is normally metabolised by conjugation with glutathione. When glutathione is depleted benzoquinone is free to interact with cellular macromolecules, leading to cellular damage.*

reported to be comparable or superior to morphine or pethidine in patients with moderate or severe pain after surgery. Ketorolac undergoes negligible hepatic first pass metabolism, and the oral bioavailability is 80–90%. There is relatively little transfer across the placenta or the blood–brain barrier. The usual precaution, applicable to all NSAIDs, should be observed when using ketorolac in the peri-operative setting. Current evidence is that the incidence of adverse effects with ketorolac is similar to that of other NSAIDs.

FURTHER READING

Bartkowski RR, McDonnell TE. Prolonged alfentanil effect following erythromycin administration. *Anesthesiology* 1990;73:566–8.

Bates JJ, Foss JF, Murphy DB. Are peripheral opioid antagonists the solution to opioid side effects? *Anesth Analg* 2004;98:116–22.

Darland T, Grandy DK. The orphanin/FQ system: an emerging target for the management of pain. *Br J Anaesth* 1998;81:29–37.

Keiffer BL. Opioids: first lessons from knockout mice. *Trends Pharmacol Sci* 1999;20:19–26.

Kurz A, Sessler DI. Opioid-induced bowel dysfunction: pathophysiology and potential new therapies. *Drugs* 2003;63:649–71.

Rossi GC, Brown GP, Leventhal L, et al. Novel receptor mechanisms for heroin and morphine-6β-glucuronide analgesia. *Neurosci Lett* 1996;216:1–4.

Varrassi G, et al. A double-blinded evaluation of propacetamol versus ketorolac in combination with patient-controlled analgesia morphine: analgesic efficacy and tolerability after gynecologic surgery. *Anesth Analg* 1999;88:611–16.

Wallace JL. Selective COX-2 inhibitors: is the water becoming muddy? *Trends Pharmacol Sci* 1999;20:4–6.

8

Cardiovascular drugs

Harry B van Wezel and Martin Pfaffendorf

Antihypertensive drugs • Anti-ischaemic therapy • Inotropic agents • Anti-arrhythmic drugs

Cardiovascular drugs can be considered under four categories: antihypertensive, anti-ischaemic, inotropic and anti-arrhythmic.

ANTIHYPERTENSIVE DRUGS

α-Adrenoceptor antagonists

Alpha-adrenoceptor antagonists inhibit the activation of α adrenoceptors by catecholamines. In the cardiovascular system these receptors are mainly located on the surface of smooth muscle cells in the walls of arteries and veins. On activation, they mediate an increase in intracellular free calcium, which induces smooth muscle contraction. Inhibition by an α antagonist causes arterial or venous vasodilatation. The postsynaptic effect is mainly mediated by α_1 adrenoceptors whereas α_2 adrenoceptors are found on the presynaptic membranes of the sympathetic neurones. Activation of α_2-adrenoceptors results in auto-inhibition of catecholamine release.

Indications

Alpha-adrenoceptor antagonists are used as antihypertensives and to reduce afterload in the treatment of heart failure. Urapidil and, to a lesser extent, ketanserin are used in the treatment of essential hypertension and acute perioperative hypertension. In contrast to other vasodilators urapidil does not increase intracranial pressure when given intravenously, making it preferable for use in neurosurgical interventions. The effects of the excessive catecholamine concentrations in patients with phaeochromocytoma can be treated by the non-selective α_1- and α_2-adrenoceptor antagonists phentolamine or phenoxybenzamine.

Contraindications

Alpha-antagonists are generally contraindicated in obstructive valvular heart disease and hepatic failure. Ketanserin should not be given to patients with AV-conduction disturbances, bradycardia or syndromes with a prolonged QT interval.

Side effects

The main adverse effects are orthostatic hypotension and reflex tachycardia due to the rapid vasodilatation. These often result in headaches and flushes. Other side effects include gastrointestinal upsets and polyuria. Ketanserin may cause dizziness, sedation, and tiredness and may inhibit serotonin-dependent platelet aggregation.

Interactions

Ketanserin should not be combined with drugs that prolong the QT interval, e.g. class Ia anti-arrhythmics, amiodarone, sotalol, erythromycin. The risk of *torsade de pointes* secondary to hypokalaemia is increased when ketanserin is combined with thiazides or loop diuretics without concomitant use of a potassium-sparing diuretic or an angiotensin-converting enzyme (ACE) inhibitor.

α_1 Antagonists

Prazosin and *doxazosin* are selective α_1 blockers with similar properties. They are competitive antagonists that can be displaced from the α_1 receptor by increases in catecholamine concentrations. This makes them unsuitable for use in the peri-operative management of phaeochromocytoma.

Urapidil is an agonist at both central α_2 and serotoninergic 5-HT_{1A} receptors, and also has antagonist actions at cardiac β_1 adrenoceptors.

Ketanserin has a complex pattern of action. It is an antagonist of 5-HT_2 receptors and peripheral α_1 adrenoceptors. Although both effects might contribute to a blood pressure lowering effect, it is likely that there is also an additional central component involved.

Non-selective α-adrenoceptor antagonists, such as *phentolamine* and *phenoxybenzamine* induce tachycardia and are not suitable for the long-term management of hypertension. This is due to their non-selective antagonism of postsynaptic α_1 receptors (which then respond less actively to noradrenaline (norepinephrine)) and presynaptic α_2 receptors that inhibit but cannot stop the release of noradrenaline. The action of noradrenaline on postsynaptic α_1 receptors is thus exaggerated, producing an increase in heart rate. In contrast, *prazosin* and *doxazosin* act selectively and do not facilitate the release of endogenous catecholamine from sympathetic nerve endings. As a result, they have a better antihypertensive action and do not cause reflex tachycardia.

Angiotensin-converting enzyme (ACE) inhibitors

The renin-angiotensin-aldosterone system is an important regulator of arterial blood pressure as well as fluid and electrolyte homeostasis. The juxtaglomerular cells in the kidney are sodium sensors that secrete the protease, renin, when the sodium content in the urine is elevated, or when renal blood flow is decreased. Renin binds with its substrate, angiotensinogen, to produce the decapeptide angiotensin I (Figure 8.1). Angiotensin I has no physiological action but acts as a substrate for angiotensin I-converting enzyme (ACE). ACE cleaves the carboxyterminal amino acids of angiotensin I to form the octapeptide, angiotensin II, the main effector of the renin-angiotensin-aldosterone system. Angiotensin II stimulates the release of aldosterone from the zona glomerulosa of the adrenal cortex. It is also a powerful vasoconstrictor and stimulates the sympathetic nervous system. A reduction of renin-angiotensin-aldosterone activity is therapeutically beneficial in patients with hypertension, heart failure or renal artery stenosis.

Inhibition of ACE inhibits the synthesis of angiotensin II. This results in vasodilatation and a lesser tendency for sodium and water reabsorption due to the reduction in aldosterone. Angiotensin II is a mediator of trophic processes responsible for cardiac and vascular hypertrophy seen in heart failure or hypertension. This can be reversed by ACE inhibition.

In addition to angiotensin I, ACE acts on other substrates, including bradykinin. In contrast to angiotensin II, which is formed by ACE, bradykinin is degraded and inactivated by this enzyme. ACE inhibition therefore leads to accumulation of bradykinin. Some bradykinin actions, like vasodilatation, actually contribute to the therapeutic effect of ACE inhibitors. Others, such as increased capillary permeability, are responsible for some of their adverse effects.

With the exception of *captopril* and *lisinopril*, all ACE inhibitors are prodrugs which have to be activated metabolically after absorption from the gut. Although there are differences in the

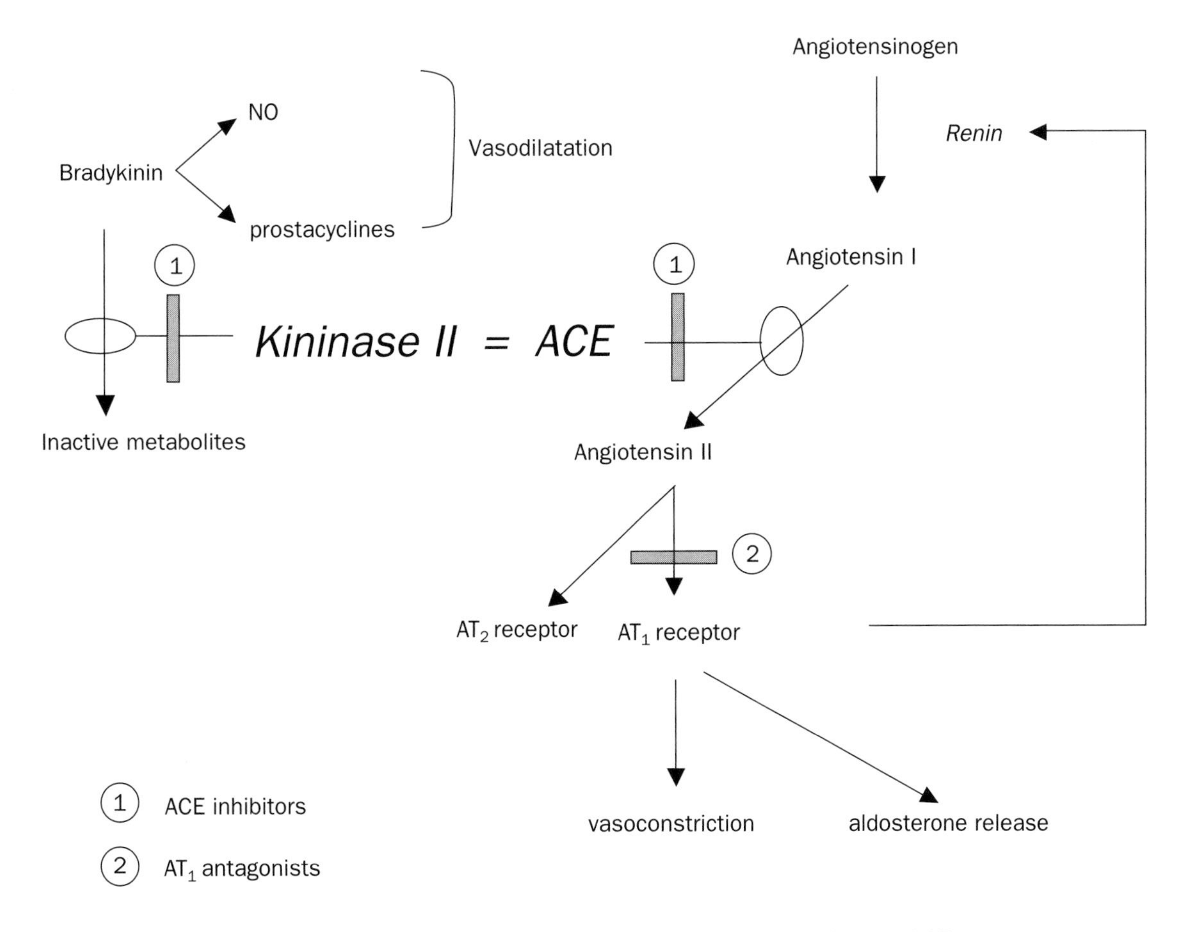

Figure 8.1 *Mechanism of action of angiotensin-converting enzyme (ACE) inhibitors and AT_1-receptor antagonists.*

affinity for the enzyme, all the available compounds share the same mechanism of action which results in qualitatively identical effects. There are differences, however, in the kinetic properties of the different drugs, such as absorption, bioavailability, distribution, route of elimination, and duration of action. *Perinopril* and *quinapril* have a very high affinity for ACE. Consequently, although both drugs have relatively short plasma half-lives their duration of action can extend to 24 hours. ACE inhibitors are contraindicated in patients with bilateral renal artery stenosis since the reduction in renal perfusion leads to renal failure, and throughout pregnancy. The oral doses of ACE inhibitors are given in Table 8.1. The active form of enalapril, *enalaprilate*, can be given intravenously. The dose for rapid control of therapy-resistant hypertension is 0.625–1.26 mg given over 5 minutes.

Side effects

Many patients experience a dry cough, especially when beginning treatment. This may be due to the accumulation of bradykinin in the bronchial mucosa. Less frequent are angioedema, xanthelasma and bone marrow suppression.

Interactions

In combination with potassium-sparing diuretics severe hyperkalaemia may occur. The elimination of lithium is prolonged. Non-steroidal anti-inflammatory drugs (NSAIDs) may reduce the antihypertensive effect of ACE inhibitors.

Table 8.1 Pharmacokinetic details of angiotensin-converting enzyme (ACE) inhibitors used for treatment of hypertension

	Absorption	*Daily dose (mg)*	*Elimination half-life (h)*	*Elimination path*
Captopril	75%	25–50	<3	Kidney
Enalapril	60–70%	5–10	11	Kidney
Fosinopril	36%	10–40	11.5	Kidney (16%) Liver (84%)
Lisinopril	25%	10–20	12.6	Kidney
Perindopril	80%	4–8	3–5	Kidney
Quinapril	60%	5–40	1	Kidney
Ramipril	50–60%	2.5–10	13–17	Kidney
Trandolapril	40–60%	2–4	16–24	Kidney

Angiotensin II (AT_1) antagonists

Blockade of angiotensin II can be achieved at the receptor level (Figure 8.1). There are two principal classes of angiotensin II receptors, referred to by confusing terminology as AT_1 and AT_2. Most of the cardiovascular actions of angiotensin II, including aldosterone release, are mediated by the AT_1 receptor. Non-peptide AT_1-receptor antagonists, which can be taken orally, have been introduced for the treatment of similar conditions as ACE inhibitors. These drugs are more specific for the renin-aldosterone system than ACE inhibitors since they are devoid of any interaction with bradykinin metabolism. This mainly affects the unwanted side effects of ACE inhibitors, such as angioedema, and possibly the dry cough.

Losartan was the first AT_1 antagonist to be used clinically. It has a complicated effect, since its major metabolite (E-3174) is about ten times more potent as an inhibitor of angiotensin II than losartan itself. *Candesartan cilexetil* is the only compound in this group which is a real prodrug. It is hydrolysed by the liver to the active form, candesartan. Differences between drugs in this class are largely accounted for by their pharmacokinetic properties (Table 8.2).

Table 8.2 Pharmacokinetic details of angiotensin-1 (AT_1) antagonists

	Absorption	*Daily dose (mg)*	*Elimination half-life (h)*	*Elimination path*
Candesartan	14%	8–16	9	Liver, Kidney
Eprosartan	13%	600–800	5–9	Liver, Kidney
Irbesartan	Good	150–300	11–15	Kidney (20%) Liver (80%)
Losartan	Good	50–100	6–9	Kidney (40%) Liver (60%)
Valsartan	23%	80–160	9	Kidney (17%) Liver (83%)

Contraindications

Hepatic failure.

Side effects

Among the rare side effects are dizziness, hypokalaemia and hypotension.

Calcium channel-entry blockers

The excitation contraction coupling in cardiomyocytes and vascular smooth muscle cells is the result of changes in membrane permeability for calcium. The influx of Ca^{2+}, the primary event for initialising contraction, is through calcium channel proteins in the cell membranes. Several types have been identified, including T-, N- and L-type calcium channels. The conformation of these channels is voltage-dependent. Membrane depolarisation opens the channels, allowing calcium influx and consequently contraction. The L-type calcium channel is the most abundant on vascular smooth muscle and cardiomyocytes. It is the activity of this channel which mainly governs vascular tone and peripheral resistance. Although skeletal muscle has abundant L-type calcium channels, it does not depend on calcium influx for contractile activity. This allows L-type calcium channel-entry blockers to be useful drugs in cardiovascular therapy. L-type calcium channel-entry blockade reduces peripheral resistance and thereby the cardiac afterload. This makes calcium-entry blockers useful in the treatment of essential hypertension.

There are three major groups of calcium channel-entry blockers: the dihydropyridines (prototype *nifedipine*), the phenylalkylamines (prototype *verapamil*) and the benzothiazepines (prototype *diltiazem*). The dihydropyridines are the largest group. They reduce peripheral resistance and cardiac afterload without affecting cardiac function directly. The first-generation drugs had a rapid onset of action that resulted in reflex tachycardia. Newer drugs have a slow onset of action, either as a result of an intrinsic property of the molecule, or through the use of 'retard' formulations. The main site of action of the phenylalkylamines is on the heart. Verapamil is typical in having effects on atrioventricular conduction, heart rate and, at higher doses, myocardial contractility. It is widely used in the treatment of cardiac arrhythmias, especially supraventricular tachycardia. Diltiazem is the only member of the benzothiazepines group that is in general clinical use. Pharmacokinetic details of the calcium channel-entry blockers are shown in Table 8.3.

Nifedipine

Nifedipine has a rapid onset of action and a short elimination half-life. A slow-release formulation allows a single daily dose to be prescribed and prevents reflex tachycardia. Newer, second- and third-generation dihydropyridines, have a slower onset and a longer elimination half-life. This makes special pharmaceutical formulations unnecessary.

Due to its light sensitivity, special precautions have to be taken when nifedipine, like other dihydropyridines, is administered parenterally. Of the members of this group, *amlodipine*, *barnidipine*, *felodipine*, *isradipine*, *lacidipine*, *lercanidipine*, *manidipine*, *nicardipine*, *nifedipine*, *nimodipine*, *nisoldipine* and *nitrendipine* are most commonly used in the therapy of essential hypertension and angina pectoris. For the latter indication they are often combined with a β-adrenoceptor antagonist. In addition to producing natriuresis, which is common with all dihydropyridines, various additional effects have been claimed for individual compounds. These include coronary selectivity (nisoldipine), renal selectivity (manidipine), cerebrovascular selectivity (nimodipine), free radical scavenging properties (lacidipine) and anti-atherogenic properties (isradipine, lacidipine). There is, however, little clinical evidence that any one dihydropyridine is superior in the treatment of essential hypertension. Nimodipine is used for various neurological disorders, such as migraine, stroke, and subarachnoid haemorrhage.

Verapamil

Verapamil does not induce reflex tachycardia. However, its short elimination half-life requires thrice-daily dosing. A slow-release formulation

Table 8.3 Pharmacokinetic details of the calcium channel antagonists

	Absorption	*Daily dose*	*Elimination half-life (h)*	*Elimination path*
Dihydropyridines				
Amlodipine	60–65%	5–10 mg	35–50	Kidney (60%) Liver (40%)
Nicardipine	10–35%	20–40 mg tid IV 0.05–0.25 mg·min^{-1}	1–12	Kidney (60%) Liver (40%)
Nifedipine Retard	50%	30–120 mg	6–12	Kidney (75%) Liver (25%)
Nimodipine	13%	10–20 mg tid (migraine)	3	Liver, Kidney
Phenylalkylamines				
Verapamil Retard	20–25%	120–240 mg	4–12	Kidney (70%) Liver (30%)
Benzothiazepines				
Diltiazem Retard	35–40%	180–360 mg	3–6	Kidney (35%) Liver (65%)

tid, 3 times a day; IV, intravenous.

is available for once-daily dosing. The main indications for verapamil are essential hypertension, angina pectoris and cardiac arrhythmias. Verapamil is a class IV anti-arrhythmic in the Vaughan-Williams classification. It slows atrioventricular conduction, and is used in the therapy of supraventricular tachyarrhythmias. The intravenous dose is 5–10 mg as a slow bolus (< 5 mg·min^{-1}). The negative inotropic action of the phenylalkylamines can precipitate cardiac failure in susceptible patients. When combined with a β-adrenoceptor antagonist there is a risk of atrioventricular block and additive negative inotropy.

Diltiazem

Although its pharmacological effects are similar to those of verapamil, diltiazem is almost exclusively used in the treatment of angina pectoris. It has a short elimination half-life that requires thrice-daily oral dosing. Diltiazem is well tolerated especially by elderly patients.

Side effects

Headache, flush, dizziness, hypotension, ankle oedema (mostly dihydropyridines), bradycardia, and impaired atrioventricular conduction (verapamil and, to a lesser extent, diltiazem), constipation (verapamil), heart failure (verapamil, rare), oesophageal reflux.

Interactions

Cardiac depressant effects may occur when verapamil or diltiazem is combined with a β-adrenoceptor antagonoist or a cardiac glycoside. Nifedipine and verapamil are metabolised by cytochrome P-450 3A4. Inhibitors of this enzyme, e.g. HIV-protease inhibitors, cimetidine, fluoxetine, ketoconazole, erythromycin, will increase plasma levels and the dose should be carefully monitored. Conversely, enzyme inducers, e.g. carbamazepine, rifampicin, phenytoin, will decrease their plasma concentrations.

ANTI-ISCHAEMIC THERAPY

Traditional long-term anti-ischaemic triple therapy for coronary artery disease consists of a long-acting nitrate, β-adrenoceptor antagonist and a calcium-entry blocker. Most of these agents are also used for the treatment of hypertension.

The nitrovasodilators

Sodium nitroprusside (SNP) and the organic nitrates are donors of nitric oxide (NO) (Figure 8.2). Their mode of action is not fully understood, but the nitrates appear to act through *S*-nitrosothiols, resulting in increased concentrations of NO and cyclic guanidine monophosphate in vascular smooth muscle. SNP can generate NO directly without any interaction with the thiol groups. Molsidomine and nicorandil are potassium channel activators which have a nitrate component. They are used in the treatment of angina pectoris and may be more tolerance resistant than the organic nitrates.

Sodium nitroprusside (SNP)

The SNP molecule consists of a ferrous core surrounded by five cyanide groups and a nitrosyl group (Figure 8.2). SNP solutions can be inactivated by trace contaminants. Products of these reactions are toxic, and are often blue,

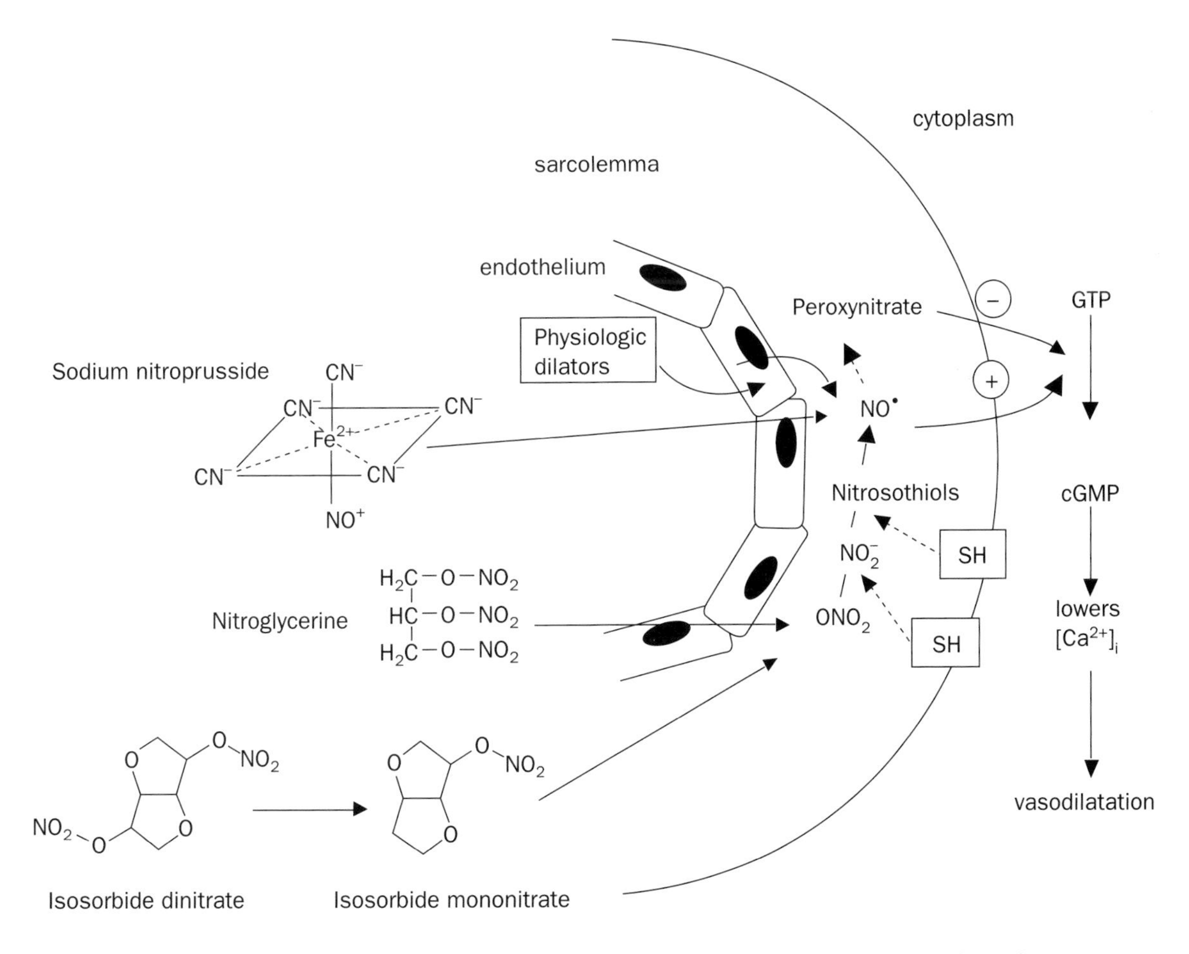

Figure 8.2 *Proposed mode of action of the organic nitrates, nitroglycerin and nitroprusside. Note that nitroprusside acts as a direct donor of nitric oxide (NO), whereas the nitrates require the presence of nitrosothiols to produce NO.*

green or red, and much brighter than the faint brownish colour of nitroprusside. Discoloured solutions should never be used. The solution should be freshly prepared and protected from light. When exposed to light SNP is hydrolysed to cyanide. SNP reacts with oxyhaemoglobin to form methaemoglobin with the release of the cyanide ions and NO. Infusion rates greater than 2 $\mu g \cdot kg^{-1} \cdot min^{-1}$ generate cyanide ions faster than the body can eliminate them, with the risk of cyanide toxicity. Relatively large quantities of SNP are required, however, to produce clinically significant methaemoglobinaemia.

In contrast to the organic nitrates, which require the presence of highly specific thiol compounds to generate NO, SNP can produce NO spontaneously, thus functioning as a direct prodrug. It causes venous and arterial vasodilatation, resulting in a reduction in blood pressure and pulmonary filling pressures, increased cardiac output, and (reflex) tachycardia. In the absence of atherosclerosis, blood flow to all organs is well maintained. However, SNP, but not the organic nitrates, may produce intracoronary shunting at therapeutic doses in patients with coronary artery disease. Because SNP is rapidly converted to thiocyanate, and its half-life is only a few minutes, it must be given by intravenous infusion. Because thiocyanate is only cleared slowly, prolonged use (> 72 h) can lead to accumulation and thiocyanate toxicity, with muscle weakness, nausea and inhibition of thyroid function.

Indications

Severe acute heart failure, hypertensive crisis, controlled hypotension during anaesthesia and severe peri-operative hypertension.

Side effects

Cyanide toxicity, overshoot hypotension, and myocardial ischaemia. Hypoxia caused by increased ventilation–perfusion mismatch due to pulmonary vasodilatation and inhibition of hypoxic pulmonary vasoconstriction. Rebound hypertension after discontinuation of SNP infusion.

Dose

Infusion rate: 0.5–2 $\mu g \cdot kg^{-1} \cdot min^{-1}$.

Organic nitrates

Glyceryl trinitrate (nitroglycerine)

This is widely used in tablet, transdermal and aerosol preparations. Its major haemodynamic effect is venous dilatation; arteriolar vasodilatation only occurs at high doses. It is also available for intravenous administration. Nitroglycerine is absorbed by polyvinyl chloride, and infusion sets made with this plastic should not be used. It is not absorbed by glass or polyethylene.

Indications

Angina pectoris, hypertension, congestive heart failure, acute myocardial ischaemia, acute pulmonary oedema, unstable coronary syndromes especially when associated with elevated filling pressures. Nitrate therapy may exaggerate outflow obstruction in hypertrophic obstructive cardiomyopathy.

Dose

Intravenous: 0.5–10 $\mu g \cdot kg^{-1} \cdot min^{-1}$.
Oral: sublingual tablets or spray, 0.4 mg for acute chest pain. Sustained-release patches give 0.4–0.8 $mg \cdot h^{-1}$.

Isosorbide

Isosorbide is available in two forms, isosorbide dinitrate (ISDN) and isosorbide mononitrate (ISDM). ISDN is rapidly metabolised in the liver to the active mononitrate. ISDM is only available in oral form. An intravenous formulation of ISDN is available, but is only used for the treatment of acute heart failure.

Newer anti-anginal agents

Molsidomine is a prodrug that is converted in the liver to metabolites which have a vasodilatory action similar to the organic nitrates. The hepatic conversion results in the release of NO. Molsidomine has been in clinical use in Europe and Japan for several years, but is not available in the UK at present (May 2002).

Nicorandil is a potent vasodilator with anti-spasmodic properties. Its cardiovascular effects are mainly characterised by dilatation of large coronary arteries in combination with reduction of preload and afterload. It has a dual mode of action, activating ATP-dependent K^+ channels and a nitrate-like effect.

β-Adrenoceptor antagonists

Beta-adrenoceptor antagonists (often referred to as β blockers) play an important role in the management of ischaemic heart disease, hypertension, arrhythmias and congestive heart failure. Two types of β adrenoceptor, β_1 and β_2, are located in cardiac sarcolemma (mostly β_1, some β_2) and bronchial and vascular smooth muscle tissue (β_2). Stimulation of β_1 receptors increase the synthesis of cyclic AMP from ATP. This leads to activation of protein kinase A, and the opening of calcium channels. The resulting Ca^{2+} influx results in positive inotropy, tachycardia, and positive dromotropy. Stimulation of β_2 adrenoceptors in bronchial and vascular smooth muscle causes bronchoconstriction and arteriolar vasoconstriction. Activation of myocardial β_2 adrenoceptors leads to activation of both stimulatory and inhibitory G proteins. This dual response may be associated with a cardioprotective (possibly anti-apoptotic) effect during myocardial ischaemia and adrenergic catecholamine stimulation. This may at least partly explain the beneficial effect of carvedilol (a combined β_1- and β_2-adrenoceptor antagonist) in patients with congestive heart failure.

Beta-adrenoceptor antagonists reduce heart rate, myocardial contractile state and cardiac output. They also produce a decrease in vascular tone (and arterial blood pressure) through decreased release of noradrenaline (norepinephrine) at vascular adrenergic nerve endings. Some β adrenoceptor antagonists are partial agonists with intrinsic sympathomimetic activity. They cause less resting bradycardia and less reduction in cardiac output. The non-cardiovascular side effects of β antagonists are primarily related to β_2 blockade. These include bronchoconstriction, cold feet and hands, sleeping disorders, dreams, fatigue and depression.

Indications

Beta-adrenoceptor antagonists are used to treat hypertension, angina pectoris, arrhythmias and secondary myocardial infarct prevention following primary infarction (timolol, metoprolol and propranolol).

Contraindications

Sick sinus syndrome, second- and third-degree AV block, hypotension, cardiogenic shock, bronchospastic pulmonary disease.

Interactions

Volatile anaesthetics, calcium channel-entry blockers, and some anti-arrhythmic drugs may potentiate the negative inotropic effect of the β-adrenoceptor antagonists. Concomitant digoxin therapy may cause AV dissociation. Potentiation of the hypoglycaemic effects of insulin and oral antidiabetic drugs may occur.

Table 8.4 summarises the currently available β-adrenoceptor antagonists, their relative β_1 selectivity, intrinsic sympathomimetic activity, and the availability of intravenous formulations.

Esmolol

Esmolol is an ultra-short-acting relatively β_1-selective β-adrenoceptor antagonist with an elimination half-life of about 9 min. After intravenous administration it is rapidly hydrolysed by non-specific esterases in the blood and tissues to a carboxylic acid metabolite. Following an intravenous infusion its haemodynamic effects are short lasting and disappear within 20–30 min. The main indication in the perioperative period is to treat tachycardia.

Labetalol

Labetalol is a non-selective β_1-, β_2- and α_1-adrenoceptor antagonist. The α_1-blocking properties (which are substantially weaker than the β-blocking activity) are largely responsible for its vasodilatory effect. Labetalol is used orally in patients with phaeochromocytoma. During

Table 8.4 Details of currently available β adrenoceptor antagonists, their relative degree of β_1 selectivity, the absence or presence of intrinsic sympathomimetic activity, and the availability of intravenous formulations

Generic name	*β_1 selectivity*	*ISA*	*Intravenous dose*
Acebutolol	$\beta_1 > \beta_2$	+	–
Atenolol	$\beta_1 >> \beta_2$	–	5 mg over 5 min; repeat 5 min later
Betaxolol	$\beta_1 >> \beta_2$	–	–
Bisoprolol	$\beta_1 >>> \beta_2$	–	–
Carvedilol	$\beta_1 = \beta_2 >> \alpha_1$	–	–
Celiprolol	$\beta_1 >> \beta_2$	+	–
Esmolol	$\beta_1 > \beta_2$	–	Initial dose: 500 $\mu g \cdot kg^{-1}$ over 2–4 min; maintenance: 50 $\mu g \cdot kg^{-1} \cdot min^{-1}$, maximum rate 300 $\mu g \cdot kg^{-1} \cdot min^{-1}$
Labetalol	$\beta_1 = \beta_2 > \alpha_1$	–	Bolus injections 0.5–2 $mg \cdot kg^{-1}$; maximum infusion 300 mg
Metoprolol	$\beta_1 >> \beta_2$	–	5 mg up to three times at 2 min intervals
Pindolol	$\beta_1 = \beta_2$	+++	
Propranolol	$\beta_1 = \beta_2$	–	1–6 mg
Sotalol	$\beta_1 = \beta_2$	–	–
Tertatolol	$\beta_1 = \beta_2$, + renal vasodilatation		–

ISA, intrinsic sympathomimetic activity.

anaesthesia it is used to induce controlled hypotension. It is also used for controlling hypertension in patients with pre-eclampsia, and during surgery for phaeochromocytoma.

INOTROPIC AGENTS

Digoxin remains the mainstay of treatment for patients with chronic myocardial failure. Other drugs with inotropic and/or vasodilator properties, including the catecholamines and phosphodiesterase III (PDE) inhibitors, are used in the treatment of acute cardiac failure. The inotropic actions of most of these drugs result from a direct or indirect elevation of $[Ca^{2+}]_i$ (intracellular Ca^{2+} concentration). This acts as a trigger for a process which leads to increased contractile state and cardiac contraction (Figures 8.3 and 8.4). Myofilament calcium sensitisers increase the sensitivity of contractile proteins to calcium. Some newer drugs, such as vesnarinone, have multiple mechanisms of action.

Cardiac glycosides

Digitalis glycosides are naturally occurring substances found in a variety of plants including foxglove. The best-known cardiac glycosides are digoxin (from *digitalis lanata*) and digitoxin (from *digitalis purpurea*). The glycosides produce only modest increases in myocardial contractility compared to the catecholamines and phosphodiesterase inhibitors.

Their mechanism of action is by inhibition of the Na^+/K^+ pump system and Na^+/K^+ ATPase,

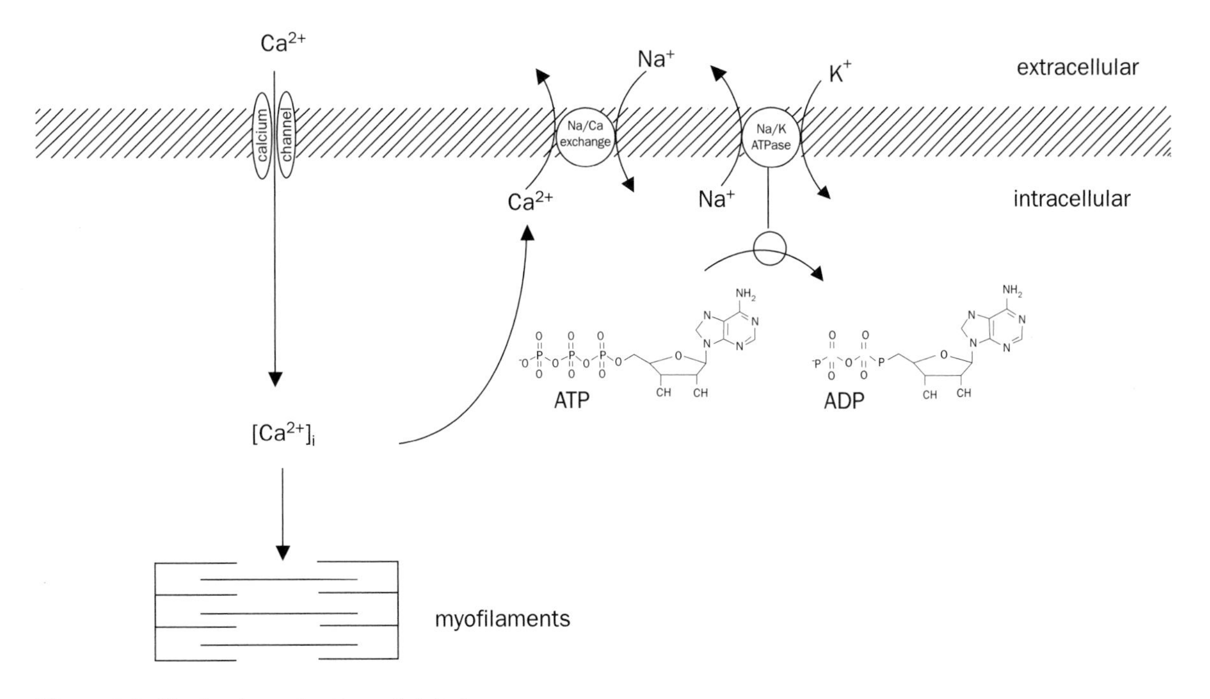

Figure 8.3 *Mechanism of action of digitalis.*

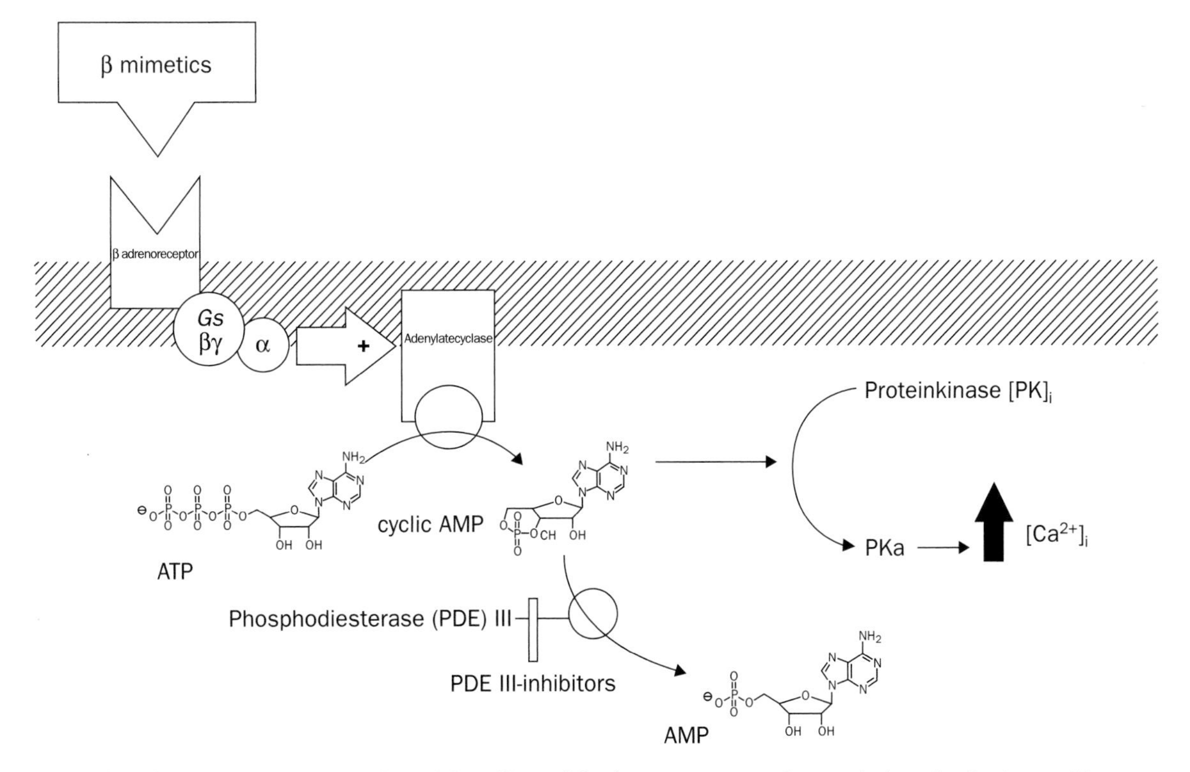

Figure 8.4 *Schematic representation of the effect of β-adrenoceptor agonists and phosphodiesterase III inhibitors.*

producing a transient increase in intracellular Na^+. This slows the removal of Ca^{2+} with an increase in the availability of intracellular Ca^{2+} during systole, thereby increasing myocardial contractility (Figure 8.3). They also have an inhibitory effect on SA and AV nodal conduction due to parasympathetic activation and mild direct depression of nodal activity. Digoxin also has an inhibitory effect on the adrenergic system, which is especially important in patients with chronic heart failure and elevated catecholamine levels. Finally, renin release is reduced because of inhibition of the renal Na^+ pump. This is associated with a natriuretic effect and mild peripheral vasodilatation.

Digoxin

The haemodynamic effects of digoxin are characterised by increased contractility, reduced heart rate and slowed atrioventricular conduction.

Indications

Congestive heart failure and arrhythmias associated with a rapid ventricular response.

Dose

Oral: loading dose: 0.75–1.25 mg; maintenance: 0.125–0.5 mg·day^{-1}.

Intravenous: loading: 0.5–1.0 mg (in a patient not previously receiving digoxin); maintenance: 0.25 mg·day^{-1}.

Side effects

Digoxin has a low therapeutic index and most side effects are related to overdose. They include headache, fatigue, malaise, confusion, anorexia, nausea, vomiting, diarrhoea and blurred vision. Cardiac side effects include a wide range of arrhythmias, especially ventricular extrasystoles, and heart block. Bradyarrhythmias can also occur. Hypokalaemia, hypercalcaemia, hypomagnesaemia and hypothyroidism increase digoxin toxicity. In patients at risk plasma concentrations should be closely monitored. A target value of 1 ng·mL^{-1} is widely advocated. In severe poisoning, digoxin can be neutralised by specific antibody fragments. These are raised in sheep and cleaved to remove the antigenic (F_c) portion of the molecule while retaining the specific antigen-binding fragment (F_{ab}).

Precautions

Concomitant use with sympathomimetic drugs, β-adrenoceptor antagonists, calcium channel-entry blockers and other cardioactive drugs may result in bradyarrhythmias, bigemini, or tachyarrhythmias. Cardiac rhythm should be closely monitored and drug dosages carefully adjusted. Digoxin is mainly excreted by the kidneys and plasma levels should be closely monitored in patients with acute renal failure and in those whose renal function is compromised.

Contraindications

Hypertrophic obstructive cardiomyopathy, Wolff-Parkinson-White (WPW) syndrome, atrioventricular block and constrictive pericarditis.

Ouabain

Ouabain is only available for intravenous administration. It has a rapid onset of action (5–10 min), which is its only advantage over digoxin. Other drugs, however, are generally preferred as the risk of toxicity is high. Its pharmacological profile is similar to that of digoxin.

Catecholamines

These are β-adrenergic agonists that act by stimulation of the enzyme, adenylyl cyclase, thereby increasing intracellular cAMP. This indirectly increases intracellular calcium, by induction of the active form of protein kinase followed by an influx of Ca^{2+} through open voltage-dependent Ca^{2+} channels (Figure 8.4).

Adrenaline (epinephrine)

Adrenaline is synthesised in the adrenal medulla and at sympathetic nerve endings from phenylalanine and metabolised by oxidation (monoamine oxidase; MAO) or conjugation (catechol *O*-methyl transferase; COMT). It is excreted in the urine as vanillylmandelic acid. Its main physiological effects are at β_1 and α adrenoceptors, with less marked effects at β_2

receptors. Its β_1 actions result in positive cardiac inotropy and chronotropy. It causes arteriolar vasodilatation in skeletal muscle and in the splanchnic circulation and constriction of vessels supplying skin and mucous membranes.

Indications

Adrenaline is used in cardiac resuscitation to convert asystole prior to defibrillation. It is also used in acute hypotensive emergencies and low cardiac output states, especially in severe sepsis or following extracorporeal circulation in cardiac surgery. In anaphylactic shock the combination of powerful α (vasoconstriction) and β_2 (bronchodilatation) effects may be life-saving (Appendix: AAGBI protocol). Adrenaline is also used to relieve bronchoconstriction in bronchial asthma and status asthmaticus.

Dose

Adrenaline may be administered intravenously via a central vein or intramuscularly. The subcutaneous route is generally unsatisfactory for a rapid effect since absorption is unreliable. The intravenous dose is 0.01–0.1 $\mu g \cdot kg^{-1} \cdot min^{-1}$ with β effects predominating in this range. At higher doses (> 0.2 $\mu g \cdot kg^{-1} \cdot min^{-1}$), such as may be used in severe sepsis, α_1 effects dominate and result in increased peripheral vascular resistance and raised systolic and diastolic blood pressure. ECG monitoring is essential during intravenous administration. The intramuscular dose for emergency treatment of anaphylaxis is 0.5–1 mg. The dose should be reduced in young children and the elderly.

Side effects

These result from over-stimulation of the sympathetic nervous system: anxiety, sweating, tachycardia, arrhythmia, hypertension, myocardial ischaemia, headache, cerebral haemorrhage, pulmonary oedema. Adrenaline may cause pupillary dilatation which must be distinguished from pupillary dilatation due to other causes, e.g. severe brain injury.

Precautions

There is a risk of inducing uterine contractions if adrenaline is used in late pregnancy. Increased oxygen demand resulting from increases in heart rate and myocardial contractility may outstrip the myocardial oxygen supply and predispose to ischaemia.

Interactions

When adrenaline is administered during halothane anaesthesia there is an increased risk of arrhythmia.

Noradrenaline (norepinephrine)

Noradrenaline is a neurotransmitter secreted by postganglionic neurones, the central nervous system, and by the adrenal medulla. It has powerful direct actions at α_1 and α_2 adrenoceptors. Its β_1 effects are similar to adrenaline but, unlike adrenaline, it has minimal β_2 effects.

Indications

Noradrenaline is used to treat shock-like conditions associated with peripheral vasodilatation, e.g. sepsis, systemic inflammatory response syndrome (SIRS), neurogenic shock. The rationale of its use in sepsis and SIRS is to counteract the vasodilatory effects of nitric oxide. Following the surgical removal of phaeochromocytoma and similar tumours, noradrenaline is often given to maintain blood pressure in the initial period. During and after cardiac surgery, it may be used to optimise haemodynamic parameters in combination with other drugs, such as phosphodiesterase inhibitors.

Dose

The drug is given into a central vein at a rate of 2–10 $\mu g \cdot min^{-1}$. Its effects are very transitory and disappear rapidly if the infusion stops. Infusions up to 0.05 $\mu g \cdot kg^{-1} \cdot min^{-1}$ increase myocardial contractility and heart rate as the result of β_1 stimulation. At doses of 0.1–0.3 $\mu g \cdot kg^{-1} \cdot min^{-1}$ vasoconstriction (α stimulation) accompanied by a reflex bradycardia predominates.

Side effects

Centrally mediated effects, such as anxiety, sweating, etc., seen with adrenaline do not occur as noradrenaline does not cross the blood–brain barrier. Skin pallor is commonly observed, due to arteriolar vasoconstriction.

Precautions

When used in high doses for long periods to treat life-threatening conditions, e.g. SIRS, it may result in peripheral ischaemia or even gangrene. Extravascular leakage my result in skin necrosis. If used in late pregnancy it may induce uterine contractions and/or reduce placental blood flow.

Isoprenaline

Isoprenaline stimulates β_1 and β_2 adrenoceptors (β_1>β_2) resulting in increased myocardial contractility and reduced peripheral vascular resistance. It does not act on α adrenoceptors. Cardiac output increases partly due to reduced afterload and an increase in heart rate. There is a diversion of blood to non-essential tissues, e.g. skeletal muscle and skin. Because of the decrease in peripheral vascular resistance arterial blood pressure and coronary perfusion pressure may decrease, which may predispose to myocardial ischaemia.

Indications

Isoprenaline occasionally has a place in the management of cardiac conditions in which bradycardia is a feature, e.g. low cardiac output associated with slow heart rate after extracorporeal circulation in patients with excessive β-blocking therapy. It may also be used in the treatment of overdose with β-adrenoceptor antagonists and for refractory bradyarrhythmias prior to cardiac pacing. Isoprenaline is used in the treatment of bronchial asthma on account of its β_2 effects.

Dose

By intravenous infusion into a central vein at 0.01–0.1 $\mu g{\cdot}kg^{-1}{\cdot}min^{-1}$. Patients with asthma may self-administer it by inhaler.

Side effects

Palpitations, angina, headache, tremor, flushed skin, sweating.

Contraindications

Myocardial ischaemia.

Dopamine

Dopamine is an endogenous catecholamine and an immediate precursor of adrenaline and noradrenaline. At low doses it stimulates vascular DA_1 dopaminergic receptors, especially those in renal, mesenteric and coronary vessels. As the dose increases it progressively stimulates β_1 and α_1 adrenoceptors. Thus, depending on the dose it may act as a renal vasodilator, a myocardial inotrope, or a peripheral vasoconstrictor. Dopamine also causes release of noradrenaline from autonomic nerve endings (DA_2 receptors).

Cardiovascular effects and doses

At lower doses (0.5–3 $\mu g{\cdot}kg^{-1}{\cdot}min^{-1}$) DA_1 effects predominate, with increases in renal blood flow, glomerular filtration rate and sodium excretion. Thus, it is useful in the treatment of low cardiac output states associated with renal compromise. At higher doses (3–5 $\mu g{\cdot}kg^{-1}{\cdot}min^{-1}$), β_1 stimulation increases myocardial contractility and heart rate with a slight reduction in peripheral vascular resistance. This dose range is probably the most suitable for treating heart failure, although the increase in heart rate is undesirable. At a dose of 5–15 $\mu g{\cdot}kg^{-1}{\cdot}min^{-1}$, β_1 effects are prominent, but at the upper range, α effects dominate due to release of noradrenaline. The result is generalised vasoconstriction, increased peripheral vascular resistance, and elevated systolic and diastolic blood pressure. Tachycardia and ventricular irritability may also occur at high doses.

Side effects

Dopamine does not cross the blood–brain barrier and so there are no CNS side effects when given intravenously. Tachyarrhythmias, myocardial ischaemia, headache, nausea and vomiting may occur.

Interactions

The effect of dopamine is prolonged and intensified by monoamine oxidase inhibitors (MAOIs). If dopamine must be administered to a patient on these drugs, the dose should be reduced to one-tenth or less of that normally used. Concomitant medication with tricyclic antidepressant drugs may also give problems and careful adjustment of the dose may be necessary.

Dobutamine

Dobutamine is a directly acting synthetic catecholamine with predominant effects at β_1 receptors. It has weak β_2 and α effects. It is a racemic mixture and both stereoisomers are β-adrenoceptor agonists. The (+) isomer is approximately ten times more potent as a β-receptor agonist than the (–) isomer, which is mainly responsible for the α-adrenoceptor activity. Unlike dopamine, dobutamine does not act by releasing noradrenaline or via dopaminergic receptors.

Cardiovascular effects

Dobutamine causes an increase in cardiac output, a decrease in peripheral vascular resistance, and a decrease in left ventricular filling pressure.

Indications

Dobutamine is widely used to increase myocardial contractility, cardiac output, and stroke volume in the peri-operative period. It is less likely to increase heart rate than dopamine. There is evidence that dobutamine can increase both myocardial contractility and coronary blood flow. This makes it particularly suitable for use in patients with acute myocardial infarction. Dobutamine is also suitable for treating septic shock associated with increased filling pressures and impaired ventricular function. Owing to the competing α and β activity there is usually little change in mean arterial pressure.

Dose

The duration of action is short and the drug is administered by continuous intravenous infusion at 2–15 $\mu g \cdot kg^{-1} \cdot min^{-1}$ depending on the response.

Side effects

Dobutamine improves atrioventricular conduction and may precipitate atrial fibrillation in susceptible patients. Hypertension and tachycardia may also occur in some patients.

Dopexamine

Dopexamine is a synthetic catecholamine with direct and indirect sympathomimetic activity. The indirect effect is caused by potent inhibition of neuronal noradrenaline reuptake. It is a potent β_2-adrenoceptor agonist with much less β_1- than β_2-receptor activity. It also has significant dopaminergic DA_1-receptor activity, with only minimal activity at DA_2 receptors and no α-adrenergic activity.

Cardiovascular effects

Dopexamine reduces afterload via β_2 and DA_1 activation and consequent renal and splanchnic vasodilatation. The β_1 activity and inhibition of noradrenaline re-uptake are responsible for its positive inotropic and chronotropic effects. It also promotes naturesis (DA_1).

Indications

Shock states associated with impaired renal function. Pulmonary hypertension.

Dose and side effects

The dose range is 1–4 $\mu g \cdot kg^{-1} \cdot min^{-1}$. Some patients respond to very low doses so careful titration is essential at the start of therapy. A reflex increase in heart rate is common and may produce angina in patients with ischaemic heart disease.

Contraindication

Unstable angina pectoris.

Phenylephrine

Phenylephrine is a potent direct α_1-adrenoceptor agonist.

Cardiovascular effects and indications

Phenylephrine is used to increase peripheral vascular resistance when cardiac output is maintained. It increases arterial blood pressure and this often results in reflex bradycardia. It is mainly used to correct anaesthesia-induced hypotension. It is also used to dilate the pupil (mydriasis) and as a nasal decongestant.

Dose

It has a very short duration of action (5–10 min), and is given as an intravenous bolus (40–100 μg) or by infusion at 0.2–0.3 $\mu g \cdot kg^{-1} \cdot min^{-1}$.

Ephedrine

Ephedrine is a sympathomimetic amine with direct and indirect effects on α, β_1 and β_2 adrenoceptors ($\beta_1 = \beta_2 > \alpha$).

Cardiovascular effects and indications

Ephedrine has positive inotropic and chronotropic effects and increases peripheral vascular resistance. It is preferable to methoxamine for maintaining blood pressure in elderly patients during spinal anaesthesia, possibly because it has less effect on coronary blood flow (less pronounced α activity). It is also less likely to impair placental blood flow than some other vasopressors, for the same reason. It is used as a bronchodilator because of its β_2-agonist effects.

Dose and side effects

Ephedrine acts both directly and indirectly on adrenoceptors, and tachyphylaxis may occur due to depletion of noradrenaline stores. The standard intravenous bolus is 5–10 mg. It can be given by intramuscular injection (15–30 mg) for a more sustained effect. Arrhythmias may occur when administered during halothane anaesthesia.

Metaraminol and methoxamine

Metaraminol is a catecholamine which acts predominantly at α_1 adrenoceptors on vascular smooth muscle, and is virtually devoid of β-receptor activity. It is used to treat hypotension during general and regional anaesthesia. Methoxamine is a vasopressor with a similar pharmacological profile.

Dose and side effects

Metaraminol has a longer duration of action than some other vasopressors and care should be taken to avoid inducing hypertension. The dose is 0.5–5 mg as a slow intravenous bolus. If necessary, 15–100 mg may be diluted in normal saline (500 mL) and given by infusion. The dose of methoxamine is 2–5 mg intravenously.

Phosphodiesterase inhibitors

Phosphodiesterases are a group of enzymes that, among other actions, hydrolyse cAMP. Phosphodiesterase inhibitors are selective for phosphodiesterase III (PDE-III) isoenzyme present in the heart. They prevent the degradation of cAMP, thereby increasing its intracellular concentration (Figure 8.4). This leads to an increase in the intracellular concentration of Ca^{2+} and an increased contractility and heart rate. PDE-III inhibitors have no adrenoceptor agonistic activity and therefore can be used in combination with other sympathomimetic drugs. They also increase cAMP levels in vascular smooth muscle, but this results in lower intracellular Ca^{2+} concentrations and thus vasodilatation.

The phosphodiesterase inhibitors include the bipyridine derivatives, amrinone and milrinone, and the imidazoline compounds, enoximone and piroximone. Several other drugs, including the methylxanthines theophylline and aminophylline, and the calcium sensitisers, pimobendan and levosimendan also have phosphodiesterase-inhibiting activity. Vesarinone, a drug with multiple modes of action including calcium sensitisation and inhibition of Na^+/K^+ ATPase, is also a phosphodiesterase inhibitor. Aminophylline and caffeine are non-selective and inhibit most isoforms of phosphodiesterase. The phosphodiesterase inhibitors are used to treat acute left and right ventricular dysfunction. They also enhance left ventricular isovolumic relaxation and improve early ventricular filling. Peripheral and pulmonary vascular resistance is reduced, and these drugs are often referred to as *inodilators*. They are valuable in the treatment of right ventricular failure associated with pulmonary hypertension. Increases in intracellular concentrations of cAMP produced by inhibition of phosphodiesterase III are associated with arrhythmogenesis. Overdosing often results in supraventricular and ventricular arrhythmias.

The first clinically used drug in this class, amrinone, had a wide variety of side effects including anorexia, abdominal pain, diarrhoea, headache, fever, liver function abnormalities, and thrombocytopenia. In contrast, milrinone and enoximone are largely devoid of these adverse effects and have replaced amrinone in the acute management of heart failure in the peri-operative period.

Phosphodiesterase III inhibitors are very useful in combination with a β_1-adrenoceptor agonist in the treatment of acute left ventricular dysfunction. The β_1 agonist increases the intracellular cAMP by activation of adenylyl cyclase, while the phosphodiesterase III inhibitor prevents degradation of cAMP. The combined effects are additive and may be synergistic in the failing myocardium.

Milrinone

Dose

Loading bolus: 0–50 $\mu g \cdot kg^{-1}$ over 10 min.
Maintenance infusion: 0.3–0.75 $\mu g \cdot kg^{-1} \cdot min^{-1}$.
Maximum daily dose: 0.75 $mg \cdot kg^{-1}$.

Side effects

Hypotension, angina pectoris, supraventricular and ventricular arrhythmias.

Contraindications

Liver disease, severe thrombocytopenia, obstructive cardiomyopathy. Acute phase of myocardial infarction.

Interactions

Hypersensitivity, sulphite allergy, excessive hypotension with disopyramide. Incompatible with dextrose and frusemide (furosemide).

Enoximone

Dose

Starting dose: 0.5–1 $mg \cdot kg^{-1}$, with a maximum rate of 12.5 $mg \cdot min^{-1}$.
Maintenance infusion: 5–20 $\mu g \cdot kg^{-1} \cdot min^{-1}$, for a maximum of 48 h.

Side effects

Hypotension, angina pectoris, arrythmias, nausea, vomiting, diarrhoea.

Contraindications

Liver disease, renal failure.

Myofilament calcium sensitisers

Myofilament calcium sensitisers are a relatively new group of drugs, which include pimobendan, sulmazole, and levosimendan, used in both the acute and chronic management of congestive heart failure. They are not dependent on an increase in intracellular cAMP or Ca^{2+} concentration for their activity. The positive inotropic effects occur by increasing Ca^{2+} binding to troponin C. This allows prolonged interaction of actin and myosin filaments during contraction resulting in a positive inotropic effect. Myofilament Ca^{2+} desensitisation occurs during myocardial hypoxia, ischaemia, and stunning, and myofilament Ca^{2+} sensitisers may be particularly useful in these conditions. In addition to producing myofilament Ca^{2+} sensitisation, many of the drugs in this class also partially inhibit vascular smooth muscle and cardiac phosphodiesterase. These actions cause arterial and venous vasodilatation and further augmentation of inotropic state.

ANTI-ARRHYTHMIC DRUGS

The rhythmic and highly coordinated action of autonomous impulse generation and conduction within the heart can be disturbed by disorders of impulse formation, impulse conduction or a combination of both. These disturbances can be due to an electrolyte imbalance, hypoxia, ischaemia and reperfusion, hormonal or neuronal disorders, chemicals and drugs, congenital or acquired malformations of cardiac tissue. The pharmacotherapy of arrhythmias is complex and anti-arrhythmic drugs form a heterogenous group of compounds with a variety of effects, sites and mechanisms of action. The most widely used classification is that of Vaughan-Williams, who grouped anti-arrhythmic drugs into four classes according to their molecular mode of action. This was later modified by subdividing group I into subclasses IA, IB and IC, incorporating effects on repolarisation (Table 8.5). The main indications for the different classes are given in Table 8.6.

Table 8.5 Classification of class I anti-arrythmic drugs

Classification	*Mechanism of action*	*Drugs*
IA	Moderate-to-marked Na^+ channel block Phase 0 conduction depression ++ Widens QRS Prolongs repolarisation, lengthens APD and QT interval	Procainamide, disopyramide, quinidine
IB	Mild-to-moderate Na^+ channel block Phase 0 conduction depression + Shortens repolarisation and QT interval	Lidocaine (lignocaine), mexiletine, tocainide, phenytoin
IC	Marked Na^+ channel block Phase 0 conduction depression +++ Little effect on repolarisation	Propafenone, encainide, flecainide, indecanidine

APD, action potential duration.

Table 8.6 Summary of main indications for different classes of anti-arrhythmic drugs

Class	*Indications*
IA	Ventricular ectopics, paroxysmal supraventricular tachycardia, atrial flutter or fibrillation, ventricular tachycardia
IB	Ventricular tachycardia, digoxin-induced arrhythmias
IC	Ventricular and supraventricular tachycardia (especially those due to re-entry phenomena), atrial fibrillation and flutter (can convert recent-onset fibrillation or flutter to sinus rhythm)
II	Paroxysmal supraventricular tachycardia, atrial or ventricular premature beats, atrial fibrillation, or flutter (slows ventricular rate)
III	Ventricular tachycardia, atrial fibrillation, and flutter (can convert recent-onset fibrillation or flutter to sinus rhythm). Amiodarone is used in the management of patients with supraventricular and ventricular arrhythmias, and arrhythmias associated with the WPW syndrome
IV	Paroxysmal supraventricular tachycardia, atrial fibrillation and flutter. Not of benefit in treatment of ventricular arrhythmias
Miscellaneous	
Atropine	Sinus bradycardia
Digoxin	Atrial fibrillation and flutter with rapid ventricular response
Adenosine	Idiopathic and re-entrant paroxysmal supraventricular tachycardia

WPW, Wolf-Parkinson-White.

Class I drugs have a local anaesthetic-like action, blocking the inward current in sodium channels. This depresses the fast depolarisation (phase 0) which initiates each action potential (Figure 8.5). This 'membrane-stabilising' effect makes them valuable for the treatment of ectopic and tachycardic arrhythmias, such as atrial and ventricular fibrillation, extrasystoles, supraventricular and ventricular tachycardia. Class I drugs also decrease contractility. A subclassification is made according to the effects on the action potential duration. Class Ia drugs lengthen and Ib drugs shorten the action potential duration. Class Ic drugs have no effect on the action potential duration, but marked phase 0 of the action potential (Figure 8.6).

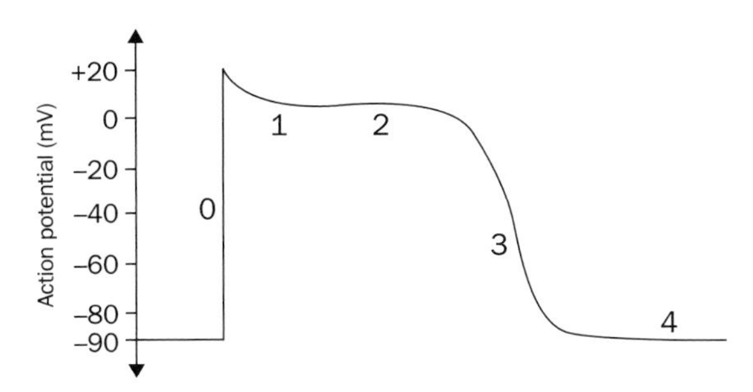

Figure 8.5 *The 5 phases of the normal cardiac action potential.*

Class II drugs are the β-adrenoceptor antagonists that suppress the sympathetic modulation of the heart action. They are used in the therapy of sinus tachycardia, supraventricular paroxysmal tachycardia and ventricular extrasystoles. Because of its rapid onset and short duration of action, esmolol is the preferred drug in this class for intra-operative use.

Class III drugs are inhibitors of the repolarising potassium currents, which lengthen the action potential duration but have no effect on the rate of depolarisation nor on the resting membrane potential. This group contains bretylium, amiodarone, ibutilide and sotalol. Sotalol is a racemic mixure; the L isomer is a non-selective β antagonist and the D isomer is a class III anti-arrhythmic. Class III drugs are used to treat tachycardia, atrial flutter and life-threatening ventricular fibrillation due to re-entry arrhythmias.

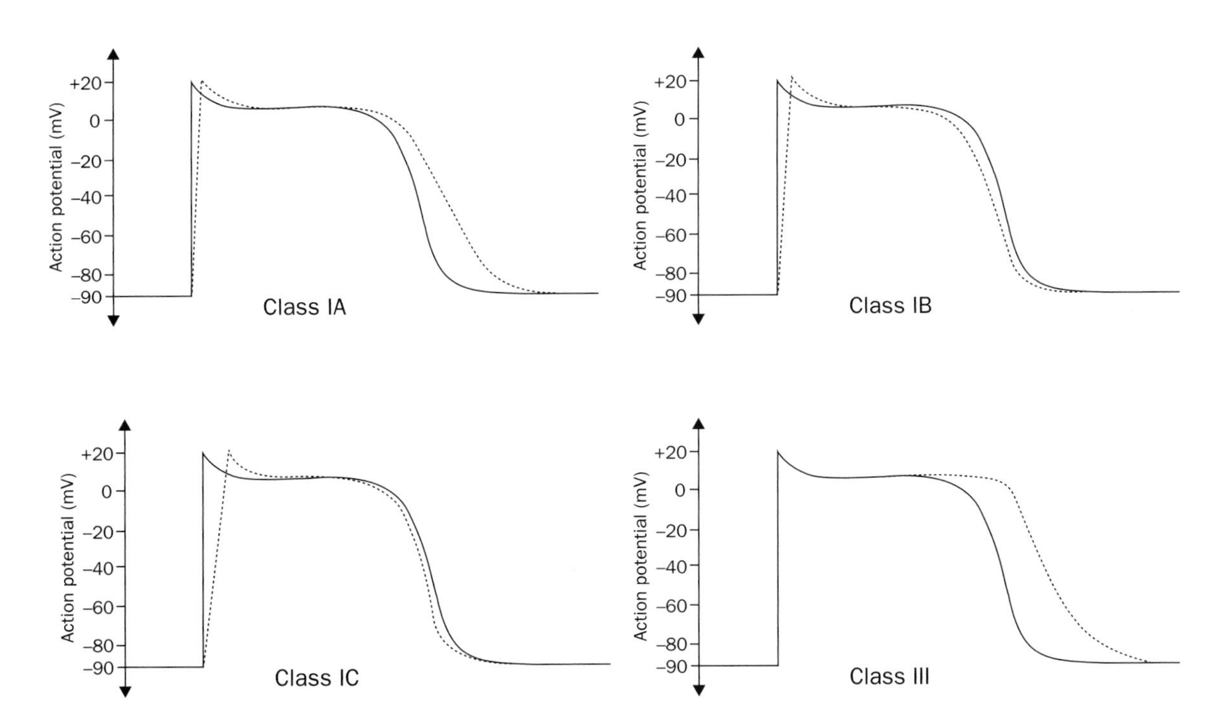

Figure 8.6 *Changes produced by class I and III anti-arrhythmic drugs on the cardiac action potential.*

Class IV drugs are calcium-entry blockers of the phenylalkylamine (verapamil) and benzothiazepine (diltiazem) type. They slow atrioventricular conduction, and are used to treat supraventricular and sinus tachycardia.

Specific drugs

Procainamide (class IA)

This is the amide analogue of procaine hydrochloride. It has an active metabolite with significant class III activity. Procainamide is particularly effective in the treatment of life-threatening ventricular arrhythmias unresponsive to other therapies. It is also used to maintain sinus rhythm following cardioversion. Intravenous administration can cause hypotension, mainly due to peripheral vasodilatation, and it should not be given faster than $50\ mg{\cdot}min^{-1}$. It should be given intravenously as a bolus of 100 mg over 2–5 min, followed by an infusion of $30–90\ \mu g{\cdot}kg^{-1}{\cdot}min^{-1}$.

Disopyramide (class IA)

This drug is only approved for oral administration in some countries. It is effective for conversion of atrial flutter or fibrillation or ischaemia-induced ventricular arrhythmias. It has significant anticholinergic properties (10% of the potency of atropine) that can offset its direct depressant effects on sinus and AV nodes. It has a pronounced negative inotropic effect and should be administered with caution to patients with a history of congestive heart failure. For acute treatment of perioperative arrhythmias it is given intravenously; $0.2\ mg{\cdot}kg^{-1}$ over 10–15 min, then $0.2\ mg{\cdot}kg^{-1}$ over the next 45 min and a maintenance infusion of $0.4\ mg{\cdot}kg^{-1}{\cdot}h^{-1}$.

Quinidine (class IA)

This agent, in addition to class IA actions, also has indirect anticholinergic properties. It is also a mild α-adrenoceptor antagonist and may cause vasodilatation when given as a fast intravenous bolus. In toxic concentrations or in combination with high digitalis concentrations, quinidine may cause sinus arrest, high-grade AV block, polymorphic ventricular tachycardia (*torsades de pointes*), and abnormal ventricular automaticity. Despite these limitations quinidine is a useful anti-arrhythmic for both supra- and ventricular arrhythmias. It can convert atrial fibrillation or flutter to sinus rhythm and maintain normal sinus rhythm. It is useful in managing re-entry supraventricular tachycardia, e.g. in the WPW syndrome, and for the suppression of ventricular ectopy.

Lidocaine (lignocaine)

This is a class IB drug used primarily for the emergency treatment of ventricular arrhythmias. It has little effect on sinus node automaticity but depresses normal and abnormal forms of automaticity in Purkinje fibres. It is generally ineffective against supraventricular and accessory pathway-induced (e.g. WPW syndrome) arrhythmias. Lidocaine is relatively safe and free from adverse cardiovascular side effects. It causes minimal cardiodepression, although high doses can cause heart block. The most common side effect is a dose-related CNS toxicity. It is given intravenously as a bolus of $1\ mg{\cdot}kg^{-1}$ followed by an infusion of $20–50\ \mu g{\cdot}kg^{-1}{\cdot}min^{-1}$.

Phenytoin (class IB)

This is primarily an anticonvulsant. Because of a wide range of toxic side effects its use as an anti-arrythmic is limited to the treatment of arrhythmias caused by digitalis toxicity. Intravenous bolus injections can cause myocardial depression, hypotension, AV block and bradycardia.

Propafenone (class IC)

This agent also has some class IA and class II effects. It is effective for the treatment of ventricular and supraventricular tachycardias (AV nodal and accessory pathway re-entry, atrial flutter and fibrillation). Propafenone is useful in converting recent-onset atrial fibrillation or flutter to sinus rhythm, and for terminating paroxysmal supraventricular tachycardia. Its pro-arrythmic and myocardial depressant effects limit its use, especially in patients with poor ventricular function.

Flecainide and encainide

These are class IC drugs with similar pharmacological profiles and with the same indication range and adverse effects. They are mainly used for the treatment of severe, life-threatening ventricular tachyarrhythmias, and non-sustained ventricular tachycardia or high-frequency premature ventricular beats. The main adverse effects are cardiovascular, including proarrhythmic actions and severe negative inotropic effects, especially in patients with impaired cardiac function. Both flecainide and encainide increase the risk of sudden death in patients with myocardial infarction and asymptomatic unsustained ventricular arrhythmias.

Amiodarone (class III)

This drug is a potent anti-arrhythmic agent with multiple cardiovascular actions. Its class III actions are due to reduction in the potassium outward current and consequent prolongation of the cardiac action potential and the QT interval in the ECG. Paradoxically, this action may also induce polymorphic ventricular arrhythmias. Amiodarone is used to treat supraventricular and ventricular arrhythmias, arrhythmias associated with the WPW syndrome, atrial flutter, and fibrillation, and for ventricular tachycardia or fibrillation after cardiac surgery or cardiac arrest. It can cause myocardial depression following rapid intravenous administration. The intravenous dose is 2–5 $mg \cdot kg^{-1}$ given over 20–120 min followed by an infusion to a maximum dose of 1000 mg per 24 h. With intravenous administration, therapeutic effects are seen within 30 min but the maximum effect may take 1–2 hours. The elimination half-life after a single oral or intravenous dose is 4–6 hours. However, with chronic oral therapy the half life is extremely prolonged, up to 40 days.

Chronic oral therapy with amiodarone is associated with several side effects, including pulmonary toxicity (fibrosis and probably immunologically mediated pneumonitis), hepatotoxicity, thyroid gland dysfunction, corneal microdeposits, blue-grey skin discoloration and neurological disturbances.

9

Respiratory drugs

JPH Fee

Factors influencing the calibre of airways • Bronchodilators • Sympathomimetic drugs • Xanthines • Steroids • Anticholinergic drugs • Respiratory stimulants

The drugs under consideration in this chapter are those that are used to relieve bronchospasm or which stimulate respiration.

FACTORS INFLUENCING THE CALIBRE OF AIRWAYS

The tone of the bronchial smooth muscle is largely regulated by the intracellular nucleotides, cyclic 3,5-adenosine monophosphate (cAMP) and cyclic 3,5-guanosine monophosphate (cGMP), which are converted from the respective triphosphates by adenylate cyclase and guanyl cyclase. An increase in cAMP leads to sequestration of intracellular calcium, bronchial smooth muscle relaxation, and bronchial dilation; a reduction in cAMP causes bronchial constriction. In contrast, an increase in cGMP causes bronchial constriction; a reduction in intracellular cGMP results in bronchial dilation. Mast cell-derived histamine and other inflammatory mediators promote broncoconstriction.

BRONCHODILATORS

Severe bronchoconstriction may present to anaesthetists either in the operating theatre during surgery or in the intensive care unit. In both situations, rapid reversal is called for and this usually requires the use of intravenous drugs. The main bronchodilator drugs are the β_2-adrenoceptor agonists, the methylxanthines and the anticholinergic drugs. Of these the selective β_2-adrenoceptor agonists may be used in combination with drugs of the other two groups for their additive effect. Steroids, both intravenous and inhaled, have a place in the management of acute asthma but their onset of action is slow. The use of prophylactic drugs, such as cromoglycate, is more appropriate for the prevention of asthmatic attacks and has no place in the management of acute attacks.

SYMPATHOMIMETIC DRUGS

The bronchi have a rich parasympathetic innervation but there is no sympathetic innervation of bronchial smooth muscle and all sympathetic effects are due to circulating adrenaline (epinephrine and noradrenaline (norepinephrine) acting on β_2 adrenoceptors. Stimulation of these receptors mediates bronchodilatation by relaxation of bronchial smooth muscle. Beta-adrenoceptor agonists also have limited anti-inflammatory actions. They inhibit mediator release from mast cells and may stimulate release of relaxant factors from bronchial epithelial cells. They may also inhibit vagal tone, increase mucous clearance by an action on the cilia, and reduce microvascular leakage thereby reducing oedema. In the past, powerful but non-selective β_2 agonists, such as isoprenaline, adrenaline (epinephrine), and ephedrine, were used for their bronchodilatating effects by inhalation and occasionally by the intravenous route. Their cardiovascular side effects, notably dangerous tachyarrhythmias, were a major disadvantage. Selective β_2 agonists, such as sabutamol or terbutaline, are now preferred. Unfortunately, their specificity is relative so that β_1 effects may occur especially at higher dosage or in the elderly.

The β_2-adrenoceptor agonists can be classified according to their duration of action into short- and long-acting drugs. The short-acting drugs include salbutamol, fenoterol, rimiterol, and terbutaline. They have an onset of action that occurs within minutes, reach their peak effect within 30–60 minutes, and provide bronchodilation for 4–6 hours (up to 8 hours with fenoterol). Rimiterol has an even faster onset, the effect appearing within 20 seconds of inhalation, and a short duration, the bronchodilatation declining after 30 min. The short-acting β_2-adrenoceptor agonists are useful in the treatment of incidental bronchospasm and are the agents of choice in the treatment of acute asthma as well as in treating bronchospasm in other chronic obstructive lung disorders.

The longer-acting agents, formoterol and salmeterol xinafoate, have a slower onset, usually 10–20 minutes, and reach their peak effectiveness in 2–4 hours. They provide bronchodilatation and bronchoprotection for up to 12 hours. The long-acting drugs are indicated for the management of asthma that reacts inadequately to treatment with steroids and for chronic bronchitis and emphysema. Long-acting β_2-adrenoceptor agonists should never be used in the treatment of acute asthma, since this may delay access to more rapid-acting β_2 agonists thus allowing potentially life-threatening bronchospasm to develop.

Salbutamol

Salbutamol is a selective β_2 agonist that may be administered by inhalation from either a pressurised aerosol delivering 100 μg per puff (standard dose 1–2 puffs) or a powder inhaler (metered dose 500 μg). The duration of action is 4–6 hours. In patients unable to use a pressurised aerosol, salbutamol-containing solution may be nebulised in a stream of oxygen using a specially designed face mask. Similarly, salbutamol-containing solution can be nebulised and introduced into the inspiratory limb of a mechanical ventilation system.

Salbutamol may be administered parenterally as an intravenous infusion at 3–20 μg min^{-1} with the dose being titrated to therapeutic effect. Side effects notably tachycardia are more common with parenteral or nebulised formulations. The drug may also be administered by the subcutaneous or intramuscular routes. Salbutamol is conjugated in the liver and excreted both in the urine as unchanged drug and metabolites, and also in the faeces.

Salbutamol inhibits uterine contractions and may be administered by intravenous infusion as a means of preventing premature labour.

Terbutaline is a similar drug that is occasionally used as an alternative to salbutamol in patients who have experienced marked sympathomimetic side effects. Other selective β_2-adrenceptor agonists include fenoterol, reproterol, and rimiterol, all of which are available as aerosols.

XANTHINES

The three methalated xanthine derivatives (methylxanthines) theophylline, theobromine, and caffeine are plant alkaloids. Theophylline is the only one of these which is widely used therapeutically. Three possible modes of action have been proposed:

1. Prevention of the breakdown of cAMP by phosphodiesterases: elevated cAMP levels may potentiate other drugs including catecholamines which stimulate cAMP production.

2. Competitive antagonism of adenosine receptors: xanthines are potent inhibitors at adenosine receptors; these may stimulate or inhibit cAMP and Ca^{2+} influx.
3. Promotion of calcium release from the sarcoplasmic reticulum augmenting muscle contraction (intercostals, diaphragm).

Theophylline is the most effective of the methylxanthines as a bronchodilator. However, it is less effective than β_2-adrenoceptor agonists, has a very narrow therapeutic window and has declined in importance for the treatment of asthma. A plasma theophylline concentration of $20\ \mu g \cdot mL^{-1}$ (the upper limit of the therapeutic range) produces 45–60% of maximum bronchodilatation compared to the 80–90% that can be achieved with β_2-adrenoceptor agonists.

The theophylline analogue, aminophylline, is administered primarily for its bronchodilating effect. Aminophylline is the ethylenediamine salt of theophylline and in the plasma dissociates to yield the parent theophylline. It has a mild stimulant action and may improve diaphragmatic and intercostal muscle contraction. Before using aminophylline it is essential to know if the patient was on medication at home with theophylline-containing drugs so that toxicity may be avoided. Aminophylline should be administered by slow intravenous injection or infusion under electrocardiogram (ECG) control and the dose titrated according to effect.

Cardiovascular system
The methylxanthines cause an increase in heart rate and contractility, decreased peripheral resistance due to smooth muscle relaxation, and, in high doses, may induce premature ventricular contractions or tachyarrhythmias.

Central nervous system
Central stimulation is common and may result in restlessness, tremor, agitation, nausea, insomnia and grand mal seizures. The therapeutic window is small and toxic side effects may occur at plasma concentrations that are only slightly above the accepted therapeutic level.

Pharmacokinetics
Theophylline is rapidly and completely absorbed following oral administration but its rapid elimination results in fluctuating plasma concentrations. Absorption from sustained release oral preparations or rectal suppositories is erratic. Theophylline is 40% bound to albumin and the volume of distribution is approximately $0.5\ L \cdot kg^{-1}$. About 10% of a dose of theophylline is excreted unchanged by the kidneys with 90% being metabolised by cytochrome P-450 pathways in the liver. After intravenous administration the plasma half-life is approximately 4–5 hours in adults and 3–6 hours in children. Theophylline clearance is reduced by cimetidine and increased by enzyme-reducing drugs, such as phenobarbital and phenytoin.

STEROIDS

Steroid therapy is indicated for the control of acute severe asthma. It is thought that the use of short-term intravenous steroid therapy may reduce the need for hospital admission. Several mechanisms have been suggested:

- An anti-inflammatory action.
- Inhibition of arachidonic acid metabolites, e.g. prostaglandins.
- Inhibition of platelet activating factor (bronchoconstrictor and pro-inflammatory actions).
- Prevention of mast cell degranulation; membrane stabilisation.
- Synergy with catecholamines. The lipid soluble steroid molecules enter cells and bind the intracellular receptors. This results in up-regulation of specific genes, changes in RNA production, and protein synthesis.

The peak response to steroids is delayed by 6–12 hours after intravenous administration. Steroid therapy may be administered by inhalation or intravenous injection. The inhaled route is unreliable in acute attacks and is most suitable for prophylaxis as a means of reducing the frequency of acute attacks. Hydrocortisone $0.5\ mg \cdot kg^{-1} \cdot h^{-1}$ or $4\ mg \cdot kg^{-1}$ intravenously 4-hourly is widely advocated although methylprednisolone 1 g 6-hourly has also been suggested. Steroid treatment is usually continued for several days usually in decreasing dosage. As the patient's condition improves the intravenous regimen may be replaced by prednisolone taken orally.

Beclometasone propionate

This steroid is widely used and is administered by pressurised aerosol (200 µg per puff) given up to three to four times a day as prophylaxis. It is often prescribed in combination with a selective β_2-adrenoceptor agonist, such as salbutamol. There are few steroid-related side effects when the inhaled route is employed at recommended dosages.

ANTICHOLINERGIC DRUGS

Parasympathetic stimulation of the bronchial tree causes an increase in guanylate cyclase activity and cGMP which in turn causes bronchoconstriction. In theory, any drug that blocks cholinergic activity may act as a bronchodilator but in practice the side-effects associated with this type of drug are unacceptable. Ipratropium bromide is possibly the only anticholinergic drug which is currently used for its bronchodilating effects. It acts through competitive inhibition at the cholinergic receptors on bronchial smooth muscle. Ipratropium is used in the management of both asthma and chronic bronchitis. It is administered by metered aerosol (20–40 µg) as one or two puffs up to four times daily. It acts fairly rapidly but its peak effect may not be seen for up to 2 hours; its duration of effect is normally 4–6 hours. These characteristics suggest that it may be more suitable for prophylaxis than the treatment of the acute condition. Ipratropium has been shown to act additively with β_2-adrenergic agonists, disodium cromoglycate, theophylline, and steroids.

Disodium cromoglycate

This drug does not have a primary bronchodilating action but protects against bronchospasm induced by allergic and other mechanisms. In asthma it acts by inhibiting the release of inflammatory mediators from mast cells. The mechanism is thought to involve the closure of calcium channels which in turn block the entry of calcium ions that are responsible for mast cell degranulation. Cromoglycate is available as an inhaled powder (Spincaps), or in a pressurised aerosol (50 µg per puff) or in a solution for nebulisation ($20\ mg \cdot 2\ mL^{-1}$). Its duration of action is 3–6 hours and it has no significant side effects.

Nedocromil sodium

Nedocromil sodium, although structurally different from cromoglycate, has similar pharmacological properties. Like cromoglycate, it has corticosteroid-sparing effects and may be particularly useful in patients with corticosteroid-dependent asthma. Nedocromil may be slightly more effective than cromoglycate, especially in younger patients.

RESPIRATORY STIMULANTS

Drugs that stimulate respiration (analeptics) have a place in anaesthetic practice but are not a substitute for mechanical ventilation. They have a direct effect on respiratory drive; they do not share a common molecular structure. Respiratory stimulation is generally better achieved by antagonising the depressant effects of the depressant drug, e.g. flumazenil for benzodiazepines; naloxone for opioids.

Doxapram

This drug stimulates the respiratory centre directly and may be used in emergencies as a single bolus ($0.5\ mg \cdot kg^{-1}$), or more usually as a bolus followed by an infusion ($1–2\ mg \cdot min^{-1}$).

After a single bolus its duration of effect is 5–10 min. It has a higher therapeutic index than other analeptics and it is unusual amongst analeptic drugs in that it acts on the carotid sinus chemoreceptors. In addition to its role as an emergency drug it has been advocated as a means of stimulating deep breathing in the peri-operative period and to reduce the incidence of apnoeic attacks in premature infants.

10

CNS drugs

Stephen J Cooper

ANXIOLYTICS AND HYPNOTICS

Anxiety is a common emotion experienced by everyone. It may be a temporary phenomenon, such as occurs before a surgical operation, or a recognised psychiatric disorder. Similarly, disturbance of sleep pattern can affect us all. It is only when these symptoms become more persistent, severe, and disabling in terms of daily functioning that actual treatment is required as opposed to temporary symptomatic management. Nine specific types of anxiety disorder are now recognised. Specific neurochemical aetiologies have not yet been identified and these may differ between different disorders. Pharmacological studies suggest involvement of the noradrenaline (norepinephrine), serotonin, and GABA systems, and possible involvement of cholecystokinin. However, the most universally effective treatment for anxiety symptoms is a benzodiazepine (BDZ).

Older drugs

Barbiturates were among the first compounds with psychotropic effects to be specifically synthesised for clinical use. Two of the group, thiopentone and methohexitone, were universally used as anaesthetic induction agents until the 1990s. Other barbiturates were used widely as hypnotics and anxiolytics until the late 1960s. The only barbiturate still used outside anaesthesia is phenobarbital, for its anticonvulsant activity. Barbiturates are potent drugs with powerful and often cumulative effects, resulting in significant impairment of psychomotor function. This potency, the rapid development of tolerance to their effects and marked induction of their own metabolism (by induction of hepatic cytochrome P-450 enzymes) led to escalation in dosing and dependence in a high proportion of patients. They are extremely dangerous in overdose, causing death by respiratory and cardiovascular depression, and largely for that reason have been withdrawn from general use in most developed countries. While at normal doses they act at the $GABA_A$-receptor site to enhance the effects of GABA (like BDZs), in overdose they can independently open the chloride ion channel, causing marked and prolonged depolarisation. This does not occur in overdose with BDZs (whose effects are always dependent on GABA). BDZs are less prone to dependence and have supplanted the barbiturates for most non-anaesthetic indications.

Propanediols (e.g. meprobamate) were also used in the 1950s and 1960s but had similar dangers to the barbiturates.

BENZODIAZEPINES

Despite some of the concerns about tolerance and dependence, BDZs remain one of the most effective and safe treatment for symptoms of anxiety. Death or serious morbidity from overdose of BDZs alone is rare and is only likely to occur if they are combined with other central nervous system (CNS) depressants. Given intravenously for sedation BZDs are generally safe provided care is taken to titrate the dose slowly according to the response. The elderly are intolerant of intravenous overdosage and profound hypotension, or worse, may result from too rapid administration. It is essential to recognise that circulation time is slowed in the elderly and that peak effect may not become apparent for many minutes. Since the use of oral BDZs as 'tranquillisers' or 'sleeping pills' fell from favour in the early 1980s there has been a marked decrease in the numbers of the people presenting with BZD overdose.

Pharmacokinetics (Table 10.1)

The pharmacokinetics of BDZs are illustrated using diazepam as the example. Absorption is generally good following oral dosing but there is considerable patient variability. In general, the intramuscular route provides slower absorption than the oral route, is painful, and should be avoided. Lorazepam, which has greater water solubility than other BZDs, is the only BDZ recommended for intramuscular use. The elimination half-life is age-dependent. The principal active metabolite of diazepam, desmethyldiazepam, has a very long elimination half-life and gradual accumulation of active metabolites is one of the principal reasons for many of these drugs, used as night time hypnotics, having 'hangover' effects through the following day. Some BDZs undergo phase I metabolism, which results in production of active metabolites, and some only phase II metabolism, resulting in inactivation.

Physiological and adverse effects

The relative anti-anxiety potencies of the different BDZs correlate with their relative potencies as agonists at the BDZ receptor. The resultant inhibitory effects in the brain are responsible for their anti-anxiety, sedative and anticonvulsant effects. Inhibition of spinal pathways results in relaxation of skeletal muscles. The therapeutic use of particular BDZs is as much related to their potency and solubility as to inherent pharmacokinetic differences.

Given orally at normal therapeutic doses BDZs have little effect on cardiovascular, respiratory or autonomic function. Respiratory depression and reduced systolic blood pressure may occur but this is seen principally with intravenous administration or overdose. Leucopenia and eosinophilia are rare. There was a suggestion in the early 1980s of increased risk of breast cancer but a subsequent large case-control study refuted this.

The more common adverse effects of BDZs are listed in Table 10.2. Sedation is common and occurs with all BDZs. Tolerance to this effect is usual on long-term treatment. Psychomotor impairment can be demonstrated in real life as well as in laboratory testing. It is partly related to sedation but also to impairment of central information-processing ability. Research is equivocal as to whether or not tolerance may develop to these impairments. The effects of BDZs on memory were first noted in 1965 when they were being used as premedication before general anaesthesia, many patients demonstrating amnesia for events which took place in the interval between drug administration and operation. This phenomenon is known as *anterograde amnesia*. Benzodiazepines do not impair memory for previous events, i.e. they do not cause retrograde amnesia. Sedation also interferes with a patient's ability to recall events accurately. Dreams and fantasies, sometimes sexual in nature, are frequently reported after intravenous BDZs and the presence of a chaperone is prudent.

It seems likely that different subtypes of the GABA-BDZ-receptor complex may mediate different actions of these drugs. The different subtypes have different anatomical distributions, although these may overlap in a number of brain regions. However, at present the available BDZs are not sufficiently specific to individual

Table 10.1 Pharmacokinetic properties of some anxiolytic and hypnotic drugs

	Biovailability (% after oral dose)	*Protein binding (%)*	*Peak concentration (min after oral dose)*	*Absorption (oral)*	*Renal excretion (% of unchanged drug)*	*Elimination life (h)*	*Elimination life of active metabolities (h)*	*Routes of administration*
Diazepam	98–99	95	30–90	Rapid	<2	20 (young adults) >30 (elderly)	>35 (*n*-desmethyldiazepam)	Oral/IV
Temazepam	95	76–96	90 (depends on formulation)	Intermediate	Very small	5.3–11.5	None	Oral
Midazolam	30–70	95	30	Rapid	<2	2–5 (young adults) up to 22 (elderly) 6–7 (neonates)	<6 (*l*-hydroxymidazolam)	Oral/IV Oral/IV/IM
Lorazepam	93	91	120	Intermediate	20	10–20	None	
Chlordiazepoxide	<95	96	2–4 h	Intermediate	<1	5–30	30–90 (*n*-desmethylchlordiazepoxide)	Oral/IV/IM
Nitrazepam	53–94	87	120	Intermediate	Small	18–57	None	Oral
Flunitrazepam	98–99	78	50–70	Rapid	<2	16–35	None clinically relevant	Oral/IV
Flurazepam	~100	97	30–60	Rapid	Small	2	36–120 (*n*-desalkylflurazepam)	Oral
Clonazepam	90	85	1–4 h	Intermediate	<2	30–40	None clinically relevant	Oral/IV
Zopiclone	80	45–80	90	Rapid	<7	3–4	3–6	Oral
Zolpidem	70	93	95	Rapid	?	2.5	None	Oral
Zaleplon	30	60	60	Rapid	<1	1	None	Oral
Alprazolam	28–33	80	60–90	Rapid	?	5–15	Very low concentration	Oral
Chlormetiazole	95	65	90	Rapid	<1	4–8 (young) 4–12 (elderly)	None clinically relevant	Oral/IV
Flumazenil	10	50	–	–	<0.2	1	None	IV

Table 10.2 Adverse effects of benzodiazepines

Common	*Occasional*	*Rare*
Drowsiness	Dry mouth	Amnesia
Dizziness	Blurred vision	Restlessness
Psychomotor impairment	Gastrointestinal upset	Skin rash
	Ataxia	
	Headache	
	Reduced blood pressure	

receptor subtypes and therefore tend to affect a number of functions.

Tolerance and dependence

The phenomena of tolerance and dependence are perhaps best illustrated by the effects of BDZs on rapid eye movement (REM) sleep. BDZ hypnotics initially suppress REM sleep from around 25% to around 10% of total sleep time after about 5 to 7 days of use. Adaptation then occurs (probably due to resetting of receptor sensitivity) and REM sleep returns to around 25% of total sleep time by around 14 days. Thus, tolerance has developed to the effect. However, if the BDZ is then suddenly stopped a rebound increase in REM sleep to around 40% of total sleep time occurs. This results in increased awakenings through the night. This increase in REM sleep takes around six weeks to return to normal.

Though tolerance appears to occur to the effects of BDZs on REM sleep it is not clear that it occurs to the hypnotic, or sleep-inducing, effects of these drugs. There is certainly evidence, using subjective measures, of effectiveness being maintained for up to six months. With regard to the other effects of BDZs, there is evidence from human and laboratory animal studies for the development of tolerance to the sedative, muscle relaxant, and anticonvulsant properties. However, evidence is equivocal with regard to tolerance to the anxiolytic and psychomotor effects. It seems clear that only some patients with anxiety disorders will begin to escalate their doses over time. Cross tolerance to other BDZs occurs.

The mechanisms underlying the development of tolerance seem to be partly pharmacodynamic, related to alterations in receptor sensitivity, but also cognitive, related to behavioural adaptation to the effects.

A withdrawal syndrome, often leading to reinstitution of use, occurs after sudden cessation of even normal therapeutic doses for six weeks or more. The symptoms of this are listed in Table 10.3, the most common being quite similar to those of the anxiety disorder for which the drug was first prescribed. Thus, withdrawal of a BDZ should be gradual, particularly if the person has been taking it for some weeks. A dose reduction by 25% every one to two weeks is recommended for long-term users. Propranolol may mitigate the symptoms of withdrawal but does not actually improve success in coming off and staying off BDZs.

Clinical use

Anaesthesia

In anaesthesia the therapeutic uses of BDZs include:

1. The symptomatic management of preoperative anxiety—oral premedication.
2. Sedation during unpleasant endoscopic, radiological, and other procedures—intravenous bolus doses.
3. Sedation in the intensive care unit—intravenous infusion.

Table 10.3 Benzodiazepine withdrawal symptoms

Anxiety type	*Disturbance of perception*
Anxiety	Hypersensitivity to stimuli
Dysphoria	Abnormal bodily sensations
Tremor	Abnormal sense of movement/body sway
Muscle pains	Depersonalisation
Sleep disturbance	Visual disturbance
Headache	
Nausea, anorexia	*Severe but rare*
Sweating	Paranoid psychosis
Fatigue	Depressive episode
	Seizures

4. Treatment of status epilepticus—intravenous boluses or infusion.

Temazepam, midazolam, and diazepam are the preferred drugs for pre-operative anxiolysis, being rapidly absorbed by the oral route and short acting after single doses. The choice of drug varies according to local practice and the availability of oral preparations. Because of concerns over its potential for abuse, temazepam in the UK is now stored under similar arrangements as those which apply to a controlled drug, such as morphine. Lorazepam is also used for pre-operative anxiolysis, particularly when it is desirable to dampen sympathetic outputs before major cardiac surgery. In these circumstances lorazepam may be given the evening before operation in addition to a second dose in the morning.

The BDZs of choice for intravenous sedation remain midazolam, diazepam (as an emulsion) and, in some European countries, flunitrazepam. These vary very little in their phamacological effects but it should be remembered that midazolam is twice as potent as diazepam and must be titrated slowly according to the patient's response.

Midazolam is the only water-soluble benzodiazepine. It is also available as a tablet and rectal suppository. It is the preferred BDZ for sedation in intensive care patients. It is particularly useful when given in combination with other drugs, such as alfentanil and propofol. Although the duration of action after bolus injection is short due to rapid redistribution, when administered for sedation as a continuous infusion for longer than 24 hours to critically ill patients, the duration of clinical effect is often prolonged, due to accumulation of midazolam and possibly also of α-hydroxymidazolam, the active metabolite of midazolam. Alpha-hydroxymidazolam is 60–80% as potent as midazolam, with an elimination half-life of about 1 hour in patients with normal renal function. The clinical effects of midazolam may be increased in patients with renal failure owing to accumulation of α-hydroxymidazolam. Following a continuous infusion of midazolam for 7 days the sedative effects of the drug may last for 2 days or longer after stopping the drug.

Diazepam is less suitable for use as an infusion on account of its longer half-life and the even longer half-life of its principal metabolite.

Given intravenously, both diazepam and midazolam are effective first-line treatments for status epilepticus. It is essential to be aware that the large doses that may be necessary to control convulsions are likely to cause respiratory depression and obtund protective reflexes. Oxygen and equipment suitable for its administration should be available. For intractable status epilepticus, clonazepam is a longer-acting alternative which can also be given by intravenous infusion.

Overdosage

Flumazenil is a competitive benzodiazepine antagonist with a half-life of approximately 1 hour. It is available only as an intravenous injection. Since its half-life is shorter than the drugs which it is used to antagonise, its beneficial effects are temporary. It is perhaps best used as a means of establishing a diagnosis before instituting appropriate supportive therapy. Flumazenil has been reported as inducing withdrawal symptoms in some habitual benzodiazepine users.

Psychiatry

In psychiatry, BDZs are used where moderate to severe anxiety symptoms arise due to acute stress. In such situations, their use should be short term, preferably for no longer than two weeks. Their main use tends to be in patients presenting with generalised anxiety disorder (GAD). Characteristically, this is a fluctuating condition with exacerbations at times of stress and chronic, milder symptoms on a longer-term basis.

Similarly, BZDs are used for insomnia but are best reserved for short-term use. They are also used to assist withdrawal from alcohol, where a long elimination half-life drug is best. In acute psychotic states short-term use of a high-potency drug, such as lorazepam, can be helpful in managing acute agitation or aggression.

OTHER ANXIOLYTIC DRUGS

Beta-adrenoceptor antagonists, particularly propranolol, have been shown to be effective for anxiety symptoms particularly in situational anxiety and GAD. Buspirone, an azaspirodecanedione, is an agonist at 5-HT_{1A} receptors and seems to have anxiolytic effects, though it is less potent than the BDZs and the effects take up to three weeks to become evident. There is high first pass metabolism and a considerable proportion of the effect is due to a metabolite (1-PP). The principal adverse effects of buspirone are nausea, gastrointestinal upset and headache. Antidepressant drugs, both the older tricyclic antidepressants and the newer drugs, have been demonstrated to have anxiolytic effects in mixed anxiety-depressive patients, GAD and panic disorder.

A number of new hypnotics became available recently (zolpidem, zopiclone, and zaleplon). These dugs, although not benzodiazepines, act via the $GABA_A$-receptor complex. They generally have shorter elimination half-lives, reduced risk of tolerance and dependence, and reduced psychomotor and hangover effects. Although clinical trials suggest similar potency to BDZ hypnotics this is not always the case in practice. The effects of zolpidem and zopiclone on sleeping patterns are not comparable with that of the benzodiazepines. They increase the time spent in deeper sleeping levels 3 and 4, and do not influence REM sleep and light sleeping levels. Side effects and contraindications to its use are similar to the benzodiazepines.

CLOMETHIAZOLE

This drug has sedative and anticonvulsant properties. Its use in anaesthesia is now almost exclusively reserved for the management of acute withdrawal syndromes in the intensive care unit. It is thought that clomethiazole enhances GABAergic transmission in the brain. At normal dosages it has little effect on the cardiovascular system.

Clomethiazole has an elimination half-life of about 4 hours after a single bolus. When administered by intravenous infusion half-lives approaching 20 hours have been reported. The drug is a very powerful inhibitor of the cytochrome P-450 system. It occasionally causes haemolysis.

BUTYROPHENONES

Haloperidol

Haloperidol is used as an antipsychotic and occasionally for control of acute agitation in the intensive care unit. It is can also be useful in the treatment of phencyclidine abuse. It produces a cataleptic state with little drowsiness and has minimal effects on blood pressure and respiration. It is a long-acting drug with a half-life of about 18 hours. It is available in oral and injectable preparations. In large doses extrapyramidal side effects may occur.

DROPERIDOL

Until quite recently, droperidol was used in combination with fentanyl to induce a state of anaesthesia which became known as *neuroleptanalgesia* or *neuroleptanaesthesia*. Droperidol induces a state of mental detachment similar to that induced by haloperidol, but its shorter half-life (1–2 hours) and powerful anti-emetic properties made it more suitable for use in anaesthesia. It was occasionally used for premedication. Unlike haloperidol, droperidol had α-blocking properties and could cause hypotension when given intravenously. Droperidol has also been associated with Q-T prolongation and ventricular arrhythmias, but this adverse effect has never been reported with the low doses used for anti-emetic therapy. Extrapyramidal side effects occur in overdosage. Sadly, in recent months the manufacturers have discontinued production of the drug.

ANTIDEPRESSANTS

Depression as an emotion is common and usually short-lived. As a symptom it can occur in most psychiatric disorders as well as other medical conditions, e.g. hypothyroidism, Parkinson's disease. As an illness, major depressive disorder (MDD), it is less common but, nevertheless, moderate to severe forms affect 5–10% of people in their lifetime and milder forms 20–30%. After a first episode, prophylaxis is required for at least 6 months and ideally 12 months to prevent relapse. This should usually be with the dose of antidepressant to which the patient initially responded. Those with recurrent episodes require prophylaxis over many years.

Classification of antidepressants

These drugs are most commonly classified according to their principal pharmacological effect rather than by specific chemical structure (Table 10.4). The exception to this is the tricyclic antidepressants which share a common chemical structure and also common pharmacological effects. The other important type of drug used in the treatment of mood disorders is the mood stabilisers (lithium compounds and some anticonvulsants) which are discussed in the next section of this chapter.

Tricyclic antidepressants

These were so named because of the three ring structure that is central to all of these drugs. However, if they were being named now they might more appropriately be called non-selective monoamine uptake inhibitors. Their principal pharmacological effects are inhibition of serotonin (5-HT) and noradrenaline (NA; norepinephrine) re-uptake into the presynaptic terminal, thus enhancing the effects of these monamine neurotransmitters at the postsynaptic receptors. Most of these drugs will also inhibit dopamine (DA) reuptake and are potent antagonists of the muscarinic cholinergic receptor, the H_1 histamine receptor and α_1-adrenoceptor. Although re-uptake inhibition occurs immediately on commencing these drugs onset of the therapeutic effect is classically delayed for around two to three weeks.

Pharmacokinetics

The tricyclic antidepressants are all lipid-soluble, are well absorbed from the gut, and are widely distributed in the body. Peak plasma levels are reached 2–6 hours after a single oral dose and elimination half-life is between 8 hours and 36 hours, generally allowing once-daily dosing. Most have active metabolites, also with relatively long half-lives. They are highly bound to plasma proteins (75–95%) and undergo extensive hepatic metabolism.

There is no evidence for a strong plasma concentration–response effect. An approximate 80–180 $\mu g \cdot L^{-1}$ 'therapeutic window' has been suggested for imipramine, with levels below this being unlikely to induce response and levels above being unlikely to induce additional improvement.

Adverse effects and toxicity

Sympathomimetic effects (from NA re-uptake inhibition) and antimuscarinic effects can cause a sinus tachycardia. Postural hypotension may occur as a result of sympatholytic α_1-adrenoceptor antagonism. With overdoses of these drugs, there is a reduced re-uptake of catecholamines, resulting in arrhythmias and hypertension. Tricyclic compounds have a high

Table 10.4 Classification of antidepressant drugs

Group	*Principal pharmacological effects*	*Examples*
Tricyclic antidepressants (TCAs)	Inhibition of re-uptake of serotonin (5-HT) and noradrenaline (NA; norepinephrine) in synapse Anticholinergic effects	Amitriptyline Clomipramine Imipramine
Selective serotonin re-uptake inhibitors (SSRIs)	Inhibition of re-uptake of 5-HT in synapse	Citalopram Fluoxetine Paroxetine Sertraline
Noradrenaline (norepinephrine) re-uptake inhibitors (NARIs)	Inhibition of re-uptake of NA in synapse	Reboxetine
Serotonin and noradrenaline (norepinephrine) re-uptake inhibitors (SNRIs)	Inhibition of re-uptake of 5-HT and NA in synapse Lack other effects of TCAs that give rise to many of their adverse effects	Venlafaxine
Atypical	Have some amine uptake inhibition but also antagonise one or more of 5-HT_2, α_1-NA, α_2-NA receptors. These receptor effects increase amine availability in the synapse	Mianserin Mirtazapine Nefazodone Trazodone
Monoamine oxidase inhibitors (MAOIs)	Inhibition of MAO types A+B and thus reduce metabolism of 5-HT and NA (These older drugs are non-selective and the effects are irreversible)	Isocarboxazid Phenelzine Tranylcypromine
Reversible inhibitors of MAO-A (RIMAs)	Inhibition of MAO-A in a competitive and reversible manner	Moclobemide

affinity for cardiac muscle. They produce a quinidine-like action on the electrocardiogram (ECG) and depressed myocardial contractility. The severity of the poisoning can be estimated from the degree of QRS widening. Once catecholamine reserves are depleted, severe cardiorespiratory depression and coma develop. Treatment includes gastric lavage, as the anticholinergic effects delay gastric emptying by 12 hours or longer. Supportive therapy should be aimed at correcting any electrolyte and acid–base disturbances as these contribute to arrhythmias. Pharmacological treatment of arrhythmias should be resisted if possible as this may potentiate the cardiotoxicity. Life-threating arrhythmias may develop even after the patient has apparently recovered from the overdose, and ECG monitoring should be continued for several days. Because of their large volume of distribution, dialysis is not helpful in reducing plasma concentrations of these drugs.

Sedation is common, particularly at initiation of treatment and is largely related to antihistamine and antiadrenergic effects. Weight gain may also be related to antihistamine effects. Some recent evidence suggests there can be impairment of psychomotor function but in the treatment of patients with depression this must be balanced against improvements in function resulting from improvement in the illness.

The antimuscarinic properties result in what are usually the most troublesome adverse effects: dry mouth, blurred vision, constipation, and (mainly in older males) urinary hesitancy and retention. Pupil size, and hence risk of glaucoma, is determined by a balance between anticholinergic (mydriatic) and sympathomimetic (miotic) effects.

These drugs lower the seizure threshold and this can occasionally result in convulsions. They should be avoided if possible in patients with cardiac disease, and are contraindicated after a recent myocardial infarction. There is no specific evidence of teratogenicity but they should be avoided if possible during pregnancy. Care is required in the elderly as they are more sensitive to the adverse effects, have a lower rate of metabolism and excretion, and are more likely to have concurrent physical disease (e.g. cardiac disease).

Tricyclic antidepressants have efficacy in other disorders besides depression. They are useful in the management of chronic pain syndromes, neuralgias, migraine headaches and sleep disorders.

Drug interactions

Co-administration with MAOIs can lead to a dangerous toxic interaction (see page 163). Though in the past such a combination might have been used for very treatment-resistant patients it would be very rare to consider it now.

Tricyclic antidepressants potentiate the pressor effects of directly acting sympathomimetic amines, such as adrenaline (epinephrine) or noradrenaline (norepinephrine), to cause hypertension. Small amounts of these, such as may be present in local anaesthetic solutions, can be dangerous. Tricyclic antidepressants will inhibit the antihypertensive effects of the older antihypertensive drugs, such as adrenergic neurone-blocking agents, e.g. guanethidine, α-methyl-DOPA, and clonidine.

Taken with alcohol they potentiate the sedative effects and impairment of psychomotor performance. Hepatic enzyme induction by barbiturates or nicotine may reduce plasma levels. Cimetidine may increase levels by enzyme inhibition. Some antipsychotic drugs may compete for similar metabolic pathways.

Selective serotonin reuptake inhibitors (SSRIs)

This is the most widely prescribed group of antidepressant drugs, essentially because of their safety in overdose and their relative lack of adverse effects in comparison to the tricyclic antidepressants. They are all inhibitors of reuptake of 5-HT with no significant effect on reuptake of noradrenaline (norepinephrine). The different potencies of the drugs currently available are illustrated in Table 10.5, together with details of other aspects of their pharmacology.

Adverse effects

Nausea and sometimes vomiting may occur because of activation of 5-HT_3 receptors. Tolerance generally develops to this within 7–10 days. A syndrome of agitation, which seems identical to the akathisia sometimes induced by antipsychotic drugs, may occur early in treatment in a small proportion of patients and is usually an indication to stop the SSRI.

Sedation is uncommon and instead many patients will find that these drugs may impair sleep, which is why the dose is best taken in the morning. There is also little effect on psychomotor function.

Occasional patients have a small reduction in heart rate but otherwise effects on the cardiovascular system are rare. Epileptic convulsions can occur but are rare and much less common than with tricyclic antidepressants. There is some evidence for potentiation of electroconvulsive therapy (ECT)-induced seizures. Sexual dysfunction is reported, principally delayed ejaculation and anorgasmia.

Drug interactions

Co-administration with other serotonergic drugs can result in development of the 'serotonin syndrome'. In this, the patient is initially restless and may have nausea or diarrhoea. Hyperthermia, rigidity, tremor, myoclonus, autonomic instability, and convulsions may

Table 10.5 Pharmacology of the SSRI antidepressants

SSRI	*Potency of 5-HT uptake inhibition*	*Metabolite activity*	*Elimination half-life (h)*	*CYP-450 1A2 inhibition (K_i)*	*CYP-450 2D6 inhibition (K_i)*
Paroxetine	+++	nil	20	++	+++
Citalopram	+++	+	36	+	+
Sertraline	++	+	25	+	++
Fluvoxamine	++	+	15	+++	+
Fluoxetine	+	++	24–72	+	++

develop with fluctuating levels of consciousness. Death may ensue. This risk is greatest with MAOI antidepressants but also exists with TCAs, lithium and L-tryptophan.

Fluoxetine and paroxetine inhibit cytochrome CYP P-450 2D6 and thus may affect metabolism of some opioids, e.g. codeine, oxycodone and tramadol, that are partly metabolised by CYP2D6, many antipsychotic drugs and tricyclic antidepressants.

Monoamine oxidase inhibitors (MAOIs)

The enzyme, monoamine oxidase, exists in two forms: MAO-A (intestinal mucosa and intraneuronally in the brain) and MAO-B (platelets and mainly extraneuronally in the brain). Serotonin is preferentially metabolised by MAO-A and noradrenaline (NA; norepinephrine), and dopamine and tyramine by both forms. The first generation MAOI antidepressants (phenelzine, tranylcypromine, and isocarboxazid) inhibit both MAO-A and MAO-B and are thought to work by increasing the availability of 5-HT and NA in the synapse—with longer-term adaptive effects occurring as for the TCAs. These MAOIs are 'irreversible', i.e. they permanently inactivate MAO. Thus, recovery of activity occurs slowly, over days, as new MAO molecules are synthesised.

Recently, drugs selective for one or other form of MAO have been developed as well as drugs that are reversible inhibitors of each form. The aim of these strategies is to develop drugs less prone to the tyramine interaction ('cheese effect') and which can be withdrawn or changed to another drug more rapidly. The only one of these in regular use is moclobemide, a reversible inhibitor of MAO-A (RIMA).

These drugs are rapidly absorbed and achieve peak plasma level two hours after a single dose. Although elimination half lives are generally short the irreversibility of the effect makes this largely irrelevant. Slow acetylators (approximately 50% of the Caucasian population) may develop toxic plasma concentrations with conventional doses.

Tyramine interaction

Tyramine acts as an indirect sympathomimetic to cause release of catecholamines from nerve terminals. It is present in a number of foods: mature cheese, yeast extracts, some red wines, hung game, pickled herrings, broad bean pods. Normally, MAO-A in the intestinal mucosa will metabolise tyramine absorbed from the gut. In patients on the older MAOIs, considerable amounts of tyramine will enter the circulation and this will lead to increased release of catecholamines stored in nerve terminals because the MAOI prevents their metabolism. For patients on RIMA drugs, high concentrations of tyramine can compete for MAO-A, thus mitigating some of the effects, and MAO-B is still available to metabolise noradrenaline (norepinephrine). MAO-B, however, has relatively much less effect on 5-HT and thus 5-HT function is still enhanced.

The clinical effect of a tyramine interaction ('cheese reaction') is a hypertensive crisis: flushing; severe throbbing headache; severe hypertension; tachycardia; pallor. There is a risk of cerebral haemorrhage. Treatment is by α_1-adrenoceptor antagonist (phentolamine or chlorpromazine) which is usually given intravenously.

Adverse effects and toxicity

These drugs are best avoided in patients with cerebrovascular, cardiovascular and hepatic disorders.

Some sympathomimetic effects may occur, mainly mild tremor and occasionally cardiac arrhythmias. Apparent 'anticholinergic' effects may also occur but these are the result of sympathetic potentiation in tissues with dual cholinergic/adrenergic innervation, e.g. pupil. Sympatholytic effects can also occur, principally postural hypotension, because of synthesis of relatively inactive 'false' transmitters, e.g. octopamine, in nerve terminals following inhibition of MAO and activation of alternative metabolic pathways.

Other adverse effects noted are restlessness, insomnia, peripheral oedema, and sexual difficulties.

Drug interactions

Tyramine-containing foodstuffs must be avoided. Hypertensive crisis has been reported during anaesthesia in patients taking these drugs. This has largely been associated with the concomitant administration of exogenous catecholamines. The administration of indirectly acting amines, such as ephedrine, are the most unpredictable in their response as degradation of monoamines at the nerve terminal is inhibited. Directly acting catecholamines are inactivated by catechol-α-methyltransferase (COMT) and are more predictable in their response than the indirectly acting catecholamines. Indirectly acting sympathomimetic amines, such as phenylpropanolamine or phenteramine, that are used as nasal decongestants or bronchodilators also pose a risk. These may be found in over-the-counter cough mixtures and will release the enhanced neuronal stores of pressor amines. There are also interactions between the tricyclic antidepressants (TCAs), SSRIs, and MAOIs, therefore combinations are therefore avoided except for occasional hospital treatment of the most treatment-resistant patients.

Hyperpyrexia and hypertension have been observed with the use of pethidine and MAO inhibitors. Pethidine is the opioid most commonly associated with an adverse reaction with MAOIs. Although only a small proportion of patients taking MAOIs will react adversely to pethidine, there is no sure way of predicting those in whom the combination could produce severe, life-threatening reactions. These can present in two distinct forms. The excitatory form is characterised by sudden agitation, delirium, headache, hypotension or hypertension, rigidity, hyperpyrexia, convulsions and coma. It is possibly caused by an increase in cerebral 5-HT concentrations due to inhibition of MAO. This is potentiated by pethidine, which blocks neuronal uptake of 5-HT. The depressive form, which is frequently severe and fatal, presents as respiratory and cardiovascular depression and coma. It is the result of a reduced breakdown of pethidine due to the inhibition of hepatic *N*-demethylase by MAOIs, leading to accumulation of pethidine. The risk of adverse reactions to pethidine may be less likely with the newer, specific MAO-A inhibitors. Interactions with other opioids, such as morphine and pentazocine, have been reported, but are less common. Other opioids appear to be safe in combination with MAOIs, with the possible exception of phenoperidine, which is metabolised to pethidine, norpethidine and pethidinic acid.

OTHER ANTIDEPRESSANT DRUGS

Other antidepressant drugs are listed in Table 10.4. Their principal pharmacological actions include inhibition of re-uptake of NA, 5-HT, or both, and they generally have some additional direct effects on specific receptors, which in theory should assist their therapeutic action.

The adverse effects of these drugs are potentially the same as for the tricyclic antidepressants but tend to be much less frequent and severe. Similarly, drug interactions are generally less of a concern.

MOOD STABILISERS

For patients with bipolar affective disorder (manic-depressive illness) lithium, usually in the form of lithium carbonate, has been the main prophylactic agent for the last forty years. However, during the last ten years certain anticonvulsants (carbamazepine and sodium valproate) have also been found to be effective.

Lithium

Lithium carbonate and lithium citrate are the most commonly used compounds. Lithium has effects on cation transport, on individual neurotransmitters (including 5-HT) and on intracellular second messenger systems. Which of these is key to its therapeutic efficacy is not entirely clear but, as for the antidepressant drugs, the net effects seem to be to enhance serotonin function and to stabilise the noradrenergic system. Once lithium treatment is established it is very important that it is not suddenly stopped as this may result in rebound hypomania.

Kinetics

Lithium is rapidly absorbed, reaching peak serum concentrations in 2–3 hours. It is not protein-bound and is excreted unchanged by the kidney at a rate proportional to the glomerular filtration rate. It is best given as a single daily dose around 22.00 hours and steady state serum levels are reached after 5–7 days of dosing, with the elimination half-life being around 10–24 hours for most people. Most proprietary formulations of lithium in current use are in the form of a slow-release preparation. There can be variations in kinetics between different proprietary brands and it is therefore best for individual patients to remain on the same brand.

Monitoring lithium treatment

Lithium has a fairly narrow therapeutic range, i.e. the gap between minimum effective serum concentration (0.4 $mmol{\cdot}L^{-1}$) and that causing toxicity (1.2 $mmol{\cdot}L^{-1}$) is low. It is therefore important to monitor serum lithium regularly. Serum concentrations above 1.2 $mmol{\cdot}L^{-1}$ must be avoided. It should also be remembered that toxicity can occur in a few patients at concentrations below 1.2 $mmol{\cdot}L^{-1}$ and that toxicity is always a clinical diagnosis.

Adverse effects

These are best considered under three headings: (1) minor, often occurring at the beginning of treatment with tolerance generally developing; (2) persistent and requiring monitoring during treatment; (3) toxicity, requiring immediate cessation of lithium. These are summarised in Table 10.6.

The management of toxicity requires monitoring of electrolytes, regular CNS observations, use of anticonvulsants should seizures occur, increased fluid intake to promote excretion (unless renal function is impaired) and cardiac monitoring. Haemodialysis should be considered if conservative measures are ineffective or serum lithium is above 3.0 $mmol{\cdot}L^{-1}$. However, it may be of limited additional value as the volume of distribution of lithium is high.

There is no final consensus on whether normal use of lithium, without any episode of toxicity (the vast majority of patients), may result in permanent renal impairment. Polyuria occurs in 20–40% and is due to inhibition of antidiuretic hormone (ADH) by lithium. It usually resolves on cessation of lithium as do any effects on glomerular function. Interference with thyroid function is due to inhibition of the action of thyroid stimulating hormone (TSH) and is easily managed by administration of thyroxine. Lithium is contraindicated during pregnancy (major vessel anomalies in fetus) and breastfeeding.

Drug interactions

Thiazide diuretics considerably reduce renal clearance of lithium and should be avoided. Loop diuretics, such as furosemide (frusemide), seem to have less likelihood of such effects but any drug affecting fluid and electrolyte balance

Table 10.6 Adverse effects of lithium preparations

Minor effects to which tolerance generally develops	*More persistent effects, some of which require to be monitored*	*Signs of toxicity that require urgent action*
Fine tremor	Polyuria and polydipsia	Dysarthria
Mild gastrointestinal (GI) upset	Hypothyroidism	Ataxia
Metallic taste in mouth	Lethargy Weight gain Persistent tremor T wave flattening on ECG Mild cognitive impairment Change in hair texture Mild leucocytosis Exacerbation of psoriasis	Coarse tremor Marked GI upset Impaired consciousness Epileptic seizures

should be used with care and with careful monitoring. Non-steroidal anti-inflammatory drugs (NSAIDs) inhibit prostaglandins and can therefore reduce sodium and lithium excretion and result in lithium toxicity. Paracetamol is safe in the correct dosage. Prolonged apnoea has been reported when patients on lithium were given succinylcholine or pancuronium. Cholinergics, such as neostigmine and pyridostigmine, are antagonised.

There are reports of interactions between lithium and carbamazepine, haloperidol, digoxin, and verapamil resulting in a variety of neurotoxic and cardiotoxic effects. These are not common interactions but clearly indicate a need for caution if such drug combinations are unavoidable.

Anticonvulsants

Carbamazepine and sodium valproate have been found effective both in the treatment of acute mania and in prophylaxis, particularly for patients with 'rapid cycling' illness (four or more episodes per year).

ANTIPSYCHOTICS

These drugs are the only effective treatment for schizophrenia, and are also used for the treatment of other psychoses. Low-dose antipsychotics are also frequently prescribed in the management of anxiety disorders.

Classification of antipsychotics

The first antipsychotic drug was chlorpromazine, introduced in 1952. This and others are listed in Table 10.7. Chlorpromazine is moderately potent in antagonism of D_1 and D_2 types of dopamine receptors but also antagonises a wide variety of other receptors—serotonergic, adrenergic, cholinergic, histaminergic—resulting in a wide variety of side effects. Other first-generation (often called 'typical') antipsychotics also had a wide spectrum of effects beyond the desired antipsychotic effect. Among the most problematic adverse effects of these drugs are the extrapyramidal side effects (EPSEs) related to dopamine receptor antagonism. Drug design to eliminate these problems is difficult because

Table 10.7 Classification of antipsychotic drugs

Drug group	*Examples*
First generation	
Phenothiazines	Chlorpromazine, thioridazine, trifluoperazine, fluphenazine
Thioxanthines	Flupenthixol, zuclopenthixol
Butyrophenones	Haloperidol, droperidol
Diphenylbutylpiperidines	Pimozide
Substituted benzamides	Sulpiride
Second generation	Amisulpride, olanzapine, quetiapine, risperidone, sertindole, ziprasidone, zotepine
Clozapine	Generally considered the prototype for other second-generation drugs but is more non-specific in its pharmacological effects and is more effective than all other drugs for treatment-resistant patients

the antipsychotic effect is primarily due to dopamine receptor antagonism.

However, there are now a number of second-generation (often called 'atypical') antipsychotics which have much reduced propensity to induce EPSEs. Most have a narrower spectrum of other receptor effects and a high ratio of 5-HT_2 to D_2 receptor antagonism. These drugs all differ from each other in chemical structure.

About 30% of patients with schizophrenia show no, or very poor response, to the drugs described above or may have unacceptable adverse effects. Around half of these will achieve better response on clozapine. Clozapine carries a 5–10% risk of neutropenia and 1% risk of agranulocytosis, hence its use is restricted to patients resistant to treatment with other antipsychotics. Regular monitoring of the neutrophil count is mandatory.

Pharmacokinetics

Antipsychotics are generally rapidly absorbed from the gut reaching peak serum concentrations in 2–4 hours. The elimination half-lives of most of the first-generation drugs are quite variable but are generally quite long—in the region of 20–30 hours, but up to 100 hours in some individuals. Many have active metabolites usually of lower potency at the dopamine receptor but often with much longer elimination half lives. Some, such as chlorpromazine, have a number of active metabolites. The second-generation drugs are also readily absorbed. Quetiapine and ziprasidone have short elimination half-lives (<10 hours) but the others have half-lives in the region of 20–30 hours. Active metabolites generally do not contribute significantly to the action of these drugs.

Adverse effects and toxicity

The number of different drugs and variety of adverse effects makes it impossible to comprehensively describe these. Table 10.8 lists the more important effects and the drugs most likely to give rise to them.

A rare, but potentially fatal idiosyncratic adverse effect is neuroleptic malignant syndrome. This can occur with any antipsychotic drug. The symptoms are rigidity, hyperthermia, autonomic lability, and reduced level of consciousness. Massively elevated levels of creatinine kinase are usually found. Prior to 1984, the mortality rate was around 25% but improved early recognition has considerably reduced this. Management is cessation of antipsychotics, appropriate conservative measures and dantrolene if necessary for muscle rigidity.

Table 10.8 Adverse effects of antipsychotic drugs

Adverse effect	*Drugs commonly causing this*
Pseudo-parkinsonism, dystonia, and tardive dyskinesia	First-generation antipsychotics
Akathisia (an unpleasant syndrome of mental and motor restlessness)	First-generation antipsychotics Clozapine
Sedation	First-generation antipsychotics Olanzapine, quetiapine, zotepine Clozapine
Anticholinergic effects (dry mouth, blurred vision, constipation, urinary retention)	First-generation antipsychotics
Weight gain	Chlorpromazine, thioridazine, olanzapine, zotepine, clozapine
Postural hypotension	Chlorpromazine, thioridazine, quetiapine, clozapine
Prolongation of QT_c interval on ECG (Though this may indicate risk of arrhythmia and sudden death)	All may cause this. Thioridazine and sertindole only available with ECG monitoring because of this
Elevated serum prolactin, galactorrhoea, and altered menstrual cycle	Varying degrees with all antipsychotics except olanzapine and clozapine. Most marked with sulpiride
Sexual dysfunction	Reported least in clinical trials with olanzapine and quetiapine
Cholestatic jaundice, skin pigmentation, skin rashes, photosensitivity	Principally seen with phenothiazines and mainly chlorpromazine

Drug interactions

Pharmacokinetics

Antacids reduce the absorption and enzyme-inducing drugs may decrease serum levels. Cimetidine and propranolol both increase serum levels. There can be competition for metabolic pathways by some tricyclic antidepressants (TCAs) and SSRIs (especially fluoxetine) which may increase serum levels.

Central nervous system

Phenothiazine-type antipsychotics will potentiate the CNS depressant action of many drugs including opiates and will potentiate the effects of general anaesthetic agents. All antipsychotics will antagonise the effect of L-dopa in Parkinson's disease, making management of this difficult where it co-occurs with psychosis.

Cardiovascular effects

Many antipsychotic drugs are α-adrenergic receptor antagonists and may thus enhance the effect of antihypertensives, including angiotensin-converting enzyme (ACE) inhibitors. On the other hand, the effects of the older adrenergic neurone blocking type of drug may be antagonised. Drugs which may also prolong QT_c interval should be avoided if possible.

11

Gastrointestinal drugs and anti-emetics

W McCaughey

Introduction • Pharmacological management • Proton pump inhibitors (H^+/K^+ ATPase inhibitors) • Mendelson's syndrome • Cytoprotectants • Mucosal protective drugs • Prokinetic and anti-spasmodic drugs • Laxatives • Anti-diarrhoeals • Nausea and vomiting • Pharmacology of anti-emetic drugs • Other substances • Non-pharmalogical therapy

INTRODUCTION

The stomach secretes acid and peptic enzymes in response to a number of neural and humoral influences:

1. *Neural*: vagal stimulation releases acetylcholine, which acts on muscarinic M_3 receptors, leading to increased cytosolic Ca^{2+}.
2. *Hormonal*: gastrin secreted by the G cells of the gastric antrum stimulates the parietal cells directly through gastrin receptors (increased Ca^{2+} as second messenger), and probably also indirectly by acting on enterochromaffin-like (ECL) cells to release histamine.
3. *Paracrine*
   - histamine acts via H_2 receptors to activate adenylate cyclase and increase cAMP
   - there also are H_3 receptors which reduce acid secretion
   - somatostatin acts via G protein-coupled receptors to *inhibit* adenylate cyclase (acetylcholine and gastrin may act in part through histamine release).

All these pathways converge to modulate the activity of the enzyme, H^+/K^+ ATPase, the proton pump of the parietal cell. This is a membrane-spanning protein, an ATP-dependent ion pump, exchanging K^+ and H^+ ions.

PHARMACOLOGICAL MANAGEMENT

Peptic ulceration has traditionally been managed by antacid therapy—drugs that raise the pH of stomach contents by directly neutralising acid, or by blocking acid production. However, mucosal protective agents are now finding a place.

In anaesthetic practice, pulmonary aspiration of gastric acid can cause a severe pneumonitis, and various drugs are used to reduce the acid content of the stomach.

Alkalis

Alkali antacids neutralise acid directly. *Sodium bicarbonate* and *sodium citrate* act rapidly, but have little buffering capacity. They are absorbed systemically, and repeated dosing may lead to metabolic alkalosis—the 'milk-alkali' syndrome characterised by hypercalcaemic alkalosis that can result from chronic intake of sodium bicarbonate along with calcium carbonate or milk. However, this is not a problem with single or a few doses given before anaesthesia. Sodium citrate is normally used as a 0.3 molar solution, in a dose of 15–20 ml. Sodium bicarbonate is very rapidly effective, but has the disadvantage that a considerable volume of CO_2 is produced, possibly increasing the chances of regurgitation.

Aluminium and magnesium salts, such as *aluminium hydroxide, magnesium hydroxide,* or trisilicate possess greater buffering capacity, and may be more appropriate for management of peptic ulcer symptoms. They are relatively unabsorbed (although absorption of aluminium increases by a factor of 10 if taken concurrently with orange juice or citric acid). These are particulate in contrast to sodium bicarbonate and citrate which are clear solutions, and aspiration into the lungs of particulate antacids can lead to damage comparable to that caused by acid gastric contents (see below).

There is evidence that antacids (particularly those containing aluminium hydroxide) have a protective effect on the gastroduodenal mucosa (see below).

Aluminium and magnesium containing antacids frequently affect absorption of other drugs, but most interactions can be avoided by giving the drug at least 2 hours before or after the antacid. These interactions may be due to reduction (Al) or increase (Mg) in gastric or intestinal motility, to adsorption of drugs to antacid molecules, or to alkalinisation of urine—so the resulting picture is complex. Magnesium (Mg) is associated with diarrhoea; aluminium (Al) with constipation.

Histamine H_2-receptor antagonists

There is a diversity of histamine receptors. The H_2, H_3 and H_4 receptors are of interest in gastrointestinal pharmacology. Histamine H_2 receptors are G protein-coupled receptors which act by increasing intracellular cAMP to stimulate gastric acid production, and blockade reduces acid secretion.

Pharmacokinetics

Histamine H_2-receptor antagonists are well absorbed orally, although concurrent antacid therapy may reduce bioavailability by up to 30%. They are widely distributed in the body, crossing the blood–brain barrier and the placenta. Cimetidine, ranitidine and famotidine are extensively metabolised in the liver, and about one-third excreted unchanged in urine, while only one-third of nizatidine is metabolised (Table 11.1). Elimination half-life is increased up to tenfold in renal failure, and doses must be adjusted.

Cimetidine and other H_2-receptor antagonists may also have an action at histamine receptors in other sites.

Central nervous system

Side effects, such as headache, dizziness, sleepiness, and even confusion and the delirium have occurred. These are rare, but most likely to occur with cimetidine which achieves the highest cerebrospinal fluid (CSF) levels.

Cardiovascular system

Histamine causes increased cardiac inotropic action and increased atrial automaticity acting through H_2 receptors in the atria. The most common side effect of H_2 antagonists, though still uncommon, is development of bradyarrhythmias following intravenous bolus or infusion of cimetidine, or less commonly another antagonist. In contrast, a slight inotropic effect of ranitidine has been described, perhaps due to action at H_2-presynaptic receptors at the sympathetic myocardial junction resulting in an increase in noradrenaline (norepinephrine) levels. An exaggerated effect of dobutamine can occur with cimetidine, due to reduced dobutamine metabolism.

Immune system

Suppressor T lymphocytes possess H_2 receptors and contribute significantly to the function of the immune system. Experimentally, cimetidine has been shown to enhance a variety of immunological functions both *in vivo* and *in vitro* because of its inhibitory effects on suppressor-cell function. This may include a degree of antitumour activity. Conversely, H_2 blockade may be deleterious in patients with organ transplant and autoimmune disorders.

Drug interaction

Cimetidine binds to cytochrome P-450 hepatic mixed-function oxidase enzymes. This leads to enzyme inhibition and reduced metabolism of

Table 11.1 Pharmacokinetics of H_2-receptor antagonists (modified from Shamburek and Schubert 1993)

	Cimetidine	*Ranitidine*	*Famotidine*	*Nizatidine*
Absorption				
Bioavailability %	60	50	45	95
Time to C_{max} (h)	1–2	1–3	1–3.5	1–3
Distribution				
V_D (L·kg^{-1})	0.8–2.1	1.0–1.9	1.1–1.3	1.2–1.6
Protein binding %	20	15	16	30
Elimination				
Plasma $t_{\frac{1}{2}}$ (h)	1.5–2.5	1.6–3.1	2.5–4	1.1–2.0
Relative potency	1	4–10	20–50	4–10

other drugs, e.g. benzodiazepines, theophylline, dobutamine, lidocaine (lignocaine), etc. Ranitidine has a 5–10-fold lesser effect, which is unlikely to be of clinical importance, and famotidine and nizatidine do not interact significantly with P-450 enzymes.

Renal clearance of creatinine, and of cationic drugs which undergo active proximal tubular excretion, is reduced by cimetidine and to a lesser extent by ranitidine.

PROTON PUMP INHIBITORS (H^+/K^+ ATPase INHIBITORS)

The membrane-bound H^+/K^+ ATPase enzyme exchanges H^+ and K^+ ions, resulting in a four million-fold gradient in $[H^+]$, between a cytosolic pH of 7.3 and an intraluminal pH of 0.8. Benzimidazole inhibitors, such as omeprazole, lansoprazole, and pantoprazole, bind covalently and irreversibly with the enzyme.

Omeprazole

This is a lipophilic weak base (pKa 4), which crosses cell membranes easily at physiological pH. It is a prodrug, which at the acidic intracellular pH in the gastric parietal cell converts to the active sulfenamide form, which is lipophobic and so is trapped and preferentially concentrated in the parietal cells. Omeprazole is highly protein-bound. Hepatic metabolism is rapid, with a plasma half-life of 0.5–1.5 h, but because of covalent binding to the H^+/K^+ ATPase enzyme, the duration of action exceeds 24 h.

Because of its pH-dependent structure, orally administered omeprazole would be prematurely converted by gastric acid and poorly absorbed, and it is therefore formulated in enteric-coated granules, and is absorbed where the pH is above 6.

As the H^+/K^+ ATPase enzyme or 'proton pump' in parietal cells is responsible for the final step in the process of acid secretion; omeprazole blocks acid secretion in response to all stimuli. Single doses produce dose-dependent inhibition with increasing effect over the first few days, reaching a maximum after about 5 days. Intragastric acidity is virtually abolished by 20–40 mg daily in most individuals, although lower doses have a much more variable effect. It is effective in healing ulcers which have failed to respond to H_2-receptor antagonists, and has been extremely valuable in treating patients with Zollinger-Ellison syndrome and reflux oesophagitis.

Side effects are few, probably mainly due to its selective concentration. Long-term use can result in hypergastrinaemia, which in animal studies has led to ECL-cell carcinoidosis, but there is growing evidence that this is of little, if any, clinical significance in patients receiving proton pump inhibitors.

Omeprazole can inhibit the metabolism of drugs metabolised mainly by the cytochrome P-450 enzyme subfamily 2C (diazepam, phenytoin), but not of those metabolished by subfamilies 1A (caffeine, theophylline), 2D (metoprolol, propranolol), and 3A (ciclosporin, lidocaine (lignocaine), quinidine). Since relatively few drugs are metabolised mainly by 2C compared with 2D and 3A, the potential for omeprazole to interfere with the metabolism of other drugs appears to be limited, but the half lives of diazepam and phenytoin are prolonged as much as by cimetidine.

Lansoprazole and pantoprazole

These agents are 'second generation' proton pump inhibitors. Their mode of action is similar to omeprazole. Structural differences give more rapid absorption and greater bioavailability of lansoprazole. Lansoprazole has less effect on P-450 enzymes, while interaction with pantoprazole is insignificant. Lansoprazole has a significant antibacterial effect on *Helicobacter pylori*.

MENDELSON'S SYNDROME

Prevention of pulmonary acid aspiration syndrome (Mendelson's syndrome) requires a combination of approaches, and only the pharmacological details will be dealt with here.

The main aim is to reduce both the volume and acidity of stomach contents. Many studies have taken a gastric volume of 25 mL and a pH of 2.5 as the 'danger level', but this is more a matter of statistical convenience than clinically proven. Vagal blockade using anticholinergics, such as glycopyrrolate, are effective in raising pH, but reduce the tone of the lower oesophageal sphincter, thus potentially increasing the risk of regurgitation. They also cause discomfort by drying up salivary secretion, and are thus not suitable in practice.

Alkali antacids are very effective at neutralising acid rapidly, but as described above, particulate antacids—especially aluminium salts, can cause pulmonary inflammation, and are no longer widely used. Non-particulate antacids, sodium citrate or bicarbonate, have not been shown to cause damage, and are used in conjunction with H_2 blockers. They will neutralise acid already in the stomach, although 'pocketing' of the stomach contents may prevent mixing with and neutralisation of all the contents.

Histamine H_2-receptor antagonists are the mainstay of prevention of Mendelson's syndrome at present. Probably the best protection is afforded by a combination of H_2-receptor blockade by ranitidine and a single oral dose of sodium citrate or bicarbonate. Because of its longer duration of action, and relative lack of enzyme inhibition, ranitidine is preferred to cimetidine for this purpose, although there is a latent period of 1–2 hours before it takes effect. Famotidine and nizatidine are probably equally effective in blocking acid secretion.

Omeprazole is more effective than H_2 blockers in producing achlorhydria when repeated doses are used in treating peptic ulceration or reflux oesophagitis. However, it is less effective than these in reducing volume and acidity of stomach contents when given as a single preoperative dose, and has no advantage over H_2 blockade in this situation.

Metoclopramide is frequently used in combination with antacid therapy. It increases the tone of the lower oesophageal sphincter, increases stomach emptying, and because of this may speed absorption of drugs absorbed from the small intestine.

CYTOPROTECTANTS/MUCOSAL PROTECTIVE DRUGS

Sucralfate

Aluminium-containing antacids exhibit cytoprotective activity or enhancement of natural mucosal defence mechanisms.

Sucralfate is a basic aluminium salt of sucrose, a complex of sucrose octasulphate and aluminium hydroxide. At acid pH (<4), it forms a very sticky gel polymer, which adheres to epithelial cells and the base of ulcer craters. It has little or no antacid activity, but more importantly has a major cytoprotective action, both protecting the mucosa from damaging influences and also causing accelerated healing. It appears to work through a number of relatively poorly understood mechanisms, enhancing several gastric and duodenal protective mechanisms—different actions may be related to its chemistry as an aluminium salt, and to the sucrose octasulphate component.

1. Interaction with local tissues. Sucralfate appears to augment the protective function of the 'mucous–bicarbonate' barrier, partly due to increased bicarbonate and mucous secretion, and partly to an interaction with the unstirred layer overlying gastric epithelium, as well as by making the mucous gel more hydrophobic. It binds bile acids and pepsin and adheres to both ulcerated and nonulcerated mucosa.
2. Increase in mucosal blood flow, with improved cell viability.
3. Stimulation of endogenous mediators of tissue injury and repair—it stimulates endogenous synthesis and release by the gastric mucosa of prostaglandin (PG) E_2, inhibits thromboxane release, and increases production of endogenous sulphydryl compounds. Sucralfate also increases binding of epidermal growth factor to ulcerated areas, stimulates macrophage activity, and also stimulates epithelial cell proliferation and repair.

Clinical use

Sucralfate is used in the management of peptic ulceration and of reflux oesophagitis, and its cytoprotective effects may be of benefit in radiation-induced mucosal damage elsewhere in the GI tract.

Prophylaxis of stress ulceration in intensive care units is the major interest to the anaesthetist. Here, it is given in a dose of 1 g every 6 hours via nasogastric tube. Several studies have shown sucralfate to be comparable in efficacy to H_2 blockers. It has been claimed, but not proved, to result in a reduction in morbidity and mortality from nosocomial pneumonias in comparison to H_2 antagonists. The latter, by raising gastric pH, eliminate the acid barrier to colonisation of the gut by pathogens, which sucralfate does not do.

Toxicity

Like other aluminium salts, pulmonary aspiration of sucralfate can lead to acute lung injury. There is some systemic absorption of aluminium, which is probably significant only in patients with renal impairment. Administration can be associated with a degree of hypophosphataemia, and there is also interference with absorption of some other drugs, e.g. quinolone antibacterials, digoxin, quinidine, and warfarin.

Misoprostol

Misoprostol is a synthetic PGE_1 analogue, which has a mild gastric acid antisecretory action, as well as increasing acid and mucus production. It promotes ulcer healing, and has a protective effect on the gastric and duodenal mucosa, reducing the incidence of non-steroidal anti-inflammatory drug (NSAID)-induced erosions, but with little effect on the renal effects of NSAIDs. Combined preparations with NSAIDs, such as diclofenac, are available. Side effects are relatively unimportant; mainly diarrhoea. However, prostaglandins do stimulate uterine contractions, and misoprostol has been widely used as an abortifacient by women in Brazil.

Bismuth compounds

Use of these as part of 'triple therapy' for eradication of *Campylobacter pylori* has been almost completely supplanted by antacid and antibiotic treatment.

PROKINETIC AND ANTISPASMODIC DRUGS

Gut motility depends on the functioning of the myenteric plexus (plexus of Auerbach), which may be regarded as a third division of the autonomic nervous system. Prokinetic drugs probably act mainly through cholinergic mechanisms, enhancing release of acetylcholine from cholinergic nerves in the myenteric plexus. This prokinetic action of metoclopramide and cisapride *may* be mediated through action at 5-HT_4 receptors in the gut wall. They have a partial agonist action at the 5-HT_4 receptors and at high dose also act as 5-HT_3 antagonists. Metoclopramide is also a potent dopamine D_2 antagonist both centrally and in the gut.

Metoclopramide and *domperidone* are discussed below in the section on anti-emetic drugs.

Cisapride

This is a serotonin 5-HT_4 agonist which acts mainly through cholinergic mechanisms. It is an oral gastrointestinal prokinetic drug chemically related to metoclopramide and domperidone, but unlike these compounds is devoid of CNS depressant or antidopaminergic effects. It has been associated with acquired long QT syndrome and ventricular arrhythmias, such as *torsades de pointes*, which produces sudden cardiac death. These cardiotoxic effects can be due to blockade of one or more types of K^+ channel currents in the human heart. These side effects are potentiated by drugs which inhibit cytochrome P-450 enzymes responsible for cisapride metabolism, such as macrolide antibiotics, leading to elevated blood concentrations of cisapride. It has been withdrawn from the UK market because of these cardiac side effects.

Anticholinergics

Atropine and related drugs act at G protein-coupled muscarinic cholinergic receptors. At least five muscarinic receptor genes have been cloned and expressed. M_1, M_3 and M_5 muscarinic receptors couple to stimulate phospholipase C, while M_2 and M_4 muscarinic receptors inhibit adenylyl cyclase. The cholinergic receptor on postganglionic intramural neurones of the submucosal plexus has recently been identified as an M_1 subtype and that on the parietal cell as an M_3 subtype. Cholinergic blockade can reduce gastric acid secretion by 40–50%. It is also used to reduce intestinal spasm, both therapeutically and to aid endoscopic procedures. Unselective drugs, such as atropine and scopolamine (hyoscine), are of limited use because of side effects, such as dry mouth and tachycardia. Selective M_1 blockade is as effective as atropine in reducing gastric secretion, and avoids side effects, but *pirenzepine*, a tricyclic antimuscarinic drug selective for the M_1 receptor, is no longer available.

Several other atropine-like drugs are used as antispasmodics. These include: homatropine, hyoscine, hyoscine-*n*-butylbromide (Buscopan), propantheline (Pro-Banthine). Some care should be exercised in their use in children and the elderly, as relative overdosage has been reported, leading to signs of hyoscine poisoning.

LAXATIVES—ESPECIALLY WITH REFERENCE TO TERMINAL CARE PATIENTS

The treatment of constipation and questions of use and abuse of laxatives are not normally of major interest to the anaesthetist. However, constipation is a particular problem in terminal care patients, especially where they are receiving opioid drugs for pain relief, and its prevention and management must be an integral part of their treatment. Both constipation and diarrhoea are problems in the intensive care patient.

A large number of drugs may contribute to constipation:

- Opioids
- Prostaglandin-inhibiting analgesics
- Anticholinergics:
  – phenothiazines, antiparkinsonian drugs, H_1-receptor antagonists, tricyclic antidepressants (anticholinergic side effects)
- Ganglion blockers
- Monoamine oxidase inhibitors (MAOIs)
- Verapamil

- Antacids containing $CaCO_3$ or $Al(OH)_3$
- Antidiarrhoeals
- Laxatives used chronically.

Two terms are often used: *laxatives* and *cathartics*. Cathartics produce prompt fluid evacuation, while laxatives produce soft-formed stools over a protracted period. Mechanisms of action vary, but the net overall effect is fluid accumulation within the bowel lumen by a hydrophilic action, an osmotic action and/or a direct action on mucosal cells to decrease absorption or to enhance secretion of water and electrolytes. Changes in Na^+/K^+ATPase, adenylyl cyclase and prostaglandins may be involved in these actions.

Bulking agents

These are mostly unrefined substances of plant origin, e.g. bran, etc. These preparations increase the bulk of stool and soften its consistency, largely by absorbing and holding water. They may diminish absorption of some minerals and drugs, but this is not usually clinically significant.

Faecal softeners

These include liquid paraffin (contraindicated if there is any risk of aspiration), and docusate sodium which is an emulsifying and wetting agent.

Saline and osmotic laxatives

Magnesium salts, e.g. magnesium sulphate (Epsom salt), sodium phosphates, and polyethylene glycol-electrolyte solutions, produce largely fluid stools, and are useful in pre-operative preparation of the bowel.

Lactulose

This is a semisynthetic disaccharide which is not absorbed from the GI tract. It produces an osmotic diarrhoea of low pH, and discourages the proliferation of ammonia-producing bacteria. It is therefore useful in the treatment of hepatic encephalopathy. Osmotic laxatives like lactulose, sorbitol, and lactilol rarely cause significant adverse effects. Glycerol suppositories are useful in softening and lubricating passage of inspissated faeces.

Stimulant laxatives

These are among the most powerful, but prolonged use can aggravate constipation. Mechanisms of action are multiple and not well studied. They include increased permeability of the mucosa leading to accumulation of water in the lumen, inhibition of intestinal Na^+,K^+-ATPase, and increased synthesis of prostaglandins and cAMP. Stimulant laxatives include the following.

Diphenylmethane derivatives

These include phenolphthalein and bisacodyl and are effective, but potential toxicity should lead to dosing being limited to 10 days. Bisacodyl is used for bowel evacuation prior to diagnostic procedures.

Anthraquinone derivatives

Danthron (1,8 dihydroxyanthraquinone) derivatives occur in senna, cascara, rhubarb. They are highly effective, and the main side effect is excessive laxative effect and abdominal pain. Danthron preparations should only be used in older patients and the terminally ill because of the risk of hepatotoxicity.

Unlike the bulk-forming laxatives, which are unabsorbed, the diphenylmethane and anthraquinone drugs are absorbed in considerable amounts, and excreted in bile, urine, and breast milk.

ANTI-DIARRHOEALS

Diarrhoea is often of infective origin, but management is generally non-specific. Diarrhoea is also common following antibiotic therapy which disturbs normal bowel flora. Replacement therapy using electrolyte solutions may be needed, and can be life-saving in severe diarrhoea, especially in children. Oral rehydration is preferred, although parenteral fluids may be required.

Other treatment is aimed mainly at decreasing discomfort. Bulking agents, such as methylcellulose, bran, etc., may be of use, but the mainstay of treatment of diarrhoea is opioid derivatives. These act mainly by an action at μ receptors, slowing transit time and thus allowing more time for absorption of fluids. They may also have an effect directly on the epithelial cells of the bowel to reduce secretion and/or increase reabsorption.

Opium derivatives, such as morphine and codeine phosphate, have been used for a long time, but the piperidine derivatives *loperamide* (Imodium) and *diphenoxylate* (Lomotil) are now preferred. Both are μ-receptor agonists, largely devoid of central opiate-like effects, and relatively insoluble in water, so that parenteral use and abuse are almost impossible.

A number of other classes of drug have shown potential in the management of diarrhoea. These include gut-specific α_2-adrenergic agonists, intestinal Cl^- channel blockers, somatostatin analogues, and calmodulin inhibitors.

NAUSEA AND VOMITING

Nausea and vomiting form a primitive reflex which developed early in evolutionary history, to detect and to expel toxic substances which have been ingested. Both central and peripheral structures are involved in the physiology of vomiting, and function together in an integrated way.

Central structures

The *chemoreceptor trigger zone* (CTZ) is located in the area postrema, close to the fourth ventricle, and is one of the four circumventricular organs which lie outside the blood–brain barrier. This allows the transfer of chemicals (endogenous and exogenous) directly into the CTZ from the cerebrospinal fluid (CSF).

The *nucleus of the tractus solitarius* and the *vagal nuclei* receive afferent input from the vagus nerve and are interconnected with the CTZ. The afferent inputs are modulated in these areas and then impulses pass to the 'vomiting centre' where, if appropriate, the emetic reflex is initiated.

The *vomiting centre* is located in the dorsolateral reticular formation of the brainstem, the Bötzinger complex. Here, the predominant transmitters (and receptor types) are serotonin (5-HT_3), dopamine (D_2), and acetylcholine (muscarinic M_3). This area coordinates all the events in the emetic reflex, which is a highly integrated physiological and protective reflex involving precise temporal coordination between autonomic and somatic motor components. The efferent stimuli pass via the vagus nerve to the upper gastrointestinal tract (GIT), the phrenic nerve to the diaphragm, and the intercostal nerves to the abdominal and intercostal muscles.

Peripheral structures

The vagus nerve is a major connection between central and peripheral components. It contains both afferent (80%) and efferent (20%) pathways from and to the upper GIT. These include both cholinergic and non-cholinergic nerve fibres; the non-cholinergic neurones may have serotonin as transmitter. Two types of vagal afferent receptors are involved in the emetic response: (1) *mechanoreceptors*, located in the muscular wall of the distal stomach and proximal duodenum, which are activated by distension or contraction of the gut wall; and (2) *chemoreceptors* located in the gut mucosa of the upper small bowel. These monitor the intraluminal contents and are activated by acid, alkali, hypertonic solutions and irritants. Serotonin is important in the transmission from these chemoreceptors. Enterochromaffin cells in the upper GIT are rich in serotonin and when stimulated release serotonin and activate the afferent vagal pathways.

There are also inputs to the vomiting centre from other sense organs, from cranial nerves and descending pathways from the cortex and hypothalamus. Stimulation of the vestibular system can cause motion sickness, and sudden movement of the head may potentiate opioid-related and post-operative nausea and so should be avoided as far as possible following surgery. The cholinergic M_3 receptor is probably dominant in this form of emesis. Behavioural and psychological inputs may also either suppress or activate the emetic response without pathophysiological stimulation. Learned responses can be important, and a memory can trigger nausea or even vomiting. Severe pain may also cause nausea and perhaps vomiting. All or any of these inputs may act together to reinforce each other.

Receptors involved in emesis

Four different receptor types have been the main focus of interest. These are muscarinic cholinergic, histamine H_1, dopamine D_2 (different from the vascular dopamine receptor), and serotonin 5-HT_3. In addition, neurokinin NK_1-receptor antagonists are undergoing early clinical trials.

Dopamine receptors are found in high concentration in the area postrema, which contains the chemoreceptor trigger zone (CTZ). Histamine H_1-receptors are concentrated in the nucleus tractus solitarius, which processes information relating to emesis, and in the dorsal motor nucleus of the vagus. This nucleus and the nucleus ambiguus also contain muscarinic cholinergic receptors, and these initiate motor components of vomiting.

In addition to these receptors, enkephalins may be involved in some parts of this process, while agents which act on gastric serotonin (5-HT_4), dopamine, and motilin receptors accelerate gastric emptying and relieve symptoms in gastroparesis.

Serotonin (5-hydroxytryptamine, 5-HT)

Serotonin is involved in a number of diverse activities, including an important role in emesis. Four main subtypes of 5-HT receptor have been discovered, each having specific roles. The 5-HT_3 receptor is a ligand-gated ion channel similar to the muscarinic acetylcholine receptor, whereas 5-HT_1, 5-HT_2 and 5-HT_4 are G protein-coupled receptors. 5-HT_3 receptors are located both pre- and postsynaptically on neurones in the central and peripheral nervous systems. In the CNS they are present in high concentrations in the area postrema, and peripherally in the upper GIT.

While the 5-HT_3 receptor is the most important in control of nausea and vomiting, others are also involved. 5-HT_4 agonists have prokinetic properties in nauseated patients with gastroparesis and functional dyspepsia. The 5-HT_{1D}-receptor agonists, such as sumatripan, are used in treatment of migraine and reduce emesis both in this condition and also in the cyclic vomiting syndrome, most likely via action on CNS sites.

Neurokinin 1, (NK_1, substance P)

Substance P (SP) is a member of the family of tachykinin peptides that also includes neurokinin A and B. Their respective receptors are tachykinin NK_1, tachykinin NK_2 and tachykinin NK_3. Substance P is best known as a pain neurotransmitter, but it also controls vomiting. In relation to emesis, its sites of localisation include the area postrema and the nucleus tractus solitarius.

Non-peptide NK_1 antagonists have shown considerable promise in alleviating emesis. The most recently developed compounds are highly selective, can cross the blood–brain barrier, and are orally bioavailable. They are effective against both chemotherapy-induced and post-operative nausea and vomiting. Unlike most other drugs, they appear to be effective in reversing established PONV and also delayed emesis following cisplatin, postoperative nausea, and vomiting and motion sickness. The first of these, aprepitant, is just entering clinical practice.

Postoperative nausea and vomiting and pre-anaesthetic fasting

Effect of anaesthetic technique

Many of the drugs used in modern anaesthetic practice have an effect on the CTZ and vomiting centre either directly or indirectly, e.g. stimulation of the vestibular apparatus, stimulation of the CTZ by opioid agonist drugs, and an anti-emetic effect of propofol or emetogenic effect of nitrous oxide.

Propofol

There is good evidence that propofol exerts an anti-emetic effect. The mechanism of this is unclear, but animal studies have shown that it may involve depleting the area postrema of serotonin as well as direct GABA-mediated inhibition, or inhibition of dopamine release in the brain. This probably requires a plasma concentration of over 350 ng·mL^{-1}, and therefore will be seen when propofol is used as an induction agent for very short cases, or when it is used as an infusion in longer cases.

Nitrous oxide

Nitrous oxide may cause gut distension and also increase middle ear pressure, leading to stimulation of the vestibular apparatus. Thus, it is associated with a very slight increase in the incidence of nausea and vomiting.

PHARMACOLOGY OF ANTI-EMETIC DRUGS

Anti-emetic drugs are used for symptomatic relief of nausea and vomiting and also in the prevention of these unpleasant symptoms in predictable situations, e.g. postoperatively or following chemotherapy and radiotherapy. A large number of differing drug groups and classes have anti-emetic effects along with other class-related side effects, e.g. extrapyramidal symptoms and signs with phenothiazine drugs. The development of more specific anti-emetics, of which the serotonin (5-HT$_3$) antagonists are the first example, has reduced the side effects of these drugs. Table 11.2 shows the broad classes of drugs with anti-emetic properties.

Anticholinergics

Hyoscine (scopolamine)

Hyoscine crosses the blood–brain barrier more rapidly than *atropine*, therefore some of the side effects are more pronounced with hyoscine. These include drowsiness, blurred vision, dizziness, dry mouth, and difficulty with micturition, while confusion may occur in the elderly. Efficacy in PONV is only moderate, and it is now rarely used. It is, however, a well-proven remedy for motion sickness, and an effect on the vestibular apparatus may contribute to its action. Here, it is given in the form of the hydrobromide (scopolamine), 1 mg of which contains 0.7 mg of the laevo-hyoscine base. Commercially available seasickness tablets usually contain 0.3 mg and one or two are recommended for protection for short journeys. Side effects preclude the long-term use of hyoscine for travel sickness.

A transdermal patch preparation is available containing 0.5 mg hyoscine. This is effective for up to 72 h, but absorption is slow, reaching a steady state plasma level only after 5 h, so that the patch needs to be applied early, i.e. 5–6 h before travel and similarly before surgery.

Phenothiazines

This group of drugs has a number of widely differing therapeutic indications. Only the phenothiazines with significant anti-emetic actions will be discussed in this section. Phenothiazine compounds share a common basic structure, and in general have similar actions and side effects. All have sedative effects and may cause extrapyramidal effects which might range from restlessness to an oculogyric crisis. The pattern of side effects will depend on the arrangement of side chains attached to the parent molecule, e.g. extrapyramidal manifestations may be greater in drugs with a piperazine ring structure. The symptoms abate with dose reduction or drug withdrawal. Occasionally, tardive dyskinesia may occur with prolonged use. Other side effects include blurred vision, urinary retention, cholestatic jaundice, blood dyscrasias, hypothermia, postural hypotension, and, rarely, neuroleptic malignant syndrome.

Table 11.2 Receptor site affinity of anti-emetic drugs (modified from Peroutka and Snyder 1982; Hamik and Peroutka 1989)

Pharmacological group	*Dopamine (D_2)*	*Cholinergic muscarinic*	*Histamine (H_1)*	*Serotonin (5-HT_3)*
Anticholinergics				
Hyosine	–	++++	+	–
Phenothiazines				
Chlorpromazine	++++	++	++++	+
Prochlorperazine	++++			
Fluphenazine	++++	+	++	–
Butyrophenones				
Droperidol	++++	–	+	+
Domperidone	++++			
Antihistamines				
Promethazine	++	++	++++	–
Diphenhydramine	+	++	++++	–
Benzamides				
Metoclopramide	+++	–	+	++
Serotonin antagonists				
Ondansetron	–	–	–	++++
Granisetron	–	–	–	++++
Tropisetron	–	–	–	++++

1. Diethyl aminophenothiazines

Chlorpromazine has direct effects on the CTZ and may also depress temperature control and prevent shivering. The effects are due to inhibition of dopamine centrally. It may potentiate the effects of hypnotics, sedatives and anaesthetic agents. It is rarely used in anaesthetic practice today.

Promethazine was first developed for its antihistamine effects but is more commonly used for its sedative/anticholinergic, anti-emetic actions, and prevention of motion-related sickness. The sedative actions are quite marked and last longer than the anti-emetic effects.

Dose: oral 10–25 mg, intramuscular or intravenous 25–50 mg.

2. Phenothiazines with a piperazine ring

Perphenazine is now only available in oral formulation. It is used less and less in anaesthetic practice, usually given with premedication (2–4 mg, 1–2 h pre-operatively). The anti-emetic effects are well recognised but there may be marked sedation. It has a role in anxiety states and in the management of psychiatric cases.

Prochlorperazine has less potentiating effects on hypnotics than chlorpromazine and does not produce lethargy and hypotension. It may be used in the treatment of migraine, Ménière's syndrome, and other labyrinthine disturbances, and is an effective choice in PONV.

Dose: oral 5–10 mg, intramuscular 12.5–25 mg; Sublingual 5 mg.

Trifluoperazine has potent anti-emetic effects but also causes marked sedation and extrapyramidal effects and is not used commonly as an anti-emetic.

Butyrophenones

Droperidol

Droperidol is the only member of this group used in anaesthesia. It is a moderately effective anti-emetic, and is used in the dose range 0.25–1.25 mg. Some studies have suggested that the lower dose is at least as effective as the higher. In the past, it was used in higher doses as part of a neuroleptic anaesthetic technique. After intravenous (IV) administration it is rapidly distributed, and eliminated mainly by hepatic metabolism, with a plasma half-life of approximately 2 h. Side effects include sedation or prolongation of recovery from anaesthesia; others are similar to those of phenothiazines. Dysphoria can occur, with restlessness and apprehension, but extrapyramidal effects are rare. A slight *α-adrenoceptor antagonist* effect may cause hypotension in some patients. It has no effect against motion sickness. Haloperidol has similar actions but a slower onset and longer duration of action.

Domperidone

Domperidone is structurally related to droperidol. It does not cross the blood–brain barrier to the same extent as droperidol so has fewer sedative side effects. It has an effect both on the CTZ and by a peripheral action on the stomach by increasing gastric emptying. Timing of the dose of drug is important for maximal efficacy.

Dose: oral 10–20 mg 6-hourly, rectal 20–60 mg 4–8 hourly.

Antihistamines

A number of antihistamine drugs also have anti-emetic properties, acting on the CTZ. They are useful in the suppression of motion-related sickness and also in emesis following labyrinthine disturbances including surgery. Most antihistamine drugs should be avoided in patients with porphyria although cyclizine and chlorphenamine are thought to be safe.

Cyclizine

Cyclizine is a piperazine derivative, with both antihistaminic and antimuscarinic effects—the latter may be responsible for most of its anti-emetic effects. (Dose: oral, intramuscular, intravenous 50 mg up to 3 times a day.) The main side effect is drowsiness and it is therefore less useful in motion sickness, although it is available as an over-the-counter remedy. Its antimuscarinic actions may cause a dry mouth and tachycardia. Although it is an old-established drug, several recent studies have suggested that its moderate efficacy and low incidence of significant side effects justify a resurgence in popularity as a first-line treatment for PONV. It is also prepared in combination with morphine (Cyclimorph = morphine 10 mg + cyclizine 50 mg) for ease of administration for the treatment of acute pain following surgery or trauma. However, there may be some risk in combining morphine with this—cyclizine has a longer half-life than morphine and tends to accumulate on repeated 6-hourly dosing. The combination has been criticised and implicated as a cause of pronounced sedation and perhaps respiratory depression, and its use has declined in the UK for this reason.

Cinnarizine is available only in oral formulation. It is useful in preventing motion sickness and reducing the symptoms from labyrinthine disorders including tinnitus and vertigo.

Dimenhydrinate has similar effects as cyclizine.

Chlorphenamine is effective in reducing pruritus from opioid drugs and may have synergistic activity with other anti-emetic drugs, although it is not primarily used as an anti-emetic.

Dose: oral 4 mg, intravenous up to 10 mg.

Benzamides

Metoclopramide

Metoclopramide is structurally related to orthoclopramide, a procaine derivative, and it can prolong the action of suxamethonium because of competition for cholinesterase. However, its common side effects are similar to those seen with phenothiazine derivatives. In high doses, a range of extrapyramidal symptoms may develop. The anti-emetic effects of metoclopramide are due to two main actions. Centrally, it blocks dopamine in the CTZ and peripherally, it hastens gastric emptying, abolishes irregular intestinal contractions, and increases the tone of the lower oesophageal sphincter. Recently, morphine-sparing affects of metoclopramide have been described. The duration of anti-emetic action is short so timing of the dose may be important and repeat doses may have to be given.

Dose: oral, intravenous 10–20 mg up to 3 times daily.

Serotonin antagonists

The development of specific serotonin antagonist drugs has added an important arm in the treatment of nausea and vomiting, whether from radiation and chemotherapy or postoperatively. The first clinically available serotonin antagonist was ondansetron, and a number of other drugs with similar activity are now available. The common side effects for this group of drugs include constipation, headache, dizziness, fatigue, headache, and transiently elevated liver enzymes. Cardiac arrhythmias, particularly prolongation of QRS, JT and QT intervals have been reported—probably related to a sodium channel blocking effect, but this is unlikely to reach clinical significance. This group of drugs has no sedative actions and does not cause extrapyramidal symptoms, in contrast to the other anti-emetics discussed above.

Ondansetron

This may be given orally, intravenously (IV) or intramuscularly (IM); the dose depends on the indication. For postoperative nausea and vomiting, common regimens are either 8 mg orally before or 4 mg IV intra-operatively. Increasing the dose does not significantly improve its efficacy. The doses used with chemotherapy are larger, especially with cisplatin therapy, e.g. 8 mg IV before, then 8 mg 2–4 hours later then 8 mg 12-hourly for 5 days.

Ondansetron is well tolerated by patients but may be less effective if vomiting is established or if the emesis is due to opioid analgesia. A number of comparative studies with other anti-emetics have appeared in the literature and ondansetron appears to be more effective than some of these drugs. However differences in efficacy from some older drugs are not always large, and advantage may lie more in a lesser side-effect profile of 5-HT_3 antagonists.

Other 5-HT_3 antagonists include *granisetron*, *tropisetron* and *dolasetron*. There are minor differences in their pharmacokinetics and doses are different, but there appears to be little difference in efficacy between them. Dolasetron has a moderate duration of action but is metabolised in the liver by a different pathway to the rest, which may be an advantage.

Cannabinoids

The cannabinoids have previously been noted to have anti-emetic properties and nabilone has been available for the treatment of emesis due to chemotherapy for some years. Recently, there have been reports of its use in preventing postoperative nausea and vomiting in gynaecological patients with some limited success.

Nabilone

This is used for control of nausea and vomiting in cancer therapy, but as yet has no licence for use in postoperative nausea and vomiting.

OTHER SUBSTANCES

Zingiber officinale **(common ginger root)**

Powdered ginger root has been used in traditional remedies for gastrointestinal complaints and is an excellent calmative. It has recently been studied in anaesthesia for day surgery, and initial reports have indicated a significant anti-emetic effect in comparison to placebo. The mechanism of action is yet uncertain, as is the active ingredient, but one constituent of ginger, galanolactone, has anti-5-HT_3 activity. Ginger appears to have effects in both motion-related and postoperative sickness.

Corticosteroids

These are used routinely in conjunction with 5-HT_3 antagonists in the management of chemotherapy-induced emesis, and more recently are becoming popular in management of PONV, most commonly dexamethasone in an adult dose of 4–8 mg, usually in combination with other antiemetics.

NON-PHARMACOLOGICAL THERAPY

Non-pharmacological techniques for the prevention and treatment of emesis include acupuncture and hypnosis. Acupuncture at the P6 or Neiguan point has been used with variable results in prevention and treatment of postoperative nausea and vomiting, and hyperemesis gravidarum. Acupressure using either digital pressure or an elastic band with a plastic stud (Sea Band) applied at the same point seems to have a limited effect. The use of hypnosis in patients with a previous history of severe postoperative nausea and vomiting has shown some effect but is not practical for mainstream practice, because of the large amount of time needed for each case.

FURTHER READING

Hamik A. Peroutka SJ. Differential interactions of traditional and novel anti-emetics with dopamine D_2 and 5-hydroxytryptamine3 receptors. *Cancer Chemotherapy & Pharmacology.* 1989;24(5):307–10.

Peroutka SJ, Snyder SH. Anti-emetics: Neurotransmitter receptor binding predicts therapeutic actions. *Lancet* 1982;i:658–69.

12

Diuretics

John P Howe

Introduction • Classification • Osmotic diuretics • Carbonic anhydrase inhibitors • Loop diuretics inhibitors of $Na^+/K^+/2Cl^-$ transport • Thiazide diuretics • Inhibitors of Na^+ channels in the collecting ducts • Mineralocorticoid-receptor antagonists • Side effects of diuretics

INTRODUCTION

Diuretics are substances that act on the nephron to increase the production of urine. True diuretics achieve this by modifying the solute content of the glomerular filtrate on its passage through the nephron. An important feature of the clinically useful agents, with the notable exception of aldosterone antagonists, is that they exert their diuretic effect from within the tubular lumen by decreasing the reabsorption of filtered solute, mostly sodium chloride. Their main uses are in the treatment of essential hypertension and oedema states. There is a wide range of drugs that can increase urinary flow, e.g. dopamine, theophylline, and digoxin, but these are not diuretics.

The two most important functions of the kidney are the elimination of waste products and the regulation of the extracellular fluid (ECF) volume. A basic knowledge of renal physiology is essential to the understanding of the actions of diuretics and should be obtained elsewhere. Some facts relevant to diuretic drugs are given in Table 12.1. The total daily solute load filtered by the kidneys is of the order of 50 mol and of this over 90% is reabsorbed throughout the nephron mostly in the form of the common cations and anions. Of the 180 litres of glomerular filtrate (essentially plasma without the protein content) produced daily about 70% is reabsorbed in the proximal convoluted tubule (PCT) secondary to the active reabsorption of Na^+ and it is the remaining 30%, still isosmotic, which is subject to the actions of diuretics. Because Na^+Cl^- is the major contributor to urine osmolality and osmolality is the major determinant of the bulk flow of urine it is not surprising that the important diuretics are naturetics that is they promote the excretion of Na^+ in the urine. As noted in Table 12.1, more than 99% of the sodium chloride and water filtered by the kidneys is reabsorbed under normal conditions.

Table 12.1 Normal values of daily solute load filtered by the kidneys

Typical 24 h indices		*Reabsorbed*
Filtered Na^+	25 mol	> 99%
Filtered Cl^-	20 mol	> 99%
Filtered HCO^-_3	5 mol	> 99%
Filtered K^+	<1 mol	> 90%
Renal blood flow	1800 L	
Renal plasma flow	1000 L	
Glomerular filtrate	180 L	
Urinary volume	2 L	

The therapeutic objective with most diuretics is to reduce the amount of Na^+ reabsorption and thereby reduce the obligatory reabsorption of water. The two exceptions to this general rule are acetazolamide and mannitol which do not act primarily on Na^+ reabsorption.

CLASSIFICATION

Diuretic agents are classified in a number of ways the simplest being in terms of efficacy. The most powerful drugs are frusemide (furosemide), bumetanide, and etacrynic acid and are described as 'high ceiling'. The thiazide and thiazide-like group are of intermediate potency. Spironolactone, amiloride, and triamterene are regarded as weak. A second and more common method of classification is by anatomical site of action on the nephron (Figure 12.1). The third method is by reference to the mechanism of action of the drug on ionic transport at the cellular level. The terms commonly used in this context are *symporter* or *co-transporter* (where two or more ions move across a barrier in the same direction) and *antiporter* (where two or more ions move across a barrier in the opposite direction). The movement of ions by a symporter or antiporter can be with or against a concentration gradient and is usually energy-dependent.

It might be anticipated that drugs acting on the PCT, where 70% of the glomerular filtrate is reabsorbed, would be potent diuretics. This is not the case because the Loop of Henle (LoH) is 'downstream' of the PCT and the LoH has a

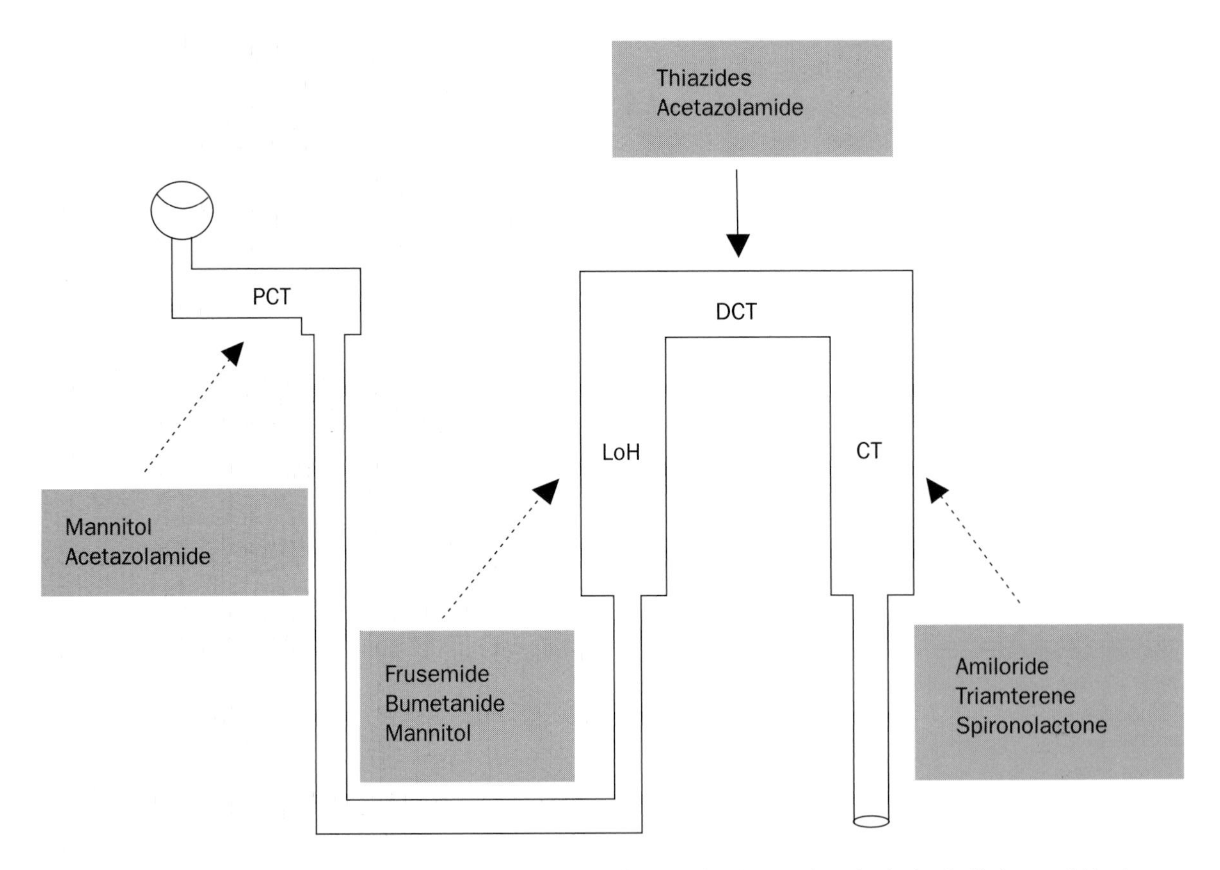

Figure 12.1 *Site of action of diuretics on the nephron. PCT, proximal convoluted tubule; LoH, Loop of Henle; DCT, distal convoluted tubule; CT, collecting tubule.*

large capacity to modify any filtrate delivered to it from the proximal tubule. The distal convoluted tubule (DCT) although 'downstream' of the LoH, lacks the same capacity to modify the filtrate emerging from the loop and therefore a loop diuretic will always be more potent than a thiazide.

As already noted, nearly all the diuretics in common use exert their effects from within the lumen of the nephron. These drugs are in general highly protein-bound and are not filtered by the glomerulus. Instead, in common with many other drugs and organic molecules, they diffuse from the peritubular vasculature across the basolateral membrane of the proximal tubular cells and from there are actively secreted into the filtrate. The efficacy of a diuretic depends not only on the mass and rate of delivery of drug to the filtrate but also on the body's state of sodium and water homeostasis.

OSMOTIC DIURETICS

These are substances that are freely filtered by the glomerulus but not reabsorbed by the tubule. They present a highly osmotic solute load to the nephron causing an obligatory loss of filtered water, sometimes referred to as 'solvent drag'. Agents available for this purpose are mannitol, urea, and glycerine although only the former is in regular use. There are probably several sites of action for osmotic diuretics with some variation among the different types. Mannitol increases the delivery of water and Na^+ out of the PCT and into the LoH and also increases the delivery of water and Na^+ out of the LoH and into the DCT. This latter action may be the more important of the two and is probably due to poorly understood interference with the transport systems in the thick ascending LoH. The pattern of electrolyte loss in the urine is similar to that of the loop diuretics following single administration namely an increased loss of Na^+, Cl^-, Ca^{2+} and Mg^{2+}.

Mannitol

This is an inert alcohol with limited clinical applications (Table 12.2). It cannot be given orally since it is not absorbed and causes profuse osmotic diahrroea. A typical intravenous dose is $0.5\ g{\cdot}kg^{-1}$ in a 10% or 20% solution. It is rapidly distributed throughout the extracellular fluid and is excreted unchanged in the urine. It has an elimination half-life of about 50 minutes. As would be expected, mannitol causes an initial expansion of the intravascular volume which may precipitate pulmonary oedema in susceptible patients. Anaesthetic use is confined to the maintenance of glomerular filtration perioperatively for example during hepato-biliary surgery and to the management of cerebral oedema. It should be used with caution in patients with suspected intracranial haematoma because of the risk of expansion due to extravasation.

CARBONIC ANHYDRASE INHIBITORS

Throughout the length of the nephron the sodium pump, Na^+/K^+ ATPase, is the driving

Table 12.2 Mannitol: indications and side effects

Indications	*Side effects*
• To reduce cerebral oedema	• Circulatory overload
• To reduce intra-ocular pressure	• Hyponatraemia
• To prevent peri-operative oliguria	• Hypernatraemia
• Forced diuresis	• Nausea and vomiting

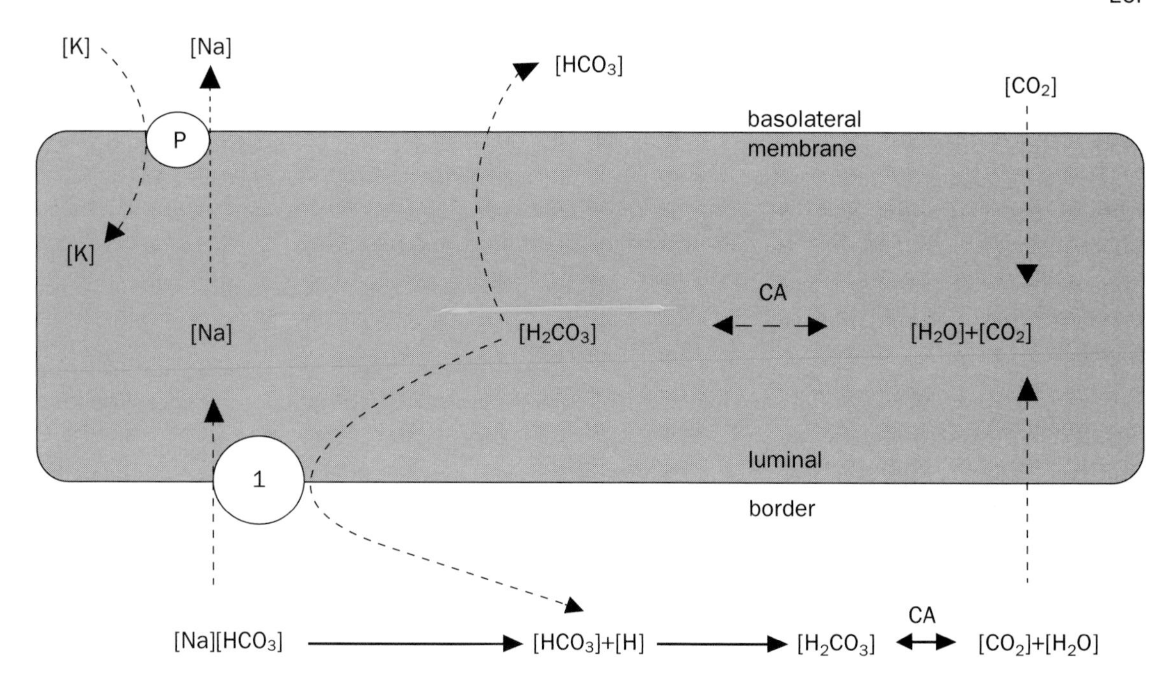

Figure 12.2 *Mechanism of action of carbonic anhydrase inhibitors on the proximal convoluted tubule. Carbonic anhydrase is an enzyme that catalyses the interconversion of CO_2 and H_2O to H_2CO_3 and is found in the luminal epithelium of the proximal, and to a lesser extent, the distal convoluted tubule. It is essential for the conservation of body base in the form of HCO^-_3. An antiporter (1) mechanism (the movement of substances across a barrier in opposite directions) exchanges filtrate Na^+ for cellular H^+. The H^+ combines with filtrate HCO^-_3 to form carbonic acid which is converted to CO_2 and H_2O in the presence of carbonic anhydrase (CA). The CO_2 is reabsorbed by the cell thereby conserving HCO^-_3. Acetazolamide inhibits the activity of carbonic anhydrase and limits the conversion of HCO^-_3 to absorbable CO_2. The concentration of HCO^-_3 in the filtrate increases as does the urinary loss. P, the sodium pump; ECF, extracellular fluid.*

force for the transfer of Na^+ ions from the filtrate to the ECF against a concentration (Figure 12.2). The pump derives its energy from the hydrolysis of ATP and the energy is used to transport Na^+ out of the cell and into the ECF in exchange for K^+. Each cycle of the pump exchanges $3Na^+$ for $2K^+$ ions.

The most important function of the proximal tubular cell is the conservation of filtered Na^+ and the reabsorption of water. The PCT is also the main site of HCO^-_3 reabsorption. This is achieved by the transfer of Na^+ and HCO^-_3 from the tubular lumen into the cell and then into the extracellular fluid (ECF) accompanied by the passive reabsorption of approximately 70% of the filtered water via the 'tight junctions' between the tubular cells. The presence of the enzyme carbonic anhydrase in the cytoplasm and luminal epithelium of the cells of the PCT allows the kidney to eliminate H^+ while simultaneously retaining HCO^-_3.

Acetazolamide

This is an inhibitor of carbonic anhydrase. It is a weak diuretic of pharmacological rather than therapeutic interest. The effect of acetazolamide is to limit the conversion of urinary HCO^-_3 ions to CO_2 thereby promoting the urinary loss of filtered HCO^-_3. The mild diuresis is due to the resultant loss of HCO^-_3 along with Na^+ in the filtrate. There is usually an increased loss of urinary Cl^- as well and the biochemical picture is that of a mild, hypochloraemic acidosis. Even though more than half the HCO^-_3 lost will be recovered elsewhere in the nephron, urinary loss of HCO^-_3 will eventually cause a decline in plasma HCO^-_3 and this becomes the rate-limiting factor. Moderate hypokalaemia occurs due to the exchange of intracellular K^+ for the increased Na^+ load in the DCT. Increased urinary excretion of phosphate is usually present.

Acetazolamide (Table 12.3) is a sulphonamide derivative and is well absorbed orally. It has a half-life of less than one hour and is metabolised in the liver. It is contraindicated in severe chronic obstructive pulmonary disease and in hepatic cirrhosis.

LOOP DIURETICS INHIBITORS OF $Na^+/K^+/2Cl^-$ TRANSPORT

The main function of the Loop at Henle (LoH) in the context of diuretics is further reabsorption and conservation of water and electrolytes from the remaining 30% of the filtrate emerging from the PCT. This is achieved by a combination of counter-current multiplier and counter-current exchange mechanisms in the LoH and the vasa recta respectively which first concentrate and then dilute the filtrate during its passage.

The thin descending part of the LoH is highly permeable to water. The progressive tonicity of the ECF from renal cortex to medulla encourages the movement of water out of the loop and into the ECF in the descending limb of the loop. The osmolality of the tubular filtrate increases as it descends through the LoH and can rise three- to fourfold by the time it reaches the most dependent part of the nephron. The thick ascending part of the loop on the other hand is relatively impermeable to water but is the site of extensive reabsorption of Na^+, K^+, and Cl^- ions which progressively dilutes the filtrate back towards isosmolality as it passes up the ascending loop. The LoH removes approximately 25% of the total filtered solute load along with an obligatory volume of water.

The reabsorption of Na^+ in the thick ascending limb is facilitated by a symporter (Figure 12.3). The symporter actively transfers $Na^+/K^+/2Cl^-$ ions into the tubular cell against a concentration gradient. The Na^+ ions are then transported out of the cell and into the ECF by the Na^+/K^+ pump as in the proximal cell.

The loop diuretics *frusemide, torasemide, bumetanide,* and *ethacrynic acid* (Table 12.4) inhibit the Na/K/2Cl symporter by occupying the Cl^- binding site. They decrease the reabsorption of Na^+ by up to 20% of the total amount filtered. These drugs are powerful naturetics; they can temporarily abolish Na^+

Table 12.3 Acetazolamide: indications and side effects

Indications	*Side effects*
• Raised intra-ocular pressure	• Metabolic acidosis
• Mountain sickness	• Nephrolithiasis
• Chronic metabolic alkalosis	• Drowsiness and paresthesia
• Epilepsy	• Allergic reactions
• Familial periodic paralysis	

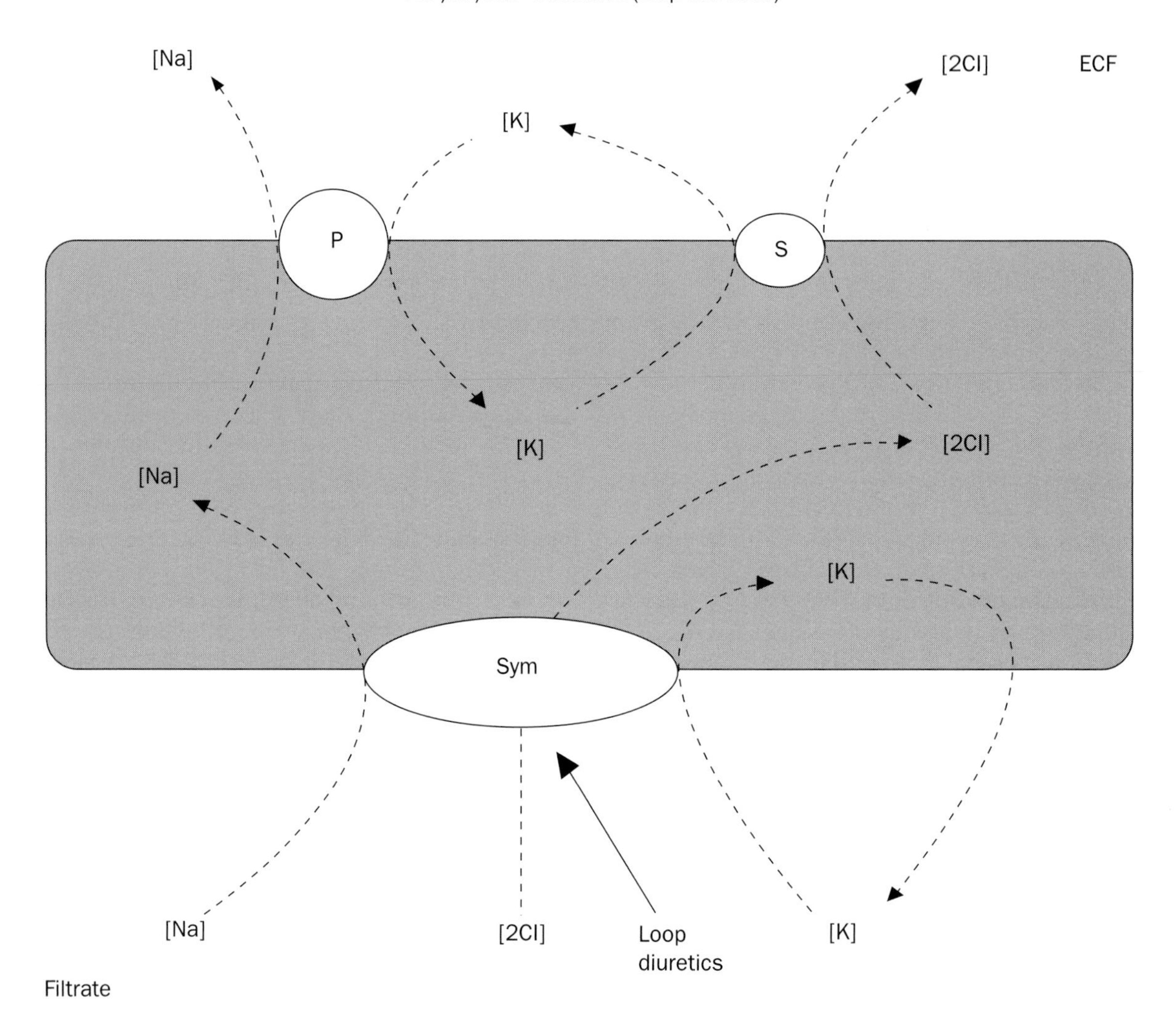

Figure 12.3 *Mechanism of action of $Na^+/K^+/2Cl^-$ symport inhibitors (loop diuretics) on the thick ascending limb of the Loop of Henle. Once again, the sodium pump (P) is the primary active transport system for the movement of Na^+ into the ECF. The symporter (Sym), also called the $Na^+/K^+/2Cl^-$ cotransporter, is the main mechanism for reabsorbing Na^+ from the filtrate in the LoH. The primary step is probably the transport of Cl^- ions. The symporter (S) is an example of secondary active transport in which K^+ leaves the cell with a concentration gradient and Cl^- leaves against the gradient. Approximately 20% of filtered Na^+Cl^- is reabsorbed in the LoH. Water moves from the filtrate through aqueous pores in the luminal and the basolateral membranes into the extracellular fluid (ECF) in response to the changing osmotic gradient produced by the movement of ions. Water can also pass via the tight junctions between the cells. Loop diuretics inhibit the $Na^+/K^+/2Cl^-$ symporter by competing for the Cl^- binding sites.*

Table 12.4 Loop diuretics: indications and side effects

Indications	*Side effects*
• Congestive cardiac failure	• Hypokalaemia
• Hypertension	• Hyperuricaemia
• Chronic renal failure	• Hyperglycaemia
• Ascites in liver cirrhosis	• Hypocalcaemia
• Nephrotic syndrome	• Hypomagnesaemia
• Forced diuresis	• Ototoxicity
• Hypercalcaemia	

re-uptake and can cause urinary Na^+ loss of up to 3 $mmol{\cdot}min^{-1}$. The increased delivery of Na^+ to the collecting tubules causes an increased exchange of Na^+ for K^+ and H^+ ions in the DCT resulting in hypokalaemic alkalosis. There is also retention of uric acid possibly due to competition between the diuretic and uric acid for the same secretory transport pathway in the proximal tubule.

Frusemide and bumetanide are derived from the sulphonamide group of drugs and have very similar pharmacokinetic profiles. Both are highly protein bound (>95%), both have a small volume of distribution (0.1–0.2 $L{\cdot}kg^{-1}$) and both have elimination half-lives of the order of 1 to 2 hours. Ethacrynic acid is not a sulphonylurea derivative but has a similar pharmacokinetic profile to bumetanide. Less than 20% of these drugs undergo metabolism in the liver, the remainder being excreted unchanged in the urine. Torasemide is a new drug and has a longer half-life of about 3 hours. The search for an ideal loop diuretic has so far failed to identify an agent that is not associated with chronic K^+ loss in the urine. Kaluresis is an inevitable accompaniment of loop diuretics (Table 12.4).

In general the loop diuretics are effective orally within an hour of administration. Given intravenously they have a peak effect at about 30 minutes and their duration of action is around 3 hours.

THIAZIDE DIURETICS

Inhibitors of Na^+/Cl^- transport

Only about 10% of the Na^+ filtered by the glomerulus is reabsorbed by the distal convoluted tubule (DCT) and therefore the capacity of the thiazide group of diuretics to influence the elimination of Na^+ in the urine is limited compared to the loop agents. Thiazides can prevent the reabsorption of up to 5% of the total filtered Na^+, whereas the equivalent figure for loop diuretics is about 20%. Thiazides can still produce a moderate naturesis and diuresis compared to carbonic anhydrase inhibitors and the K^+-sparing agents. Most thiazides are ineffective at low glomerular filtration rates. They also hinder the ability of the kidneys to produce a dilute urine.

The benzothiadiazides and the newer thiazide-like diuretics antagonise the absorption of Na^+ and Cl^- in the DCT by inhibition of the Na^+/Cl^- symport mechanism in the luminal membrane (Figure 12.4). They do not have any effect on the LoH. Some of the thiazides are thought to have a minor action on the PCT but this is minimal and is not due to inhibition of the Na^+/Cl^- symporter. It may be due to carbonic anhydrase inhibition which is a feature of sulphonamide-derived drugs.

The most frequently used drug is bendrofluazide and there are other very similar agents, including benzthiazide, hydrochlorothiazide,

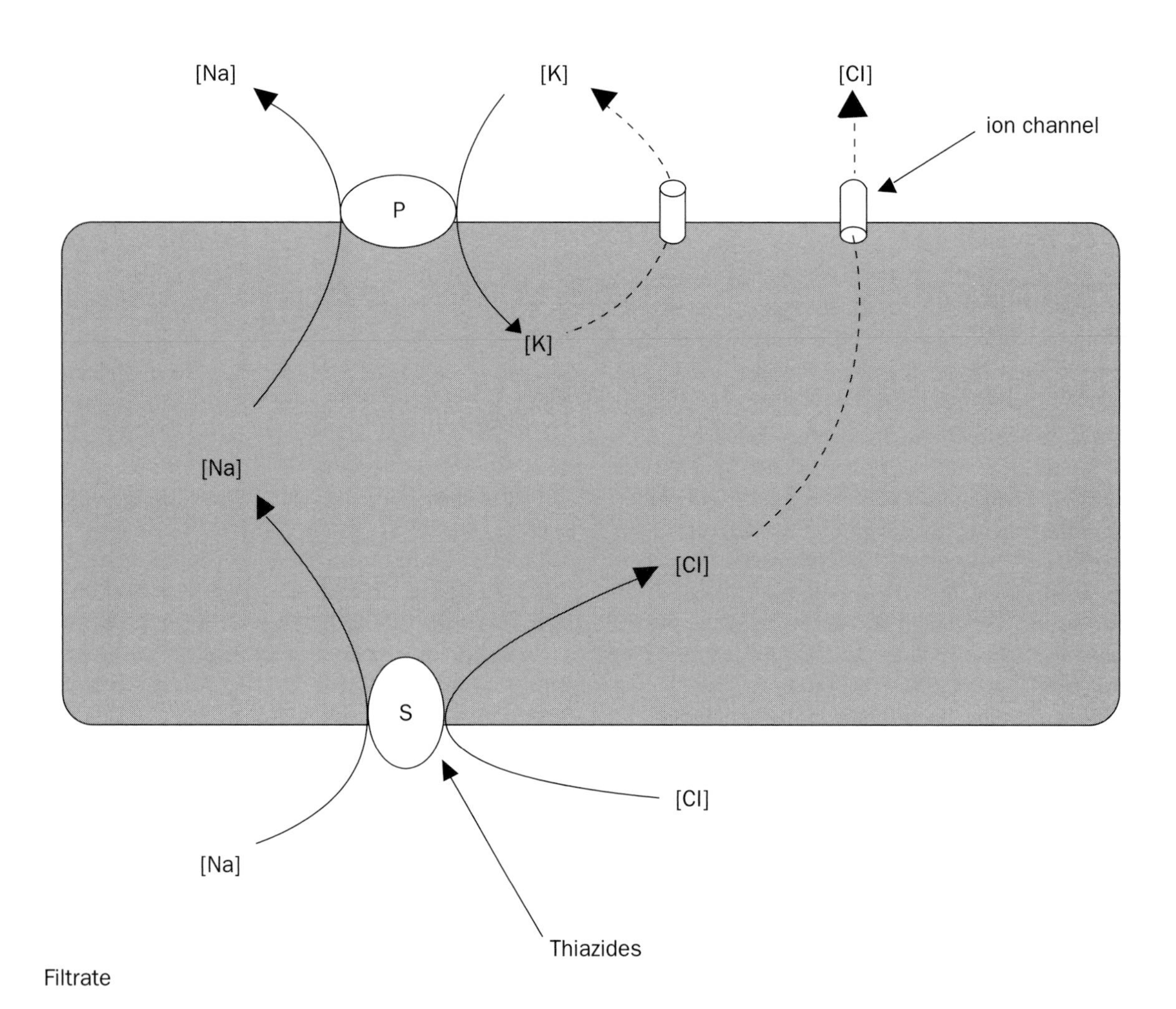

Figure 12.4 *Mechanism of action of Na^+/K^+ symport inhibitors (thiazides) on the distal convoluted tubule. As in the other parts of the nephron, Na^+ movement is powered by the energy-requiring sodium pump (P) in the basolateral membrane which exchanges intracellular Na^+ for K^+ in the extracellular fluid (ECF). The transport of Na^+ and Cl^- into the cell from the filtrate against the prevailing electrochemical gradient is facilitated by the symporter (S). The Na^+ ions are then transported by the pump mechanism described above and the Cl^- ions diffuse passively into the ECF through ion channels in the basolateral membrane. Thiazide diuretics inhibit the symporter by disabling the Cl^- binding site with the loss of Na^+ and Cl^- in the urine.*

and hydroflumeththiazide. They act within 1–2 hours of oral administration and have a duration of action of 12–24 hours with elimination half-lives of 5–20 hours. Chlortalidone is a thiazide-related compound with a longer duration of action and a half-life of several days. Indapamide is one of the newer thiazide-like drugs and is related to chlortalidone. It has a half-life of about 15 hours and has high bioavailability and high protein binding. The most common use of these drugs is in the treatment of essential hypertension where they have a dual action in modifying the volume and Na^+ content of the ECF and in decreasing systemic vascular resistance. The early decline in systemic blood pressure is due to volume depletion of the ECF but the long-term decline is due to vasodilatation. The newer thiazide-like drugs, such as indapamide, have a larger vasodilator component than the older drugs. The vasodilator effect is due to potassium channel activation of vascular smooth muscle and is a general property of all thiazide drugs.

The thiazides have a wide safety margin and serious side effects are uncommon (Table 12.5). Less serious side effects, on the other hand, are very common and among these hypokalaemia is one of the most troublesome. Hyperglycaemia is also frequent (see later). By their nature these drugs are often administered along with other non-diuretic drugs. Numerous interactions have been reported, including reduced efficacy of oral anticoagulants, uricosurics, and insulin. Thiazide efficacy is reduced in the presence of non-steroidal anti-inflammatory agents (NSAIDs). An unusual but potentially fatal interaction occurs in combination with quinidine when ventricular tachycardia has been reported.

INHIBITORS OF Na^+ CHANNELS IN THE COLLECTING DUCTS

Under normal circumstances only about 2% of the filtered Na^+ reaches the collecting tubules, the final regulators of the Na^+ and water content of the urine (Figure 12.5). There are two types of tubular cell in the collecting tubules, principal cells and intercalated cells. The principal cell is the site of Na^+ and H_2O reabsorption and K^+ secretion and the intercalated cell is the site of H^+ secretion. The principal cells are impermeable to Na^+ in the absence of aldosterone and impermeable to H_2O in the absence of antidiuretic hormone (ADH).

Amiloride and triamterene

These agents inhibit the Na^+ ion channel in the luminal epithelium. This causes hyperpolarisation of the luminal membrane and limits the transfer of cations across the luminal surface. Hyperpolarisation not only prevents the reabsorption of Na^+ but also reduces the excretion of intracellular cations such as K^+, Ca^{2+}, H^+ and Mg^{2+}. The ability of sodium ion channel inhibitors to reduce the excretion of K^+ is used to conserve body K^+ in patients who are taking thiazide or loop diuretics and for this reason they are more commonly known as the K^+-sparing diuretics. They are rarely used alone because their diuretic action is weak, instead they are administered in combination with thiazide or loop diuretics for their antikaluretic effect. Combination therapy is also synergistic when used in the treatment of hypertension.

Amiloride and triamterene (Table 12.6) are administered orally and have a relative potency of ten to one. Amiloride is poorly absorbed

Table 12.5 Thiazides: indications and side effects

Indications	*Side effects*
• Hypertension	• Hypokalaemia
• Congestive cardiac failure	• Metabolic alkalosis
• Chronic renal failure	• Hyperuricaemia
• Hepatic cirrhosis	• Hyponatraemia
• Nephrogenic diabetes insipidus	• Hypercalcaemia
• Calcium nephrolithiasis	• Hypomagnesaemia

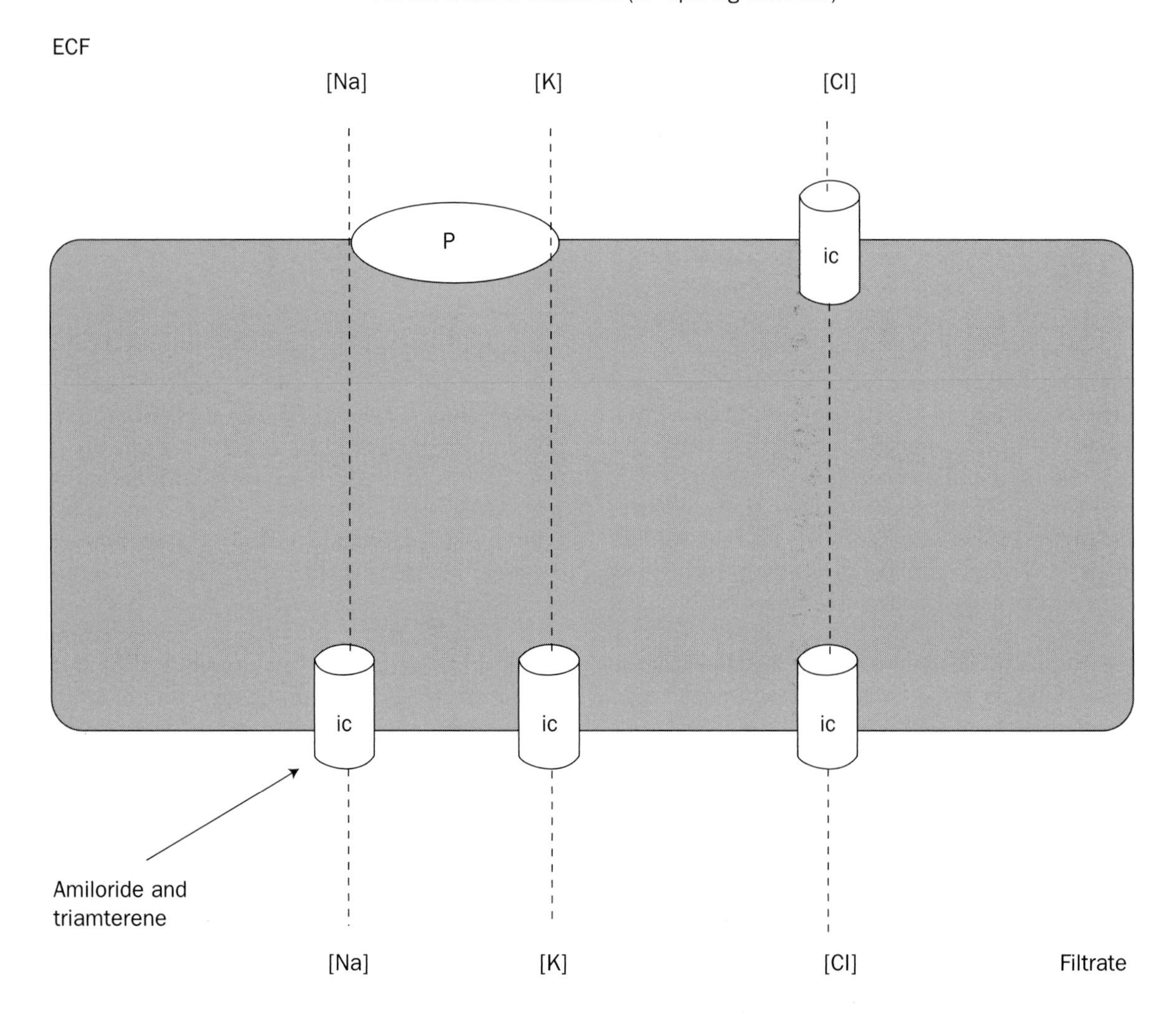

Figure 12.5 *Mechanism of action of sodium channel inhibitors (K^+ sparing diuretics) on the collecting tubule. The luminal epithelium of the principal cell of the collecting duct has an ion channel (ic) for Na^+. The high Na^+ permeability of the membrane, under the influence of aldosterone, allows filtered Na^+ to pass through and along the electrochemical gradient to the ECF established by the Na^+/K^+ pump (P). This causes voltage changes in the luminal membrane that aid the passage of K^+ out of the cell through a selective ion channel and into the filtrate. Amiloride and triamterene block the Na^+ ion channel resulting in a failure to reabsorb urinary Na^+ and a failure to excrete intracellular K^+. The precise nature of the channel inhibition is unknown. The reabsorption of H_2O from the filtrate occurs via luminal membrane channels under the influence of ADH. The secretion of H^+ by the adjoining intercalated cell (not shown) is aided by a proton pump. The H^+ is derived from metabolic CO_2 under the influence of carbonic anhydrase and is responsible for the acidification of the urine.*

Table 12.6 Na^+ channel inhibitors (K^+-sparing diuretics)

Indications	*Side effects*
• Antikaluretic	• Hyperkalaemia
• Combination diuretic	• Metabolic acidosis
• Pseudoaldosteronism	• Interstitial nephritis
• Cystic fibrosis	• Nephrolithiasis (triamterene)
• Lithium-induced diabetes insipidus	

orally, has a peak action at about 6 hours and a duration of effect of about 24 hours. The relative half-lives are approximately 20 and 5 hours, respectively. Amiloride is excreted unchanged in the urine. Triamterene is partly metabolised in the liver yielding an active metabolite, which is equipotent with the parent compound. It is excreted partly unchanged in the urine.

Hyperkalaemia, not surprisingly, is the most important side effect of these drugs and can be dangerous in patients who are taking K^+ supplements or other K^+-sparing diuretics. Concomitant use of angiotensin-converting enzyme (ACE) inhibitors and NSAIDs can also exacerbate hyperkalaemia.

MINERALOCORTICOID RECEPTOR ANTAGONISTS

Aldosterone is a mineralocorticoid hormone of the adrenal gland that stimulates retention of salt and water by the epithelium of the late DCT and CD (Figure 12.6). Aldosterone also increases the permeability of the tight junctions between tubular cells to H_2O molecules. Hyperaldosteronism is characterised by hypernatraemia, hypokalaemia, alkalosis and fluid retention.

Spironolactone

This is an aldosterone antagonist. It enters the cell by the basolateral membrane and forms a drug–receptor complex with the mineralocorticoid receptor. This complex fails to generate the aldosterone-induced protein (AIP) and therefore the dormant sodium ion channels and sodium pumps remain inactive. As a result Na^+ is lost in the urine and K^+ and H^+ are retained by the cell. The pattern of urinary electrolyte loss is essentially similar to that of the Na^+ channel inhibitors, amiloride and triamterene. Water loss also occurs by a decrease in the permeability of the tight junctions.

Spironolactone is well absorbed orally, is subject to significant first pass metabolism, and undergoes enterohepatic recirculation. It is highly protein-bound and has a very short half-life of the order of minutes. It is likely that the active component is a metabolite, canrenone, which has a half-life of 15 hours. The drug is most commonly used in conjunction with other diuretics as a K^+-sparing agent in the treatment of hypertension and oedema. It is the drug of choice in conditions where fluid retention is associated with secondary hyperaldosteronism, such as hepatic cirrhosis, nephrotic syndrome and chronic heart failure (Table 12.7).

Side effects are similar to the Na^+ channel inhibitors, i.e. hyperkalaemia and metabolic acidosis. Side effects like gynacomastia and impotence are related to the steroid origin of the drug. It is contraindicated in patients with peptic ulceration.

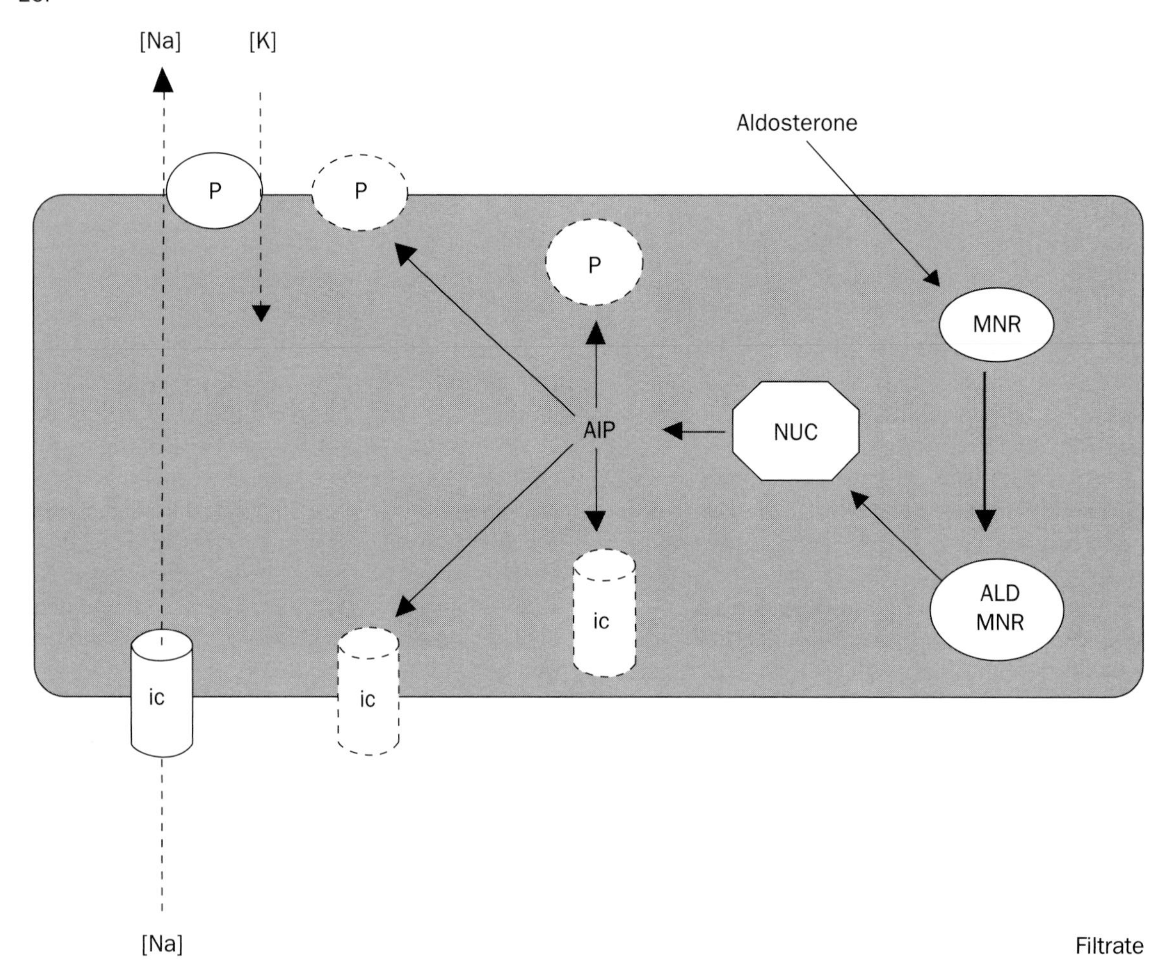

Figure 12.6 *Mechanism of action of mineralocorticoid receptor antagonists in the collecting tubule. Aldosterone enters the tubular cell by the basolateral surface and binds to a specific mineralocorticoid receptor (MNR) in the cytoplasm. The hormone receptor complex triggers the production of an aldosterone-induced protein (AIP) by the cell nucleus (NUC). The AIP acts on the sodium ion channel (ic) to augment the transport of* Na^+ *across the basolateral membrane and in to the cell. An increase in AIP activity leads to the recruitment of dormant sodium ion channels and Na pumps (P) in the cell membrane. AIP also leads to the synthesis of new channels and pumps within the cell. The increase in* Na^+ *conductance causes electrical changes in the luminal membrane that favour the excretion of intracellular cations, such as* K^+ *and* H^+*. Spironolactone competes with aldosterone for the binding site on the MNR and forms a complex which does not excite the production of AIP by the nucleus.*

Table 12.7 Aldosterone antagonists

Indications	*Side effects*
• K^+-sparing diuretic • Primary aldosteronism • Secondary aldosteronism	• Hyperkalaemia • Metabolic acidosis • Gynacomastia • Gastric erosion

SIDE EFFECTS OF DIURETICS

Diuretics are among the most commonly used drugs and are often administered over lengthy periods. Side effects are frequent, particularly in the elderly but tend not to be dangerous. Many of them are common to the different drug groups.

Volume depletion of some degree occurs with all diuretics following prolonged use. This can cause problems, such as postural hypotension, in those with poor cardiac function. Volume depletion also causes a fall in glomerular filtration that can trigger homeostatic reflexes such as increased aldosterone and antidiuretic hormone secretion. This contributes to electrolyte disturbances, such as hypokalaemia and metabolic alkalosis.

Hyponatraemia is common with the thiazides and to a lesser extent with the loop diuretics. It occurs when the osmolality of the urine persistently exceeds that of the fluid intake and is associated with the inability of the kidney to produce a dilute urine. It is not usually severe. The origin is multifactorial and involves unrestricted fluid intake and increased ADH activity due to volume depletion. Co-administration of dipsogenic drugs, such as the tricyclic antidepressants, or those with ADH-like effects, such as chlorpropamide, can exacerbate the problem. There are rare occasions when hyponatraemia (Na^+ concentration less than 100 $mmol{\cdot}L^{-1}$) can be of sufficient severity to be life threatening.

Hypokalaemia is very common and can occur with any diuretic except the K^+-sparing agents. Thiazides are more kaluretic than loop diuretics. A fall in total body K^+ is very common and a fall in plasma K^+ also occurs in more than half the patients taking thiazides. Normal K^+ loss is of the order of 1 $mmol{\cdot}kg^{-1}day^{-1}$ but can rise by as much as tenfold during diuretic therapy. Once again the origin is multifactorial. The delivery of larger than normal amounts of Na^+ to the distal portion of the nephron promotes an exchange for intracellular K^+ across the basolateral membrane. Unrestricted Na^+ intake will have a similar effect. Volume depletion stimulates aldosterone secretion leading to Na^+ conservation and K^+ loss in the DCT. The increase in urinary flow also attracts an obligatory K^+ loss. Prevention of hypokalaemia can be achieved with the aid of K^+ supplementation and K^+-sparing diuretics. The incidence of hypokalaemia is reduced in patients taking ACE inhibitors and NSAIDs and in those on restricted Na^+ intake.

Hyperkalaemia occurs occasionally with K^+-sparing agents and can be dangerous. It is most likely to occur in those on concomitant drug therapy, which raises serum K^+. It is also more likely in those with a low GFR.

Calcium and *magnesium* homeostasis is altered by chronic diuretic therapy. Loop diuretics increase the urinary excretion of Ca^{2+} and can lead to stone formation. Thiazide administration, on the other hand, has the opposite effect and causes frank hypercalcaemia in some patients. Both thiazide and loop drugs increase the urinary loss of Mg^{2+} and this has been associated with cardiac arrythmias in the elderly.

Acidosis and *alkalosis* are infrequent. Metabolic acidosis is a side effect of acetazolamide therapy and is due to bicarbonate loss in the PCT. All the K^+-sparing diuretics can cause metabolic acidosis by H^+ retention in the cells of the collecting duct. Metabolic alkalosis is associated with the loop and thiazide drugs. Reflex responses to volume depletion cause reabsorption of HCO^-_3 in the PCT and H^+ secretion in the collecting tubule.

Hyperuricaemia is very common with chronic diuretic therapy but frank gout is not. Uric acid reabsorption in the PCT is increased and is related to activation of the ACE system secondary to volume depletion. Diuretics and uric acid also compete for the same secretory mechanism in the PCT.

Glucose intolerance is seen with thiazide and to a lesser extent the loop diuretics. It appears to be dose-related and is more common with the long-acting agents, such as chlortalidone. The K^+-sparing drugs do not have this problem. The mechanism is a combination of peripheral insulin resistance and depressed insulin secretion. The condition is associated with derangement of K^+ homeostasis. Activation of K^+ channels, a feature of thiazides, is associated with insulin resistance. Glucose intolerance is reversible on withdrawal of the drug. A hyperosmolar non-ketotic syndrome has been associated with the joint administration of thiazide and loop drugs.

13

Drugs acting on the endocrine system

Vesna Novak-Jankovič and Adela Stecher

Introduction • Hypothalamo-pituitary function • Anterior pituitary hormones • Posterior pituitary hormones • Adrenal cortex • Adrenal medulla • Thyroid • Pancreas

INTRODUCTION

Pathology of the endocrine system (and especially diabetes mellitus) is relatively common in patients presenting for surgery. Patients with pre-existing endocrine disease are at an increased risk for developing multiorgan dysfunction in the peri-operative period. Anaesthetists should therefore have a knowledge about the physiology of the endocrine system, underlying endocrine disease and concomitant therapy. The physiology of the endocrine system is covered in detail in our companion volume, Physiology for Anaesthesiologists (Wallace 2004), and only the essential details will be summarised here.

HYPOTHALAMO-PITUITARY FUNCTION

The hypothalamus plays a central role in the coordination of homeostatic mechanisms, receiving and integrating information from peripheral sources. It influences the pituitary gland through polypeptide-releasing factors that cause the release of a variety of pituitary hormones (Table 13.1).

ANTERIOR PITUITARY HORMONES

Human growth hormone (HGH)

HGH, released in a pulsatile fashion with secretory peaks occurring every 3–4 hours, stimulates growth of all tissues, including linear bone growth. After epiphyseal closure, excess secretion of growth hormone, usually from adenomas, produces acromegaly. Acromegaly is characterised by enlargement of the hands, feet, nose, and jaw with thickening of the tongue, which may cause practical problems for the anaesthetist. Diabetes mellitus, hypertension and cardiac problems are also common. The primary treatment is surgery, then irradiation and drug therapy. HGH secretion by adenomas can be suppressed by a dopaminergic agonist, such as bromocriptine. Long-acting analogues of somatostatin, such as octreotide, are more effective than bromocriptine, but the need for parenteral administration limits their use. Bromocriptine is also used in the treatment of hyperprolactinaemia resulting from pituitary tumours.

Adrenocorticotrophic hormone (ACTH)

ACTH stimulates the adrenal cortex to secrete glucocorticoids, mineralocorticoids and

Table 13.1 Hypothalamic and pituitary hormones

Hypothalamic hormone	*Pituitary hormone*	*Source*	*Principal effects of pituitary hormone*
Human growth hormone-releasing hormone and -inhibiting hormone (somatostatin)	Human growth hormone (HGH)	Anterior pituitary	Stimulates body cell growth
Prolactin-releasing factor and -inhibiting factor	Prolactin	Anterior pituitary	Stimulates breast growth and secretion of milk
Luteinizing hormone-releasing hormone	Luteinizing hormone (LH); Follicle-stimulating hormone (FSH)	Anterior pituitary	Promotes gametogenesis and gonadal steroid hormone production
Corticotropin-releasing factor (CRF)	Adrenocorticotrophic hormone (ACTH); Melanocyte-stimulating hormone (MSH); β-lipotropin and endorphins	Anterior pituitary	Stimulates adrenal cortex to secrete glucocorticoids, mineralocorticoids, and androgens; stimulates melanocytes; endorphin synthesis
Thyrotropin-releasing hormone	Thyroid-stimulating hormone (TSH)	Anterior pituitary	Stimulates secretion of thyroid hormones
–	Antidiuretic hormone (ADH) (vasopressin)	Posterior pituitary	Promotes water retention and vasoconstriction
–	Oxytocin	Posterior pituitary	Stimulates ejection of milk and uterine contractions

androgens. Increased plasma concentrations of cortisol inhibit ACTH release by a negative feedback mechanism (Figure 13.1). ACTH secretion is inhibited by increased cortisol concentrations and with chronic administration of corticosteroids. Chronic corticosteroid therapy leads to functional atrophy on the hypothalamic-pituitary-adrenal axis. The clinical condition resulting from excess ACTH production by a pituitary adenoma is called Cushing's disease.

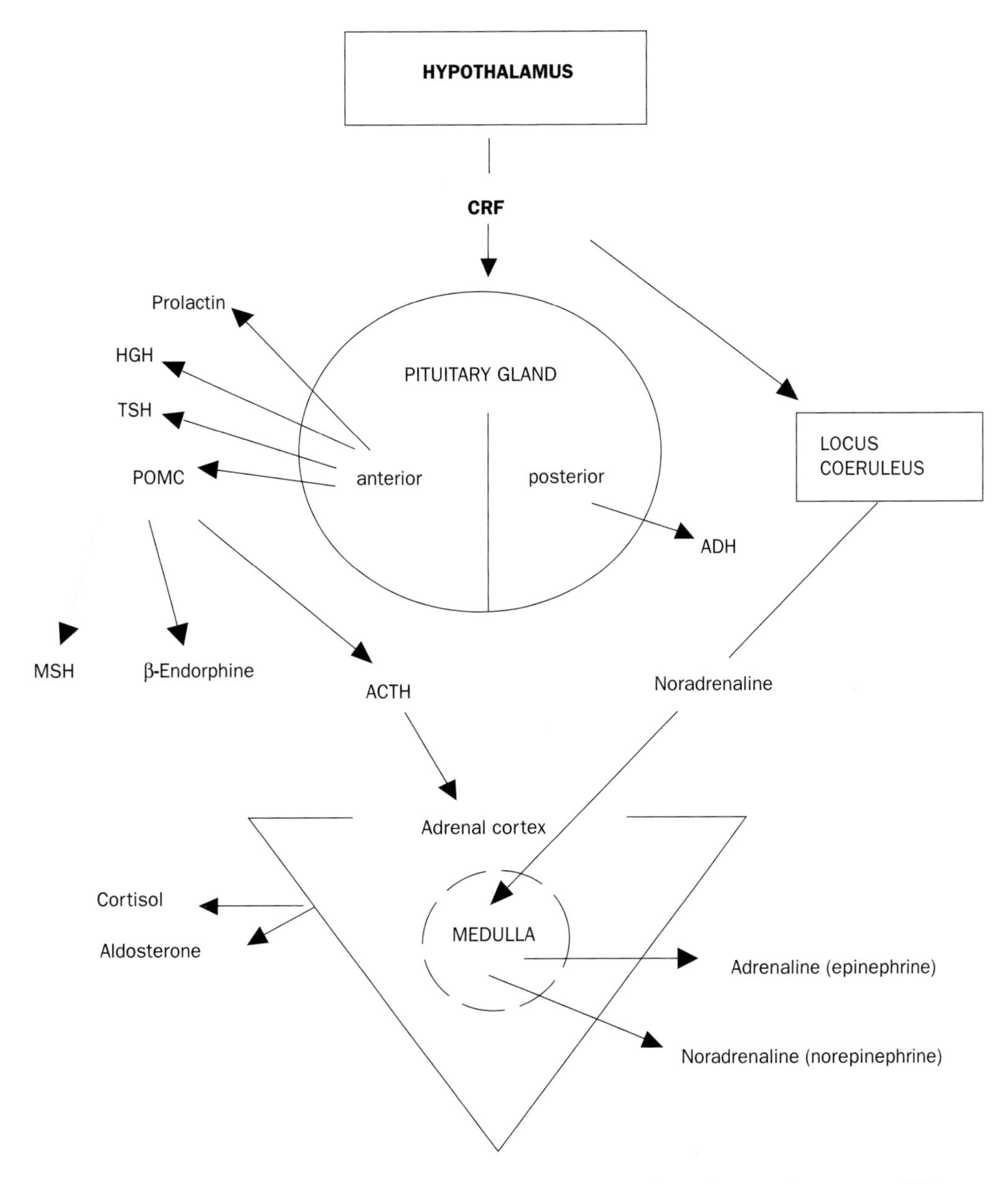

Figure 13.1 *Schematic outline of the hypothalamo-pituitary-adrenal axis and stress hormones. CRF, corticotrophin-releasing factors; ADH, antidiuretic hormone; HGH, human growth hormone; TSH, thyroid-stimulating hormone; POMC, proopiomelanocortin; MSH, melanocyte-stimulating hormone; ACTH, adrenocorticotrophic hormone.*

POSTERIOR PITUITARY HORMONES

Antidiuretic hormone (ADH)

Antidiuretic hormone (vasopressin) is synthesised in the supra-optic nuclei of the hypothalamus then transported in secretory granules along axons to the posterior pituitary. The main stimuli for vasopressin secretion are raised plasma osmolarity and decreased intravascular volume. ADH secretion is inhibited by decreased plasma osmolarity, ethanol and clonidine administration. Vasopressin is an extremely potent generalised vasoconstrictor, mediated via V_1 receptors, and involves mobilisation of intracellular calcium concentration via IP_3 receptors. It is used in the treatment of patients with bleeding oespohageal varices, but octreotide, a long-acting octapeptide analogue of somatostatin, is sometimes preferred. Vasopressin is occasionally valuable in treating hypotension in patients using angiotensin-converting enzyme (ACE) inhibitors, especially after cardiac surgery. Hypotension in these patients is often poorly responsive to conventional vasoconstrictors, such as phenylephrine or noradrenaline (norepinephrine). The renal effects of ADH are mediated through V_2 membrane receptors in the distal tubules and collecting ducts. ADH increases the permeability of the membrane to water, allowing water conservation by producing a concentrated urine. This action, which occurs at much lower concentrations than those producing vasoconstriction, involves activation of adenylyl cyclase and increased cAMP production.

Several synthetic analogues of ADH of vasopressin have been developed. Desmopressin (1-deamino-8-D-arginine vasopressin), which is selective for the V_2 receptor, has 12 times the antidiuretic action of vasopressin and minimal vasopressor effects. It can be administered subcutaneously, intravenously or intranasally to treat central diabetes insipidus. Administration is guided by urine output; repeat doses are typically required every 6–18 hours. Desmopressin is also used for the treatment of type I von Willebrand's disease, mild factor VIII deficiency (haemophilia A), and intrinsic platelet function defects (see Chapter 17). Felypressin (Phe^2-Lys^8-vasopressin) is a short-acting V_1-selective analogue sometimes added as a vasoconstrictor to local anaesthetics to prolong their effects.

Diabetes insipidus

Diabetes insipidus is a condition resulting from a relative or absolute deficiency of ADH. Central diabetes insipidus can occur from trauma, infections, tumours or vascular accidents. The kidneys produce a high volume of dilute urine (urinary output of 2–5 litres daily is common), and this can lead to hypovolaemia and hypernatraemia. Patients with adequate access to water avoid severe dehydration by marked increases in water intake. Patients to whom access to water is restricted, e.g. after surgery, are at risk of hypovolaemia. Anaesthetic management of patients with diabetes insipidus consists of close monitoring of fluid status. In ambulatory patients, allowing unrestricted access to water may be sufficient. Nephrogenic diabetes insipidus is caused by failure of the renal V_2 receptors to respond to ADH. Differentiation between central and nephrogenic causes is important as central diabetes insipidus may be treated with hormone replacement therapy. Nephrogenic diabetes insipidus is difficult to treat, although thiazide diuretics may produce a paradoxical fall in urine output. Chlorpropamide (an anti-diabetic drug) and carbamazepine (an anti-epileptic drug) potentiate the actions of ADH and are also used in the treatment of diabetes insipidus.

Syndrome of inappropriate antidiuretic hormone secretion

The syndrome of inappropriate antidiuretic hormone (SIADH) secretion is a condition in which secretion of ADH continues despite serum hypo-osmolarity. This results in fluid retention and hyponatremia that can lead to brain oedema, mental confusion and coma. The causes are hypothalamic-pituitary tumours or an ectopic vasopressin-secreting tumour, particularly lung small cell (oat) and pancreatic carcinoma. Stroke, head trauma, neurosurgery, and infectious disease of the central nervous system (CNS) are other causes of SIADH.

The mainstay of medical treatment is fluid restriction, but this may not be appropriate in the surgical and critical care patient population. Severe (< 120 mmol·L^{-1}) or symptomatic hyponatraemia (mental status changes, seizure) requires more aggressive therapy to reduce cerebral oedema. Infusion of hypertonic saline to increase plasma sodium concentrations to 120–125 mmol·L^{-1} alleviates symptoms. Adjunct therapy with demeclocycline (600 mg·day^{-1}) may assist management in resistant SIADH. Demeclocycline is a tetracycline antibiotic which inhibits the actions of ADH at the renal tubules.

Oxytocin (syntocinon, pitocin)

Oxytocin is a nonapeptide which is structurally related to vasopressin. It stimulates rhythmic uterine contractions and is widely used by intravenous infusion of a diluted solution to induce labour and to treat postpartum bleeding. In large doses, it may cause relaxation of vascular smooth muscle causing hypotension in patients with cardiac disease or who are dehydrated. It has water-retaining properties and when given for prolonged periods to patients whose intake is electrolyte-free it causes overhydration and hyponatraemia. This may result in convulsions in the newborn with the risk of cerebral damage.

ADRENAL CORTEX

Anterior pituitary ACTH stimulates the adrenal cortex to secrete glucocorticosteroids, mineralocorticoids and androgens. Glucocorticosteroids bind with cytoplasmatic receptors and activate transcription of target genes for synthesis of new proteins which are responsible for the physiological effects. In humans, cortisol (hydrocortisone) is the main glucocorticoid and aldosterone is the main mineralocorticoid. Other naturally occuring corticosteroids are cortisone, corticosterone and desoxycorticosterone. The terms *glucorticoid* and *mineralocorticoid* derive from their respective roles in carbohydrate metabolism and electrolyte balance. Mineralocorticoids act on the distal tubules and collecting ducts of the kidney to increase reabsorption of sodium and the urinary excretion of both potassium and hydrogen. The glucocorticoids have profound effects on carbohydrate and protein metabolism, as well as anti-inflammatory and immunosupressive effects. Glucocorticosteroids have a wide range of actions on the immune system. They are used in the management of autoimmune and chronic inflammatory diseases, such as rheumatoid arthritis and asthma. They prevent organ rejection after transplantation.

Glucocorticosteroids

Synthetic glucocorticoids are prednisolone, prednisone, methylprednisolone, dexamethasone, betamethasone and triamcinolone (Table 13.2). Hydrocortisone is available as either succinate or phosphate salts for oral and intravenous administration. It is the drug of choice when a rapid effect is required, e.g. acute adrenal insufficiency, or as peri-operative replacement therapy. Prednisolone can also be given intravenously. It has about 0.8 of the mineralocorticoid activity of hydrocortisone. Prednisone is a prodrug that is converted to prednisolone in the body. For chronic therapy, synthetic steroids without mineralocorticoid activity are preferred, such as dexamethasone, betamethasone or triamcinalone. Beclometasone passes membranes poorly and is more active topically than when given orally. It is used as an aerosol for chronic rhinitis and asthma, and topically in severe eczema. Fludrocortisone is a synthetic halogenated derivate of cortisol that is used for its mineralocorticoid effect.

Adverse effects

Long term use of glucocorticoids is associated with several adverse effects. High circulating

Table 13.2 Relative potencies of various corticosteroids

Corticosteroids	*Anti-inflammatory potency*	*Sodium-retaining potency*
Hydrocortisone	1	1
Cortisone	0.8	0.8
Prednisone	4	0.8
Prednisolone	4	0.8
Methylprednisolone	5	0.5
Triamcinolone	5	0
Betamethasone	25	0
Dexamethasone	25	0
Fludrocortisone	10	125

concentrations of glucocorticoids for prolonged periods will result in Cushing's syndrome. The most common causes are glucocorticoid drugs, an adrenal tumour, ectopic production of ACTH associated with a neoplasm or pituitary tumour. Lung cancer is the most frequent malignancy associated with ectopic ACTH production. Increased protein catabolism leads to muscle weakness and wasting. The skin becomes thin leading to striae and the gastric mucosa becomes susceptible to ulceration. Altered carbohydrate metabolism leads to hyperglycaemia, glycosuria and diabetes mellitus. Bone catabolism leads to osteoporosis. Body fat is redistributed with the classic appearance of so-called 'moon facies' and 'buffalo hump'. Water and salt retention may cause oedema, hypertension and cardiac failure. Chronic Cushing's syndrome is a secondary cause of diabetes mellitus with its attendant complications. Hypokalaemia may predispose the patient to dysrhythmias. In patients in whom Cushing's syndrome develops from corticosteroid therapy, adrenal function is completely suppressed. Despite their cushingoid appearance, these patients require continued therapy with corticosteroids.

Chronic corticosteroid therapy results in negative feedback on the hypothalamus, pituitary and adrenal glands (Figure 13.2). The adrenal gland becomes atrophic and remains so for many months after treatment has stopped. As a result, the adrenal cortex cannot produce sufficient endogenous cortisol when exogenous glucocorticoids are stopped abruptly or when demands are increased during periods of stress and surgery. If supplementary hydrocortisone is not administered peri-operatively this can lead to hypotension or cardiovascular collapse. The adrenal cortex produces about 20–30 mg cortisol daily. A typical regimen of oral administration of cortisone is 25 mg in the morning and 12.5 mg in the late afternoon. Increased amounts are required to prevent adrenal crisis during surgical stress. For moderate surgical stress hydrocortisone requirement is about 50–75 mg daily for a period of two days. For major surgical procedures hydrocortisone 100 mg intravenously 8 hours prior to induction of anaesthesia, at induction and 8 hours following surgery is recommended.

Although glucocorticoids have only weak mineralocorticoid activity, chronic use can result in fluid retention. They act on the distal renal tubule, leading to sodium retention and potassium excretion, causing oedema, hypertension and cardiac failure. Mineralocorticoid activity is greatest with hydrocortisone and least with methylprednisolone and dexamethasone. Steroid therapy is associated with an increased incidence of neurosis and psychosis. In children, steroid therapy can inhibit normal growth.

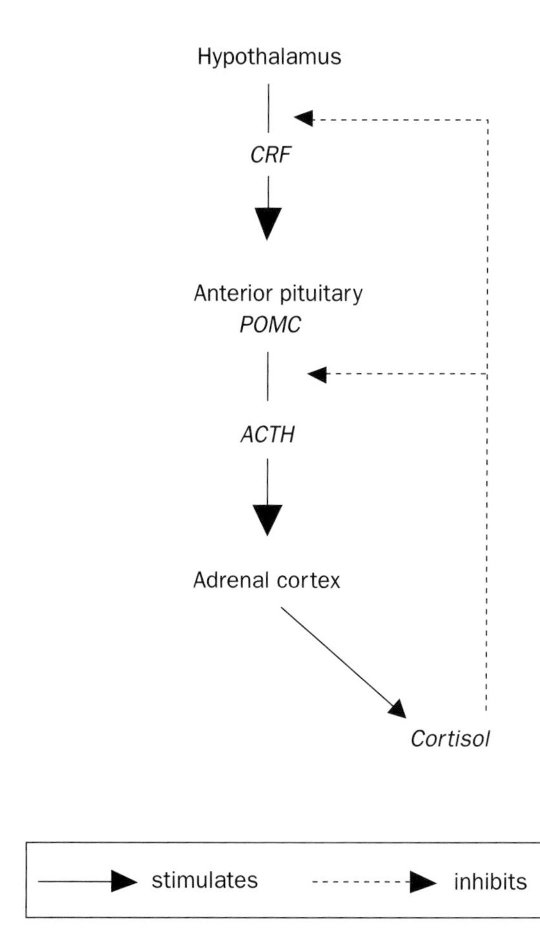

Figure 13.2 *Overview of the negative feedback affecting corticosteroid production.*

ADRENAL MEDULLA

Phaechromocytoma

Phaechromocytoma is a rare tumour arising from chromaffin cells in the adrenal medulla or in other paraganglia of the sympathetic nervous system. The tumour secretes the catecholamines, noradrenaline (norepinephrine) and adrenaline (epinephrine), which are responsible for the clinical signs and symptoms. Hypertension is the commonest presentation and headache is the most common symptom. High circulating noradrenaline concentrations cause vasoconstriction with a decrease in circulating blood volume. Catecholamines increase blood glucose concentration as a result of increased glycogenolysis. Excessive secretion of adrenaline causes paroxismal tachycardia with palpitations, sweating and fear.

Anaesthetic management

Two primary goals must be satisfied prior to surgery: haemodynamic stability and replacement of intravascular fluid volume. Blockade of α_1-adrenergic response is achieved with a variety of α_1-adrenoceptor antagonists, including the non-selective antagonist, phenoxybenzamine, and selective α_1 antagonists (e.g. prazosin, doxazosin and terazosin). The disadvantage of phenoxybenzamine is that it also blocks α_2 adrenoceptors, so that the release of noradrenaline (norepinephrine) at cardiac sympathetic nerve endings is uninhibited, which can lead to cardiac arrhythmias. Labetalol is popular because it antagonises both α and β adrenoceptors. Selective β_1-adrenergic antagonists (e.g. metoprolol and atenolol) are the drugs of choice for prevention of tachyarrhythmias (Table 13.3).

If a β-adrenoceptor antagonist is administered prior to sufficient α_1-adrenoceptor blockade, a hypertensive episode may be precipitated with cardiac failure and pulmonary oedema. Most intravenous anaesthetic agents have been used safely, but ketamine is contraindicated. Sodium nitroprusside can be used to achieve arteriolar dilation. Esmolol, a β_1-selective antagonist with very short duration of action, is administered intravenously to prevent cardiac arrhythmias intra-operatively. After tumour removal, volume administration should be aggressive to maintain haemodynamic stability, and a noradrenaline infusion may be required.

THYROID

The thyroid gland secretes two iodinated hormones, thyroxin (T_4) and triiodothyronine (T_3). The thyroid contributes only about 20% of the unbound circulating T_3. The remainder is produced by the peripheral conversion of T_4 to T_3. T_3 and T_4 bind extensively to plasma proteins, mainly thyroxine-binding globulin (TBG). Binding increases the pool of circulating

Table 13.3 α- and β-Adrenergic receptor antagonists

Antagonist	*Receptor subtype*	*Dose*	*Route*	*Half-life*
Phenoxybenzamine	α_1; α_2	0.5–1.0 $mg \cdot kg^{-1}$	Oral	24 h
Prazosin	α_1	2–20 $mg \cdot day^{-1}$	Oral	2–3 h
Doxazosin	α_1	2–8 $mg \cdot day^{-1}$	Oral	10–20 h
Terazosin	α_1	4–20 $mg \cdot day^{-1}$	Oral	12 h
Labetalol	α_1;	0.5–2.0 $mg \cdot kg^{-1}$	IV	
	β_1; β_2	0.5–1.0 $mg \cdot kg^{-1} \cdot h^{-1}$	Infusion	4–6 h
		15–300 mg	Oral	
Metoprolol	β_1	50–200 $mg \cdot day^{-1}$	Oral	3–4 h
Atenolol	β_1	100 $mg \cdot day^{-1}$	Oral	5–8 h
Esmolol	β_1	50–300 $\mu g \cdot kg^{-1} \cdot min^{-1}$	Infusion	9.2 min

hormones, delays their clearance, and perhaps, modulates hormone delivery. The secretion of T_3 and T_4 is controlled by thyroid-stimulating hormone (TSH), released from the anterior pituitary. Thyroid hormones bind to nuclear α and β receptors, both of which are expressed in most tissues. T_3 binds to the receptors with about 10–15 times greater affinity than T_4, which explains its greater potency. Receptor binding triggers increased synthesis of proteins, increased gluconeogenesis, and increased metabolism. In addition, thyroid hormones regulate differentiation and proliferation of cells, influence the myelination of nerves, and reduce the concentration of cholesterol in liver and blood.

Hypothyroidism

Hypothyroidism, a condition in which the circulating concentrations of thyroid hormones are too low, is the most prevalent thyroid disease. Primary hypothyroidism, the commonest form, is an autoimmune disease (Hashimoto's thyroiditis) often associated with goitre. Like other autoimmune diseases, it is more prevalent in women (4 per 1000) than in men (1 per 1000). Other causes include thyroidectomy, radioactive ablation and, in some countries, iodine deficiency. Hypothyroidism can also be caused by several drugs, including lithium, interleukin-2 and interferon. Secondary hypothyroidism is a disease caused by decreased secretion of TSH by the pituitary.

Severe hypothyroidism manifests as non-pitting oedema (myxoedema), thick puffy features, ascites, pleural, and pericardial effusions. Progression leads to mental status changes (lethargy, somnolence) and eventually myxoedema coma. A large tongue may make airway management difficult. A hoarse voice may indicate vocal cord oedema. Cardiac involvement results in bradycardia and decreased cardiac output. The electrocardiogram (ECG) can show low voltage and altered T wave. Adrenal cortex suppression exacerbates haemodynamic changes.

Treatment of hypothyroidism

The only effective treatment is replacement therapy with thyroid hormones. *Levothyroxine*, a synthetic levoisomer of thyroxine (T_4), is the drug of choice since it is stable, relatively inexpensive, free of antigenicity, and of uniform potency. It results in a pool of thyroid hormone that is rapidly converted into the more potent T_3. Levothyroxine can be administered orally or intravenously. With oral administration, the therapeutic effect only becomes apparent in 1–3 weeks. When given intravenously, onset occurs within 8 hours and the maximum effect is reached in 24 hours. The half-life of levothyroxine is 9–10 days, that of T_3 is 1–2 days. The dose of levothyroxine has to be adjusted in older patients and in patients with heart disease, because of the risk of arrhythmias. *Liothyronine* is a synthetic T_3 preparation. Because of the higher incidence of adverse cardiac effects associated with its use, it is usually reserved for the emergency treatment of the rare myxoedema coma, when the more rapid onset of action is an advantage.

Hyperthyroidism (thyrotoxicosis)

In thyrotoxicosis, there is excess activity of the thyroid gland. Hyperthyroidism has multiple causes, including diffuse toxic goitre (Graves' disease), pituitary tumours, pregnancy, excess iodine ingestion, and excessive thyroid hormone therapy. Graves' disease is the most common cause of hyperthyroidism. It is an autoimmune disorder in which an antibody that mimics TSH (an 'imposter' TSH) binds to the TSH receptors stimulating thyroid hormone production and the hyperthyroid state. The clinical signs of hyperthyroidism are a high metabolic rate, an increase in temperature, sweating, tremor, tachycardia, and an increased appetite associated with weight loss. The changes in the cardiac system are the most relevant to anaesthesiologists. Sinus tachycardia is common, and atrial fibrillation and premature ventricular contractions are frequently associated arrhythmias. Hyperthyroidism can result in high-output cardiac failure where oxygen delivery is unable to meet tissue metabolic demands. Patients are susceptible to dehydration from the hypermetabolic state.

The most serious complication of hyperthyroidism is thyroid storm (thyrotoxic crisis). This is an acute exacerbation of hyperthyroidism with marked tachycardia, fever, mental status changes and haemodynamic collapse. It is usually precipitated by acute illness, trauma, parturition or surgery, especially of the thyroid gland. The mortality rate is 20–30%, even with aggressive treatment, due to cardiac failure, arrhythmias or hyperthermia.

Nonsurgical treatment of hyperthyroidism

Iodine

Radioactive iodine (^{131}I) is concentrated in the thyroid gland. Because the radioactivity (β particles) only penetrates about 0.5 mm into the surrounding tissue, the thyroid gland alone is affected without damage to surrounding tissues. The half-life of ^{131}I is 8 days and radioactivity will have disappeared by 2 months. It is used for the initial treatment of hyperthyroidism and for treating patients for relapse after oral antithyroid therapy. ^{131}I is given in a single dose, but the effect on the gland is delayed for 1–2 months, and reaches a maximum effect in 3 months. Treatment with ^{131}I results in hypothyroidism in 10–30% of patients in the first year of treatment; and in a further 3% of patients it occurs later. The use of ^{131}I is contraindicated during pregnancy and in mothers who are breastfeeding.

Iodine was the first form of therapy for thyrotoxicosis, but is no longer used alone because of the unreliable effect. Potassium iodide, given orally as concentrated drops, is occasionally used in combination with one of the thioureylenes, because of its fast onset of action, within 1–2 days. It acutely blocks thyroid hormone release, inhibits hormone synthesis, and decreases the size and vascularity of the gland. It may also interfere with the iodination of thyroglobulin. In high doses, it is used in the preparation of patients for thyroidectomy to reduce the vascularity of the hyperactive thyroid. Treatment needs to be started 7–14 days preoperatively. It is also used for protection of the thyroid gland during treatment with radioactive isotopes. The other main indication is in the management of thyrotoxic crisis (thyroid storm).

Thioureylenes (thioamides)

These are the most important of the antithyroid drugs. The main compounds are *propylthiouracil*, *carbimazole*, and its active metabolite, *methimazole*. They all contain a thiocarbamide group (S=C—N) which is essential for their activity. They inhibit thyroid peroxidase, preventing the oxidation of trapped iodine and its subsequent incorporation into T_4 and T_3. They also inhibit the coupling of mono- and diiodothyronine to form T_4 and T_3. Propylthiouracil also inhibits the removal of an iodine molecule from T_4 to form T_3, although this is of minor benefit. They also reduce thyroid antibodies by a mechanism that is unclear. The thioureylenes are well absorbed from the gastrointestinal (GI) tract and are actively concentrated in the thyroid gland so that there is a disparity between their relatively short plasma half-lives and their effectiveness on once-daily oral dosing. The half-life of methimazole is 5 hours but because it accumulates in the thyroid the effect lasts 40 hours. The thioureylenes may take 3–4 weeks to achieve an effect, partly because of the long half-life of thyroxine but also because the thyroid has large stores of preformed hormones, which must first be depleted. Between 1% and 5% of patients experience rash, urticaria, fever and arthralgia. The main adverse effect is agranulocytosis, trombocytopenia, pancytopenia and aplastic anaemia due to inhibition of myelopoiesis, but these are rare (incidence $< 1\%$) and reversible when the drug is stopped. The incidence is greater with propylthiouracil than carbimazole. Propylthiouracil can cause liver necrosis, hepatitis or cholestatic jaundice.

Emergency treatment of thyroid storm

Therapy begins with large doses of propylthiouracil, 300 mg every 6 hours, orally, as crushed tablets through a nasogastric tube or rectally. Inhibition of the conversion of T_4 to T_3 by propylthiouracil makes it the agent of choice. Two hours thereafter potassium iodide is started, 40–80 mg every 12 hours. Beta-adrenergic antagonists should be given to reduce tachycardia and other adrenergic manifestations. Propranolol is often preferred since it decreases the conversion of T_4 to T_3. This action is caused by the *d*-propranolol isomer, which has no β-antagonist activity. The active *l*-propranolol has little or no effect on T_4 to T_3 conversion. Additional measures include cooling, intravenous fluids and steroids.

PANCREAS

The pancreas secretes numerous enzymes that break down carbohydrates and proteins and thus facilitate their absorption through intestinal mucous membranes. The most important endocrine function of the pancreas is secretion of insulin and glycogen. Insulin is a 51 amino acid polypeptide consisting of an α and a β chain linked by two disulphide bonds. It is stored in the β-islet cells of the islets of Langerhans as a precursor molecule, proinsulin. When secreted from the pancreas, proinsulin is enzymatically cleaved to insulin and C peptide. Daily 40–50 units of insulin are released into the bloodstream, which is about 25% of the total quantity of insulin stored in the pancreas. Secretion of insulin regulates the level of glucose in the blood. Insulin binds to specific receptors on the surface of cell membranes, especially those of muscle and fat tissue, and facilitates the transport of glucose, amino acids, potassium, magnesium and inorganic phosphates into the cells. Although insulin has no influence on the transport of glucose through the membrane of liver cells—the membrane is entirely glucose-permeable—insulin influences numerous liver enzyme processes. In the liver, glycogen synthesis and inhibition of protein catabolism is promoted. The brain, heart and kidney rely on insulin to preserve cellular energy and oxidative metabolism. Insulin is both metabolised by hepatic mechanisms and excreted by the kidney.

Diabetes mellitus

Diabetes mellitus is one of the commonest endocrine disorders. Type 1 diabetes mellitus (insulin-dependent diabetes) usually develops in the first two decades of life and accounts for 5–10% of all diabetics. It is characterised by a specific cell-mediated T lymphocyte immune process leading to destruction of the pancreatic islet β cells, absolute lack of insulin and dependence on insulin therapy. Patients are prone to ketoacidosis if insulin is withheld. Type 2 diabetes mellitus is the commonest form and usually affects patients over 30 years of age. It is associated with (partial) retention of endogenous pancreatic insulin production but there is a defect in insulin secretion, almost always with a major contribution from insulin resistance. Diabetes mellitus type 2 is often asymptomatic until clinical signs of late complications occur. These include diabetic retinopathy, nephropathy, polyneuropathy, ulcers of lower extremities and joint deformities. Other less common types of diabetes are those due to monogenetic defects in β-cell function and diabetes associated with pregnancy.

Treatment of diabetes mellitus

Insulin

Insulin preparations are of bovine, porcine or human origin. Bovine and porcine insulin differ from human insulin by three and one amino acid residues, respectively. Bovine insulin is more antigenic than pork or human insulin despite high purification. Human insulin, produced by recombinant DNA technology, is used for most patients. Insulin potency is determined by bioassay against an international standard and expressed as units of activity per volume. All insulin preparations require refrigeration for storage. Prior to use, the bottle should be gently rolled to ensure even re-suspension. Insulin is administered subcutaneously, intramuscularly or intravenously. Because of destruction by digestive juices it is ineffective orally. The half-life of insulin in plasma is 9 minutes. Insulin is available in short-, intermediate- and long-acting preparations.

Short-acting insulins

Soluble (regular) insulin is a rapidly acting form that can be administered by subcutaneous or intravenous routes. When given subcutaneously, onset of action occurs in 20–30 minutes with a peak at 1–3 hours and a 6–8 hour duration. Subcutaneously, absorption is slow because the insulin must dissociate into monomers in the tissue before absorption. This often results in hyperglycaemia occurring 1–3 hours after a meal due to inadequate insulin levels, and possibly excessive insulin levels a few hours later with the risk of hypoglycaemia. When given intravenously the onset is within a few minutes and the duration is approximately 30 minutes, and it is frequently administered as a continuous infusion as a 1 unit·mL^{-1} solution. Insulin has variable adsorption to glass and plastic intravenous lines. Priming the tubing may help eliminate initial delivery variance. *Insulin Lispro* is a monomeric insulin analogue, produced by recombinant DNA technology, in which a lysine and a proline amino acid have been switched. It is more rapidly absorbed than soluble insulin but has a shorter duration. When injected at mealtimes it results in earlier bioavailability of insulin and thus more effective control of blood glucose.

Intermediate- and long-acting insulins

These are made by precipitating insulin with protamine or zinc to form amorphous, relatively insoluble crystals which are injected as a suspension from which the insulin is slowly absorbed. Since all intermediate- and long-acting insulin preparations are suspensions, not solutions, they cannot be given intravenously as this would result in drug microembolization.

Semilente insulin is a suspension of amorphous insulin zinc. The onset is 1–3 hours after subcutaneous administration, reaches maximum effect in 5–10 hours and the effect lasts 10–16 hours. *Isophane insulin* (NPH; Neutral solution, Protamine, Hagedorn's laboratory insulin) is an intermediate-acting preparation prepared with protamine. The maximum effect is reached in 4–12 hours and lasts 8–26 hours. Patients using these preparations who present for cardiac surgery are at increased risk for anaphylactic reactions to protamine. *Ultralente insulin* is a long-acting preparation formed with zinc rather than protamine. Zinc retards the release of insulin and these preparations have a duration of up to 36 hours. Protamine zinc insulin, which contains both protamine and zinc, has a duration of 28–36 hours.

Oral hypoglycaemic drugs

The main groups of oral hypoglycaemic drugs are the biguanides and sulphonylureas. Newer drugs include thiazolidinedione derivatives, the meglitinides, and α-glucosidase inhibitors. The oral hypoglycaemic drugs are only effective in patients with some endogenous insulin secretion, i.e. type 2 diabetes mellitus.

Sulphonylureas

These drugs, which are structurally related to sulphonamides, act mainly by stimulating insulin release from β-islet cells of the pancreas by inhibiting ATP-sensitive potassium channels. The decrease in K^+ flux partially depolarises the β-cell membrane, leading to an increased influx of Ca^{2+} through voltage-sensitive calcium channels and release of insulin. Insulin sensitivity is also increased, possibly due to up-regulation of insulin receptors. They enhance the effect of insulin to stimulate glucose uptake into muscle and fat cells.

The first-generation sulphonylureas were *tolbutamide*, *chlorpropamide*, *tolazamide* and *acetohexamide*. Second- and third-generation drugs include *glibenclamide*, *glipizide*, *gliclazide* and *glyburide*. They are 10–100 times more potent than the first-generation drugs, but their maximum hypoglycaemic effects are similar. Because they have less potential for interactions with other drugs they are preferred over the first-generation compounds. Newer formulations, such as glipizide-GITS and glimepiride, are long acting (24 hours) so need only be taken once daily to achieve control of fasting blood glucose and improvement of meal-related insulin secretion. The sulphonylureas are rapidly and completely absorbed after oral administration, with peak effects within 2–4 hours. They are predominantly (90–95%) metabolised by the liver to inactive or only weakly active metabolites that are excreted in the urine. Chlorpropamide has an active metabolite. All are highly protein-bound (> 90%), mainly to albumin. For the first-generation drugs this binding is ionic and thus they can be readily displaced from protein binding sites by other binding drugs such as NSAIDs, coumarins, and some uricosuric drugs, e.g. sulfinpyrazone. This interaction can result in severe hypoglycaemia. Because the protein binding of the second-generation drugs is non-ionic they are less readily displaced.

Tolbutamide is a short-acting drug, with a half-life of 5 hours, and is given in divided daily doses. It is the least likely of the sulphonylureas to cause hypoglycaemia. Chlorpropamide has a long duration of action, with a half-life of 35 hours, so that a single morning oral dose is sufficient. It is much more likely to cause hypoglycaemia than tolbutamide, and hypoglycaemia can be prolonged. For this reason, it should be avoided in the elderly and in patients with impaired renal function. Glibenclamide should also be avoided in these patients because of the risk of hypoglycaemia since it has several metabolites that are moderately active and are excreted in the urine.

Meglitinides

This is a relatively new class of oral antidiabetic drugs, introduced in the late 1990s. Like the sulphonylureas, they act via ATP-dependent K^+ channels, but bind to different subunits than the sulphonylureas. In addition to stimulating pancreatic insulin production they modulate hepatic glucose production. At the moment there are only three drugs in this class, *meglitinide*, *repaglinide* and *mitiglinide*. They are ultra-short acting and can be taken with meals to stimulate insulin secretion to coincide with the meal.

Insulin sensitisers

These improve the action of insulin at target cells, thus correcting one of the fundamental defects in patients with type 2 diabetes. There are two classes, biguanides and thiazolidinediones. The only biguanide currently available is *metformin*. Metformin stimulates the tyrosine kinase activity of the intracellular portion of the β subunit of human insulin. Since it does not increase insulin production it has little potential for hypoglycaemia, and is effective in patients with non-functioning β-islet cells. Metformin is well absorbed from the gastrointestinal tract and is excreted unchanged by the kidneys. The half-life is about 3 hours. With chronic use metformin can interfere with the absorption of vitamin B_{12}.

Accumulation of metformin can occur in patients with renal insufficiency, and interference with pyruvate metabolism can lead to severe lactic acidosis. Lactic acidosis is more likely in situations associated with anaerobic metabolism, and metformin should not be given to patients with renal disease, liver disease, or severe pulmonary or cardiac disease predisposing to hypoxia. It is recommended to switch patients taking metformin to another oral hypoglycaemic prior to cardiac or other major surgery.

The thiazolidinediones (or glitazones) specifically target insulin resistance without directly stimulating insulin secretion. Type 2 diabetes mellitus is characterised by both resistance to insulin and reduced insulin secretion in response to glucose. The first of these compounds to become available for clinical use was *troglitazone*, but was withdrawn from the market in March 2000 due to its association with idiosyncratic hepatotoxicity and acute liver failure. Currently two thiazolidinediones, *rosiglitazone* and *pioglitazone*, are approved for treatment of type 2 diabetes. It remains unclear whether or not hepatotoxicity is a class effect or is related to the unique tocopherol side chain of troglitazone. However, current clinical evidence supports the conclusion that rosiglitazone and pioglitazone do not share the hepatotoxic profile of troglitazone. In addition to beneficial effects on glucose metabolism, they also have profound effects on circulating lipids. These drugs improve insulin sensitivity by binding to specific nuclear receptors known as the peroxisome proliferator-activated receptors (PPARs). This results in increased expression of proteins encoded by these genes that enhance cellular insulin activity on glucose and lipid metabolism thereby improving glucose sensitivity.

α-Glucosidase inhibitors

Alpha-glucosidases are enzymes located on the surface of the small intestinal microvilli that digest dietary carbohydrates into monosaccharide, a process that is necessary before they can be absorbed. *Acarbose*, *miglitol* and *voglibose* are reversible inhibitors of α glucosidases. Acarbose was the first of these drugs to be used in the management of patients with type 2 diabetes who are inadequately controlled by diet with or without other oral hypoglycaemic drugs. Acarbose competes with dietary oligosaccharides for α glucosidases, and has a higher affinity for the enzymes. Because binding is reversible, digestion and absorption of complex carbohydrates after a meal is slower than usual but not prevented. There is, therefore, a reduced rise in blood glucose after a carbohydrate meal. Postprandial insulin levels are also reduced but fasting insulin is generally unchanged. Acarbose can also be used in insulin-dependent diabetic patients to improve glycaemic control. The delayed digestion and absorption of carbohydrates allows better synchronisation of insulin pharmacokinetics with changes in glucose levels after a meal.

FURTHER READING

Wallace WFM. The endocrine system. In: Fee JPH, Bovill JG (eds) Physiology for Anaesthesiologists. London, Taylor & Francis 2004, Chapter 4.

14

Therapy for infection

Ronan McMullan and Amit Bedi

Introduction • Antibacterial agents • Other antibacterial drugs • Antifungal drugs • Antiviral therapy

INTRODUCTION

Pharmacological therapy for infection began in 1867 when Joseph Lister, Professor of Surgery in Glasgow, used carbolic acid to cause lysis of bacteria present in wounds and in the surgical environment. The subsequent discovery of penicillin by Alexander Fleming and Howard Florey in 1929 introduced the modern antibiotic era. The key to antimicrobial therapy is exploitation of differences in metabolic pathways between microorganisms and humans. This chapter considers antibacterial, antiviral and antifungal drugs; antiprotozoal and anti-helminthic agents are not included in this discussion.

ANTIBACTERIAL AGENTS

The antibacterial drugs can be divided into three categories according to their mechanisms of action (Figure 14.1):

1. Inhibition of the bacterial cell wall synthesis.
2. Inhibition of bacterial DNA (nucleic acid) synthesis.
3. Inhibition of bacterial protein synthesis.

β-Lactam antibiotics

This group of drugs prevents cross-linking between peptide chains of the peptidoglycans which form the bacterial cell wall by inhibiting a transpeptidase enzyme. They possess a β-lactam ring; this shares structural homology with the amide bond of the bacterial cell wall which it impersonates. *Penicillin* was discovered in 1929 and underwent clinical trails in the 1940s. It is an extremely effective bactericidal antibiotic and has given rise to a family of natural, synthetic and semi-synthetic derivatives. *Benzyl penicillin* was the first of this family and still remains a useful drug. It is largely degraded by gastric acid and so must be given parenterally. It has a short half-life (~30–60 min) and should be administered at least 4-hourly. *Phenoxymethyl penicillin* has a similar antimicrobial spectrum and, although active orally, has variable (usually poor) bioavailability.

Many bacteria produce a β-lactamase or penicillinase which opens the β-lactam ring rendering some β-lactams ineffective. The problem of β-lactamase-producing bacteria can, in part, be overcome by the addition of a β-lactamase inhibitor such as *clavulanic acid* (as in co-amoxiclav).

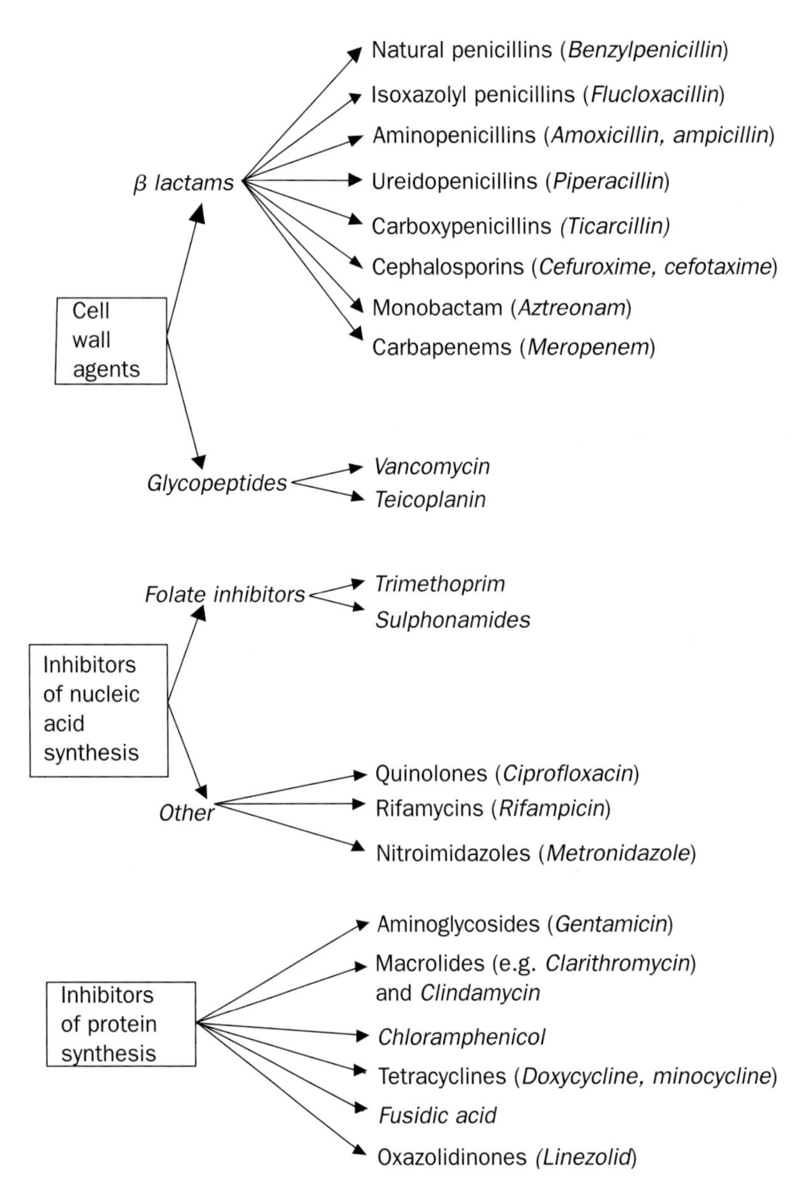

Figure 14.1 *Classification of commonly prescribed antibacterial drugs according to mechanism of action.*

Flucloxacillin is a semi-synthetic compound in which an isoxazolyl group prevents the bacterial enzymes accessing the β-lactam ring. The spectrum of activity of flucloxacillin is narrow and its main indication is staphylococcal infection.

In contrast, *amoxicillin* and *ampicillin* have broad spectrums of activity, being active against non-β-lactamase producing Gram-positive bacteria and also Gram-negative bacteria into which they diffuse more readily than benzyl penicillin. Generally, however, these antibiotics are effective against only the more sensitive strains of Gram-negative pathogens and are therefore rarely appropriate for treating nosocomial infection.

Synthetic derivatives of the penicillins include the *ureidopenicillins*, e.g. azlocillin and piperacillin, and the *carboxypenicillins* (ticarcillin). These compounds have the additional advantage of being active against *Pseudomonas aeruginosa*, an important cause of Gram-negative pneumonia and septicaemia in ventilated patients. The *cephalosporins* have a similar mechanism of action to the penicillins and reasonably broad spectrums of activity. Since these drugs are chemically closely related to the penicillins a proportion, often quoted as 10%, of patients who have had a hypersensitivity reaction to a penicillin will also have an allergic reaction to cephalosporins. There are now several generations within this class and each has specific benefits in various clinical settings. In general terms, first- and second-generation cephalosporins have better antistaphylococcal activity whereas the third and fourth generations have better activity against Gram-negative organisms.

Other agents which contain the β-lactam ring include *aztreonam* and the *carbapenems*. Aztreonam is an unusual β-lactam for two reasons; its antibacterial activity is exclusively Gram-negative and it is reported to carry very low risk of anaphylaxis in individuals who are penicillin-hypersensitive.

The carbapenems are not affected by β-lactamases and penetrate the cell wall effectively due to their compact structure. They have extremely broad spectrum activity against Gram-positive and Gram-negative bacteria, including anaerobes, with the notable exceptions of MRSA (methicillin-resistant *Staphylococcus aureus*), some enterococci, and a small number of multiresistant Gram-negative organisms (e.g. *Stenotrophomonas maltophilia*). As a result, meropenem is used as a second-line agent in the treatment of several life-threatening infections in the intensive care unit (ICU). Its major adverse effects include seizures, neutropaenia, pseudomembranous colitis, diarrhoea and nausea. Of note, patients with penicillin allergy may also develop reactions to carbapenems, but the extent of co-existing allergy and the associated risks are not well characterised.

Glycopeptides

Vancomycin and *teicoplanin* are soluble polypeptide antibiotics which interfere with cell wall synthesis at an 'earlier' stage than β-lactams by preventing the formation of the long chains of peptidoglycan polymer. Their antimicrobial action is further enhanced by altering the permeability of the cytoplasmic membrane and interfering with RNA synthesis. Glycopeptides are active against almost all Gram-positive bacteria and are eliminated by the kidney. Vancomycin causes both nephrotoxicity and ototoxicity although much less commonly than is seen with aminoglycosides. As it is often used in patients who are predisposed to acute renal failure the monitoring of serum concentrations, and maintaining these within therapeutic limits, is recommended. Teicoplanin is of lower toxicity than vancomycin, but serum concentrations must be monitored in serious infections to avoid underdosing; regular monitoring adds significantly to the cost of using these drugs. Suggested reference ranges for glycopeptide serum levels are given in Table 14.1.

Table 14.1 Suggested reference ranges for serum levels of aminoglycoside and glycopeptide antibiotics

Group	*Antibiotic*	*Trough range*	*Peak range*
Aminoglycosides	Gentamicin	< 1 μg·mL^{-1}	> 10
Once-daily dosing			> 50
regimen only			
	Amikacin	< 5 μg·mL^{-1}	regimen
Glycopeptides	Vancomycin	5–10 μg·mL^{-1}	20–40 μg·mL^{-1}
	Teicoplanin	20–60 μg·mL^{-1}	

Aminoglycosides

Aminoglycosides bind both the 30S and 50S ribosomal subunits and have an inhibitory effect on the translocation of messenger RNA (mRNA). This group of antibacterial drugs has potent bactericidal effects against many Gram-negative and some Gram-positive organisms. They act synergistically with β-lactams against these organisms. Their selective action on bacteria is enhanced by their active uptake into the bacterial cell, a process requiring aerobic metabolism. Aminoglycosides are, therefore, inactive against anaerobic bacteria.

Aminoglycosides are most useful for bacteraemias (especially Gram-negative septicaemia) since their volume of distribution is relatively low. With the exception of patients with renal failure or endocarditis they should be administered once-daily. This is because they exhibit a *dose-dependent* pharmacodynamic effect. This means that bactericidal activity is determined more by the peak plasma concentration than by the time that the plasma concentration is above the minimum required to achieve bacterial killing. The converse is true of β-lactams, which exhibit *time-dependent* bacterial killing.

The adverse effects of this group are nephrotoxicity, ototoxicity and neuromuscular blockade. These correlate, generally, with duration of tissue exposure either as a result of prolonged therapy or failure to achieve low trough concentrations. The measurement of pre-dose serum concentrations is, therefore, of great importance and in the context of single daily dosing, measuring the peak level is not always necessary. Suggested reference ranges for serum levels are given in Table 14.1.

Aminoglycosides interfere directly with renal tubular function and indirectly with glomerular filtration; no substantial differences in toxicity among the commonly prescribed aminoglycosides have been demonstrated. Of patients, 3–5% will develop nephrotoxicity using standard dosing regimens; this is greater with co-administration of loop diuretics, vancomycin, and amphotericin B, or when the kidneys are otherwise challenged by, e.g., underperfusion or inflammatory mediators as a result of sepsis syndrome. The toxic effect is greater when the daily dose is divided because of higher trough concentrations. High peak serum concentrations are not considered to be a risk factor for toxicity because there is a saturable movement of aminoglycosides into the renal tubular cell.

Risk factors for aminoglycoside-induced cochlear and vestibular damage, which are typically irreversible, include:

- Age (≥ 60 years).
- Pre-existing ear disease.
- Elevated plasma trough concentrations.
- Prolonged therapy or repeated treatment with aminoglycosides.
- Concomitant use of loop diuretics or other ototoxic drugs.

The mechanism of neuromuscular blockade with aminoglycosides is by inhibition of calcium internalisation into the presynaptic region of the axon. This process is essential for the release of acetylcholine. The effect is rapidly reversed by administration of calcium gluconate. The risk of potentiation of neuromuscular blockade is greatest in patients who are receiving non-depolarising neuromuscular-blocking drugs. Myasthenia gravis, hypocalcaemia, and hypomagnesaemia, have also been associated with increased risk.

Quinolones

The quinolones prevent DNA gyrase forming supercoiled DNA from relaxed DNA in bacteria. *Ciprofloxacin* has excellent antibacterial action against the aerobic Gram-negative organisms (including *Pseudomonas* spp.) and some Gram-positive pathogens. Other members of this group (e.g. moxifloxacin) have better Gram-positive activity.

Within the critical care environment, ciprofloxacin may form part of a regimen for hospital-acquired pneumonia and it has been recommended for anthrax prophylaxis. Care must be taken when co-prescribing ciprofloxacin with warfarin or theophyllines as the metabolism of both is decreased in its presence. The quinolones, being GABA antagonists, may give rise to convulsions and ciprofloxacin has been associated with achilles tendonitis and rupture in patients receiving systemic corticosteroid therapy.

Sulphonamides and trimethoprim

The sulphonamides were discovered in 1935 and were the first drugs to be effective in the treatment of systemic infections. Both they and trimethoprim prevent the production of tetrahydrofolic acid which is used by bacteria to produce purines for DNA synthesis. The sulphonamides act by competitively inhibiting the synthetase which converts *p*-aminobenzoic acid into dihydrofolic acid. Trimethoprim acts at the next step of the conversion of this compound to tetrahydrofolic acid. These two compounds are, therefore, synergistic. Cotrimoxazole contains both sulfamethoxazole and trimethoprim in a ratio of 5:1. This drug is particularly useful in the treatment of *Pneumocystis carinii* pneumonia and some hospital-acquired infections due to multiresistant Gram-negative pathogens (e.g. *Stenotrophomonas maltophilia*). Due to interference with folate metabolism, the sulphonamides may cause agranulocytosis, haemolytic anaemia (especially in patients with glucose-6-phosphate deficiency), and also Stevens-Johnson syndrome. Skin rashes are common and sulphonamides displace bilirubin from plasma proteins which, in the neonate, may lead to kernicterus. Consequently, these drugs should not be used in late pregnancy.

OTHER ANTIBACTERIAL DRUGS

Macrolides, of which *erythromycin* is the prototype, inhibit RNA-dependent protein synthesis at the 50S ribosome, and are most commonly used in the setting of penicillin hypersensitivity or for the treatment of infection caused by 'atypical' pulmonary pathogens (e.g. *Legionella pneumophila*, *Mycoplasma*). They frequently cause gastrointestinal upset and are best administered orally since intravenous formulations require dilution in large volumes and cause thrombophlebitis. An additional effect of erythromycin is a prokinetic action on gastric emptying, even at low dose, which is often useful in the intensive care setting. The macrolide antibiotics are potent inhibitors of the cytochrome P-450 enzyme, CYP 3A4. This enzyme is responsible for the metabolism of several drugs used in anaesthesia, notably midazolam and alfentanil. The use of these antibiotics has been implicated in cases of prolonged sedation after midazolam administration and respiratory depression by alfentanil.

Clindamycin also acts by binding the 50S ribosomal subunit and thereby inhibiting protein synthesis. Oral bioavailability and tissue penetration are extremely good; it is active against many Gram-positive organisms and most anaerobes. The major adverse effect of clindamycin is diarrhoea which is reported to occur in as many as 30% of patients receiving the drug, however, it is usually self-limiting with only a small proportion of patients developing *Clostridium difficile*-associated colitis.

Tetracyclines have broad-spectrum activity against Gram-positive and Gram-negative bacteria as well as *Mycoplasma*, *Chlamydia*, *Rickettsia*, and anaerobes. They act on the 30S subunit of the bacterial ribosome and inhibit its binding with aminoacyl-transfer RNA. Adverse effects include nephrotoxicity, hepatotoxicity, nausea, diarrhoea, and the permanent discoloration of the teeth in pre-adolescent children. The use of tetracyclines should, therefore, be avoided in both young children and breast-feeding mothers.

Chloramphenicol also has broad-spectrum activity against anaerobic organisms as well as Gram-positive and Gram-negative aerobes. It prevents transfer RNA binding to the 50S ribosomal subunit and, hence, the transfer of amino acids to the protein chain. Its metabolism is hepatic and it potentiates the action of several agents including the sulphonylureas, warfarin and phenytoin. This drug is well absorbed after oral administration and penetrates tissues, including the central nervous system, well. Rarely, chloramphenicol can cause bone marrow aplasia which may be either an irreversible, idiosynchratic, reaction or a reversible, dose-dependent, effect. In neonates, it may give rise to the grey baby syndrome (pallor, collapse and abdominal distension). Its few licensed indications in the UK are meningitis (when β-lactams are contraindicated), epiglottitis and typhoid.

Metronidazole, a nitroimidazole, is effective only against anaerobic bacteria since its mechanism of action involves the generation of toxic metabolites in a milieu of low redox potential. It is well absorbed when administered orally and, apart from disulfiram reactions when co-administered with alcohol, is well tolerated. It is indicated in infections in which anaerobes have a major role, such as intestinal or biliary tract sepsis, and is the first-line agent for *C. difficile*-associated colitis.

Rifampicin is an inhibitor of transcription which acts by inhibiting DNA-dependent RNA polymerase. It has activity against Gram-positive and some Gram-negative organisms as well as having antituberculous properties. Although it has frequently formed part of many regimens for treating MRSA infection, its use should be limited to preserve its antituberculous potency and help to reduce the growth in incidence of multidrug-resistant tuberculosis. Rifampicin often causes transient hyperbilirubinaemia, when therapy commences, because of competition for hepatic excretion; similarly, it causes an elevation in hepatic transaminases which usually resolves while on treatment. However, it is an hepatotoxic agent and may produce severe hepatitis and jaundice; liver enzymes should, therefore, be carefully monitored on therapy.

Linezolid is a novel oxazolidinone antibiotic with exclusively Gram-positive activity (including MRSA) which acts at the level of the 30S and 70S ribosomal subunits by a unique mechanism; it inhibits protein synthesis by preventing formation of initiation complexes. Linezolid has excellent oral bioavailability and tissue penetration; the most important adverse effect is marrow suppression which is usually reversible. Its major indications are soft tissue infections and nosocomial pneumonia, although these will probably expand in the future.

Selecting appropriate antibacterial therapy

The cornerstone of this process requires identification of an agent with good activity against the likely pathogens (Table 14.2) which is

Table 14.2 Examples of medically important bacterial pathogens

	Gram-positive (aerobes)	*Gram-negative (aerobes)*	*Anaerobes*
Cocci	Streptococci, e.g. *Streptococcus pyogenes* Staphylococci, e.g. *Staphylococcus aureus*	*Neisseria meningitidis*	Anaerobic streptococci, e.g. *Peptostreptococcus* spp.
Bacilli	*Listeria monocytogenes*	*Escherichia coli* *Salmonella* *Campylobacter* *Proteus* *Klebsiella* *Pseudomonas* *Haemophilus*	*Bacteroides fragilis* (Gram-negative) *Clostridium difficile* (Gram-positive)

capable of accessing the site of infection in an adequate concentration. One must, therefore, remember that many antibiotics are poorly absorbed and/or distributed to various tissues. Furthermore, some drugs are inactive in certain settings, e.g. macrolides and aminoglycosides have poor activity in a low pH environment, such as an abscess. The potential adverse effects, especially in susceptible patients (Table 14.3) as well as cost, prior antibiotic therapy, and other co-prescribed medications also figure in the selection process.

An additional consideration is the role of excessive prescription of broad-spectrum antibacterial drugs in the generation and proliferation of resistant organisms. While it may seem best for the individual, at the time, to prescribe the most potent, broad-spectrum, agent possible such practice is likely to disadvantage future patients and the wider community.

Figure 14.2 illustrates the major antimicrobial activity of commonly prescribed antibiotics; with this in mind selecting therapy is more straightforward. For example, soft tissue

Table 14.3 Clinical syndromes associated with adverse reactions of commonly prescribed antimicrobial drugs

Adverse effect	*Details and exemplar drugs*
Nephrotoxicity	**Pre-renal failure,** e.g. hypotension following β-lactam-induced anaphylaxis **Obstructive nephropathy,** e.g. crystal deposition following cephalosporin administration **Direct tubular damage,** e.g. aminoglycoside, vancomycin, tetracycline, amphotericin
Hepatotoxicity	**Cholestasis,** e.g. fusidic acid **Direct hepatocellular injury,** e.g. antituberculous drugs (e.g. rifampicin), erythromycin, high-dose penicillins (e.g. flucloxacillin), fluconazole and flucytosine
Haemopoietic abnormalities	**Granulocytopaenia,** e.g. high-dose penicillins/cephalosporins **Immune thrombocytopaenia/Coombs positive anaemia,** e.g. penicillins, cephalosporins **Aplastic anaemia,** e.g. chloramphenicol **Marrow aplasia due to decreased nucleic acid synthesis**, e.g. sulphonamides, ganciclovir
Rashes	**Allergy:** mainly β-lactams **Non-specific itching rashes,** e.g. sulphonamides, penicillins, ampicillin in infectious mononucleosis **Erythema multiforme ± Stevens-Johnson syndrome:** sulphonamides **'Red-man' syndrome** (vasodilatation-hypotension due to histamine release) characteristic of rapid administration of vancomycin
Phlebitis	Vancomycin, fusidic acid, macrolides and amphotericin all cause irritation to veins when administered intravenously

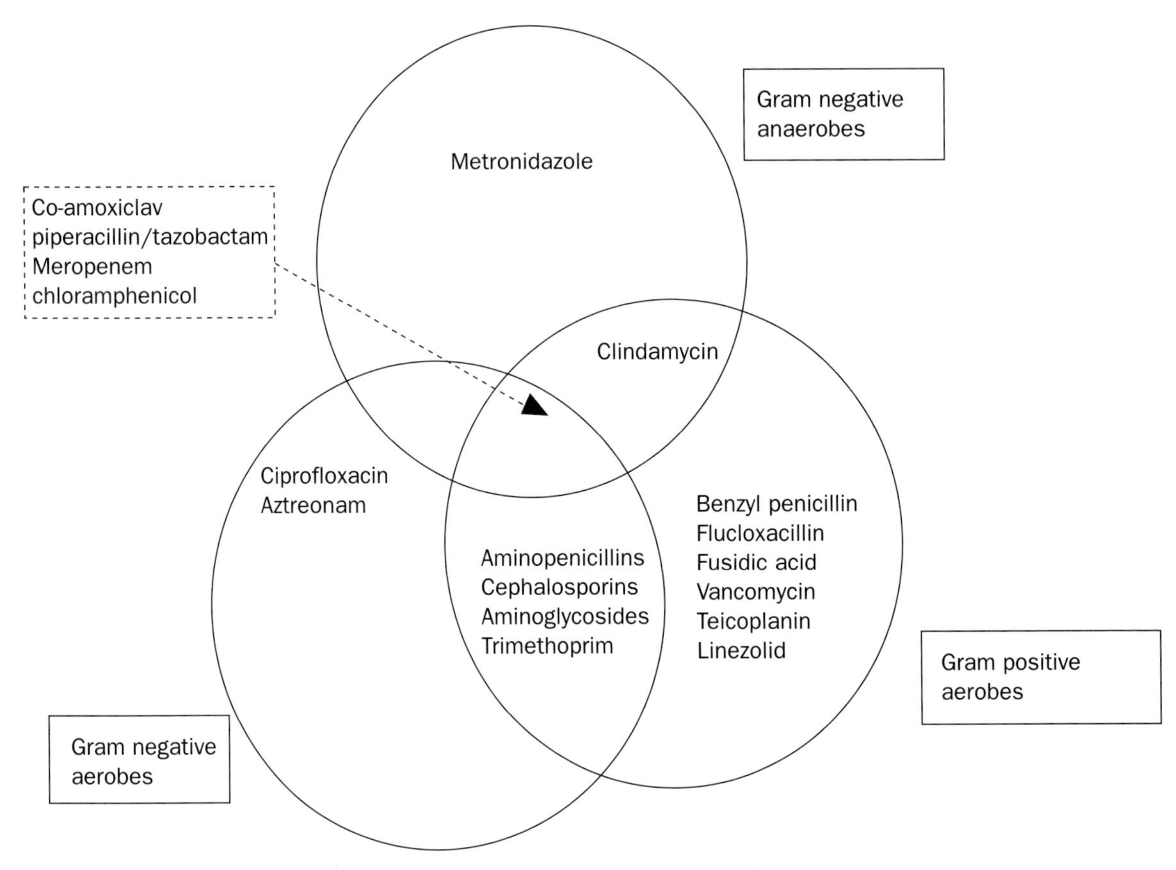

Figure 14.2 *Main antimicrobial activity of commonly prescribed antibiotics.*

infections are most commonly due to β-haemolytic streptococci and *Staph. aureus*. Benzyl penicillin and flucloxacillin provide appropriate, narrow-spectrum, activity as well as reasonably good delivery to the site, have few adverse effects and are inexpensive. Nosocomial pneumonia is likely to be caused by Gram-negative aerobes and *Staph. aureus* and an appropriate regimen might consist of flucloxacillin with ciprofloxacin. These would provide a focused spectrum of activity and good penetration to pulmonary tissue. In contrast, when managing septicaemic shock, it is important to select a regimen with broad spectrum and low likelihood of failure. It is also an advantage to incorporate an aminoglycoside for potent bacterial killing and synergy with a co-prescribed broad-spectrum β-lactam. An exemplar regimen might consist of piperacillin (± tazobactam, as in tazocin) and gentamicin.

Antimicrobial resistance

Antimicrobial resistance (AMR) is a major, worldwide problem with implications for mortality, morbidity, and consumption of healthcare resources. It is likely that the increase in AMR in recent years is attributable, to a large extent, to overuse of antimicrobial drugs in both humans and animals. Furthermore, it appears that prescribing patterns favouring *lower* doses of antibiotics for *longer* durations contribute more towards AMR.

Mechanisms which may facilitate bacterial AMR can sometimes be produced following only a single mutation and, in some cases, without cost to the virulence of the organism. Such mechanisms include:

- Impermeability of the bacterial membrane to the antibiotic.

- Absence of cellular binding site for the antibiotic.
- Reduced uptake of antibiotic.
- Active efflux pump removing antibiotic which passes into the cell.
- Switching on metabolic pathways alternative to those inhibited by the antibiotic.
- Production of enzymes to degrade the antibiotic, e.g. novel β-lactamases, extended-spectrum β-lactamases, or aminoglycoside-modifying enzymes.

In the presence of antimicrobial selection pressure, due to antibiotic exposure, organisms that have resistance determinants to that antibiotic will proliferate while their competitors without these decline. The situation is made more complex by the potential for transmission of genetic material that codes for resistance determinants between organisms; this may occur between the same species, different species and, in fact, also between different genera. Hence, a bacterium that is initially susceptible to an antimicrobial drug may become resistant by acquisition of resistance determinants from another organism. Mechanisms of transferring genetic material between bacteria are:

- **Transformation**: one organism sheds 'naked' DNA fragments into the environment which are taken up by another organism and incorporated into its genome.
- **Transduction**: DNA fragments are taken up by a bacteriophage and transferred to a second organism when the phage infects it.
- **Conjugation**: this involves the direct transfer of DNA fragments between two conjoined organisms.
- **Transposition**: occurs when transposons (genetic elements capable of moving between bacteria, plasmids or between chromosomal DNA and plasmids) migrate to confer resistance determinants to another organism.

Methicillin-resistant Staphylococcus aureus *(MRSA)*

Strains of *Staph. aureus*, perhaps the most renowned resistant pathogen, which are resistant to methicillin (and, hence, flucloxacillin), are a problem for physicians treating patients in the critical care environment. MRSA is resistant to all β-lactam agents, including cephalosporins and carbapenems. Many strains are still susceptible to quinolones, trimethoprim/sulfamethoxazole, aminoglycosides, fusidic acid, or rifampicin. However, because of the rapid emergence of resistance during therapy, neither rifampicin nor fusidic acid should be used as monotherapy for MRSA infections. The treatment options are limited with vancomycin often being an essential therapy for serious infections in the critically ill patient, although, teicoplanin, and, perhaps, linezolid may be reasonable alternatives.

Control of spread of MRSA and other multiresistant organisms is of great importance, particularly in a setting where patients are susceptible to infection, as in the ICU. Important resistant nosocomial pathogens and their major mechanisms of proliferation are outlined in Table 14.4. Infection control measures to limit the spread of such pathogens in hospital include:

- Treatment of infected patients.
- Decolonisation of colonised patients in some cases, e.g. MRSA.
- Environmental cleaning of contaminated materials/surfaces.
- Rigorous hand-washing practices.
- Barrier nursing techniques.
- Careful use of aseptic techniques of carrying out procedures, including simple procedures, such as handling central venous catheters.

Selective decontamination of the gastrointestinal tract

Selective decontamination of the gastrointestinal tract was conceptualised with a view to preventing nosocomial infection (mainly due to enterobacteriaciae), specifically ventilator-associated pneumonia, in intensive care units. Protocols typically included the prescription of an intravenous cephalosporin with good activity against such Gram-negative pathogens (e.g. cefotaxime) with co-prescribed, poorly

Table 14.4 Mechanisms of proliferation and spread of resistant strains of some nosocomial pathogens

Organism	*Main mechanisms of proliferation*
Methicillin-resistant *Staphylococcus aureus* (MRSA)	Transmission of resistant clones of bacteria from patient to patient
Vancomycin-resistant enterococci (VRE)	Transmission of resistant clones of bacteria from patient to patient Spread of resistance genes between organisms
Enterobacter cloacae	Organisms with mutation for resistance in patient's flora selected for by antibacterial therapy
Acinetobacter baumanii	Transmission of resistant clones of bacteria from patient-to-patient *and* via environmental reservoirs Organisms with mutation for resistance in patient's flora selected for by antibacterial therapy

absorbable, oral antibacterials and, often, an antifungal agent.

While several trials demonstrated efficacy of such interventions in reducing the incidence of pneumonia, no convincing impact on mortality or length of hospital stay was demonstrated. In fact, the implications of these practices for development of antimicrobial resistance are so great that selective decontamination is not favoured and is, generally, not practised.

ANTIFUNGAL DRUGS

Serious fungal infections have dramatically increased during the past few decades. This is probably because of an increase in numbers of critically ill patients. Patients who, in the past, would have died are now surviving for long enough to acquire a fungal infection because of advances in cancer therapy, surgical interventions, and intensive care practices. The increased use of broad-spectrum antibacterial drugs has been one of the main aetiological factors. Four main categories of antifungal drugs useful for treating systemic mycoses exist: azoles, polyenes, flucytosine, and echinocandins.

Azoles

These block a methylation step in the synthesis of ergosterol, an essential component of the fungal cell membrane. *Fluconazole*, the best known of these, is a well absorbed and generally well tolerated drug. Occasionally, it may cause hepatic transaminitis. It is active against most *Candida*, *Histoplasma* and *Cryptococcus* spp. *Itraconazole* has extended action against *Aspergillus* and is available for intravenous administration. The drug can also be taken by mouth although absorption by this route is variable. *Voriconazole*, a novel azole, has a very broad spectrum of antifungal activity incorporating the fluconazole-resistant *Candida* spp. *Aspergillus* and *Penicillium* spp.

Polyenes

These bind sterols in the cell membrane causing leakage and, hence, cell death. *Amphotericin B* is the most important member of this group and is active against almost all medically important fungi. However, its limitations are mandatory parenteral administration and toxic reactions that include headache, vomiting, anaemia, thrombophlebitis and nephrotoxicity. Many of these may be overcome by incorporation into lipid carriers such as liposomes; these preparations are, however, very expensive.

Flucytosine

Flucytosine is converted into the antimetabolite 5-fluorouracil that inhibits thymidilate synthetase, thereby disrupting DNA synthesis. It also interferes with protein synthesis by incorporation of fluorouracil into RNA in place of uracil. Although active against most *Candida* species, its spectrum of antifungal activity, overall, is narrow. Since resistance can develop rapidly it is usually co-administered with another agent and its main value is that it facilitates a reduction in the dose (and, presumably, the toxic effect) of amphotericin when co-prescribed in this way. The main adverse effects are marrow aplasia and hepatotoxicity.

Echinocandins

Members of this group, the main example of which is *caspofungin*, irreversibly inhibit glucan synthesis in the fungal cell wall. Since this is a novel target, it is likely that this agent will be active against fungi that are resistant to fluconazole or amphotericin, although its spectrum of activity remains incompletely understood. Its major limitation is lack of an oral formulation. Echinocandins are likely to have a future role in the management of critically ill patients.

ANTIVIRAL THERAPY

The replication of viral particles is intimately linked to the human cell which hosts these parasites; they are intracellular organisms that rely on many of the host cell synthetic processes. Therapeutic options for viral infections are, therefore, limited. In the immunocompetent patient such therapy may be unnecessary and may even cause difficulty in establishing an accurate diagnosis. The antiviral agents may be considered in the following three categories depending upon mode of action:

1. Inhibition of viral replication.
2. Prevention of viral entry to the human cell.
3. Protease inhibitors.

Inhibition of viral replication

Acyclovir, *ganciclovir* and *zidovudine* belong to this class. The most useful of these agents is acyclovir (a guanosine analogue) which has an inhibitory effect on the replication of both the herpes simplex and varicella zoster viruses. These viruses both contain a thymidine kinase which phosphorylates acyclovir. This phosphorylated compound inhibits DNA polymerases of both type 1 and type 2 herpes simplex virus and also of the varicella and Epstein-Barr viruses, albeit at higher concentration. Uninfected cells do not create sufficient phosphorylated compound to interfere with normal human cell synthesis facilitating a selective effect. This drug is useful intravenously and also topically for the treatment of herpes infections. Ganciclovir has a similar mechanism of action.

Zidovudine is a thymidine analogue which has action against the human retro viruses, particularly HIV. After phosphorylation, the drug binds with great affinity to reverse transcriptase, preventing viral replication. Unfortunately, its use is limited by severe side effects including nausea, myalgia, and depressed red and white blood cell counts. Resistance to this drug develops over time.

Drugs preventing the entry of virus into the human cell

Amantidine and *rimantidine* belong to this class. Both are synthetic derivatives of the tricyclic amines and were noted by chance to have antiviral activity. Both agents destroy intracellular vesicles involved in the uptake of virus to host cells. They inhibit the myxoviruses, rubella, respiratory syncytial, and influenza A viruses. Their clinical use is, however, confined to the treatment of the influenza A. Prevention of transmission of this disease by vaccination is obviously preferable to antiviral treatment of established infection.

Protease inhibitors

This class of antiviral drugs, which includes *saquinavir*, *ritonavir*, *indinavir* and *nelfinavir*, interferes with a virus-specific protease involved in post-translational processing of viral precursor polypeptides. They are used in the treatment of HIV infection and AIDS. Since this protease does not occur in the host it is a good target for chemotherapeutic attack. Their use, in combination with reverse transcriptase inhibitors, has been a major advance in the treatment of HIV. They are all given orally, and can cause a variety of gastrointestinal upsets and increases in liver enzymes. All inhibit cytochrome P-450 enzymes, and the doses of benzodiazepines and alfentanil should be reduced in patients taking these drugs.

15

Histamine and histamine antagonists

JG Bovill

Introduction • Histamine receptors • Histamine H_1-receptor antagonists • H_2-receptor antagonists

INTRODUCTION

Histamine is a basic amine that acts as a neurotransmitter, a regulator of inflammatory and immunological reactions, and gastric acid secretion. It also plays an active role in the pathophysiology of allergy and anaphylaxis. Histamine is widely distributed throughout the animal kingdom and is present in many venoms, bacteria and plants. Injection of histamine intradermally causes a combination of effects known as the 'triple response', first described by Sir Thomas Lewis in 1927. This consists of a reddening of the skin and a wheal with a surrounding flare. The reddening is due to dilatation of the small arterioles and precapillary sphincters and the wheal is caused by local oedema due to leakage of fluid from postcapillary venules made more permeable by histamine.

In mammals, most histamine is synthesised and stored in secretory cytoplasmic granules of mast cells in the tissues and the basophils in the blood. Within these granules it is positively charged and held as an ionic complex with negatively charged constituents, such as heparin and proteases. The release of histamine, and many other mediators, from mast cells and basophils is common during allergic disorders. Glucocorticoids inhibit the release and synthesis of histamine. Histamine is present in all human tissues with the highest concentrations in the lungs, skin, the gastrointestinal tract and blood vessel endothelium, sites corresponding to the highest density of mast cells. The concentration of histamine in the plasma is normally low ($< 1\ ng \cdot mL^{-1}$) but may reach $40\ ng \cdot mL^{-1}$ or higher during anaphylactic or anaphylactoid reactions. Concentrations above $12\ ng \cdot mL^{-1}$ are associated with severe hypotension, bronchospasm, and ventricular arrhythmias.

HISTAMINE RECEPTORS

The biological effects of histamine (Table 15.1) are mediated via three receptor subtypes, H_1, H_2 and H_3 that are linked to G protein but activate different cell-signalling systems. The histamine H_1 receptor is associated with the phospholipase C-catalysed formation of inositol 1,4,5-triphosphate (IP_3) and 1,2-diacylglycerol (DAG). The H_2-receptor is coupled to adenylyl cyclase, increasing the production of cAMP. The cellular messenger system involved in H_3-receptor activation has not been fully defined, but it may couple to N-type Ca^{2+}-channels. The genes encoding for H_1 and H_2 receptors have been cloned. A mutation of the human H_2 receptor has been linked to schizophrenia.

Table 15.1 Pharmacological activity associated with individual histamine receptors

H_1	Vasodilatation
	Increased vascular permeability and oedema
	Pulmonary artery vasoconstriction
	Coronary artery vasoconstriction
	Activation vagal afferent nerves in airways
	Bronchospasm
	Gut contraction
	Adrenaline (epinephrine) release from adrenal medulla
	Stimulation of cutaneous nerve endings, pain and itching
H_2	Controls gastric acid secretion
	Increased lower airway mucous secretion
	Relaxation vascular smooth muscle
	Positive inotropy
	Slows AV conduction
	Increased atrial and ventricular automaticity
	Bronchodilation
	Suppression of lymphocyte proliferation
	Suppression of antibody production by B lymphocytes
	Relaxes stomach and gallbladder smooth muscle
H_3	Modulation of histamine synthesis and release
	Inhibits vagally mediated bronchoconstriction
	Vasodilatation
	Tonic inhibition of gastric acid secretion
	Inhibits gut contraction by inhibition of acetylcholine at nicotinic synapses in autonomic nerve terminals
	Presynaptic regulation of neurotransmission processes in CNS

H_1 receptors are widely distributed throughout the body, including the central nervous system (CNS), airway smooth muscles, the gastrointestinal tract, and the cardiovascular system. In the adrenal medulla they elicit the release of adrenaline (epinephrine) and noradrenaline (norepinephrine). Histamine is involved in maintaining wakefulness, and this may explain the sedating properties of some H_1 antagonists. In the heart, histamine acting via H_1 receptors produces a negative inotropic effect and reduces heart rate. In contrast H_2-receptor stimulation results in a positive chonotrophic and inotropic effect. Histamine typically induces a contraction in non-vascular smooth muscle in the bronchi, gut, and the uterus, mediated via H_1 receptors. Guinea pigs are exquisitely sensitive to histamine, and they die from asphyxia due to severe bronchospasm after even small doses of histamine. The contraction of the guinea pig terminal ileum formed the basis of the original bioassay for histamine.

Most of the important effects of histamine in allergic diseases, including bronchoconstriction and contraction of the gut, are mediated through H_1 receptors. Other effects, including the cardiovascular responses, involve both H_1 and H_2 receptors. In man the predominant cardiovascular effect is vasodilatation and a lowering of blood pressure. This response is also responsible for the cutaneous flushing commonly observed with histamine release. The vasodilator effects of histamine are mediated by H_1 receptors on the vascular endothelial cells and H_2 receptors on vascular smooth muscle. Activation of H_1 receptors results in the local production of nitric oxide. In the pulmonary circulation H_1 receptors mediate vasodilatation while H_2-receptor agonists cause vasoconstriction. The hypotension and shock associated with anaphylaxis are secondary to increased vascular permeability and vasodilatation.

Although H_1 receptors are dominant in human bronchial smooth muscle, H_2 receptors are also present where they have a dilatatory function. However, H_2-mediated bronchodilatation is probably minimal and of little clinical consequence. Patients with asthma tolerate H_2 antagonists well. In humans, other mediators, such as leukotrines, are probably more important in producing bronchospasm than histamine. Histamine H_2 receptors play an essential role in the regulation of acid secretion by gastric parietal cells. Histamine interacts with acetylcholine and gastrin via H_2 receptors to control acid production. H_2-receptor antagonists are potent inhibitors of gastric acid secretion.

The H_3 receptor is a presynaptic receptor that regulates the release and synthesis of histamine (autoreceptor). H_3 receptors are highly sensitive to histamine, and are activated at histamine concentrations two orders of magnitude lower than those required to activate H_1 or H_2 receptors. H_3 agonists antagonise gut contractions caused by H_1-receptor stimulation. In the gastric mucosa, H_3 receptors have a tonic inhibitory role in the regulation of basal acid secretion. In the lungs, H_3-receptor activation inhibits cholinergic neurotransmission and vagally mediated bronchoconstriction. Cholinergic mechanisms are important in airway diseases, such as asthma, and H_3 agonists offer potential therapeutic benefit. The coronary vasodilatation caused by histamine is mediated by both H_2 and H_3 receptors, and this is nitric oxide (NO)-dependent. At the present time no drugs acting specifically at the H_3 receptor are clinically available, although several H_3-receptor agonists have been synthesised in recent years, and some are undergoing the early phases of clinical trials.

Histamine H_1-receptor antagonists

Numerous compounds capable of antagonising the effects of histamine are available. The main therapeutic role of these drugs is in the treatment of allergic diseases involving IgE-mediated hypersensitivity, such as allergic rhinitis, hay fever, and urticaria (Table 15.2). The main

Table 15.2 Clinical uses of H_1 antagonists

Prophylaxis and treatment of allergic disorders (second-generation non-sedating drugs preferred)
- Allergic rhinitis
- Hay fever
- Urticaria
- Asthma
- Anaphylactic and anaphylactoid reactions (in combination with an H_2 antagonist)

As anti-emetics
- Motion sickness
- Labyrinthine disorders, e.g. vertigo, Ménière's disease
- Drug-induced, including post-operative emesis

Mild forms of Parkinson's disease

For sedation

beneficial effect is blockade of H_1 receptors on postcapillary venule smooth muscle, resulting in decreased vascular permeability, exudation, and oedema. Antagonism of histamine on type C nociceptive nerve fibres also results in decreased itching and sneezing. Although histamine is not a major mediator in asthma, it contributes to the pathogenesis of the disease and antihistamines, particularly the newer non-sedating drugs, have a role in its therapy. H_1 antagonists, in combination with an H_2 antagonist, are also used in the prophylaxis and treatment of anaphylactic and anaphylactoid reactions.

Many of the older, first-generation drugs, e.g. chlorphenamine (chlorpheniramine), are small, lipid-soluble compounds that cross the blood–brain barrier. This accounts for many of their side effects, which are not directly related to antagonism of the H_1 receptor, but may be caused by agonism at other receptors such as the muscarinic cholinergic, 5-HT_3 or α_1-adrenergic receptors. Some, particularly the phenothiazines, produce a high incidence of sedation, which limits their clinical usefulness. Several have marked antimuscarinic effects causing dry mouth, blurred vision, and constipation. Because of these properties the first-generation H_1 antagonists are seldom used specifically for their antihistamine effects, but are used for their actions at non-histamine sites. Some of the phenothiazines, e.g. promethazine and trimeprazine, are used for premedication. Those with antimuscarinic effects, such as promethazine, diphenhydramine, and cyclizine, are useful as anti-emetics. Where a specific antihistamine effect is wanted the second-generation, non-sedating H_1 antagonists are preferred.

First-generation (sedating) H_1-antagonists

The first-generation H_1 antagonists form a heterogeneous group of chemical compounds with two aromatic rings connected by a two- or three-atom chain to a tertiary amino group. The aromatic rings confer lipophilicity so that they can readily enter the CNS. Sedation or drowsiness is a common adverse effect of the classical antihistamines. The incidence is dose-related and varies among the various chemical classes. Ethanolamines and phenothiazines generally have marked sedative effects, while the alkylamines cause only mild sedation (Table 15.3).

Ethanolamines

The prototype antihistamine of this group is diphenhydramine. It has antimuscarinic and pronounced central sedative properties and also an antitussive effect. The mechanism of the latter is unclear, but diphenhydramine is a common ingredient of propriety preparations for the treatment of coughs and colds. It is an effective anti-emetic, especially useful for prevention and treatment of motion sickness. Because of its anticholinergic properties it is occasionally used in the treatment of mild forms of Parkinson's disease. It is also of use in the treatment of drug-induced extrapyramidal effects.

Piperazine derivatives

Cinnarizine is an H_1-receptor antagonist and a calcium channel blocker used for the treatment of vertigo and emetic symptoms due to Ménière's disease and related labyrinth disorders. It is also effective in motion sickness. It is used for peripheral and cerebral vascular disorders, because of its calcium channel blocking properties.

Cyclizine has antimuscarinic properties and is a potent anti-emetic, effective for the control of postoperative and drug-induced nausea and vomiting. It has been used to prevent motion sickness, although diphenhydramine and promethazine are more effective. It is available in oral and parenteral formulations. In contrast to many other first-generation antihistamines sedation is not marked. It is available in tablet form as the hydrochloride and in injectable form as the lactate. Because of its anticholinergic action, blurred vision and dry mouth are associated with clinical doses. When given by rapid intravenous injection tachycardia may be a problem. Meclozine is a related drug which, like cyclizine, is used primarily for motion sickness.

Alkylamines

The prototype drug in this class is chlorphenamine (chlorpheniramine) maleate. It is a very potent H_1 antagonist with only weak

Table 15.3 Pharmacological characteristics of some first-generation H_1 antagonists

Drug	*Sedation*	*Antimuscarinic effects*	*Presystemic metabolism*	*Active metabolites*	*Dose*	*Half-life (hours)*
Ethanolamines						
Diphenhydramine	+++	+++	70%	No	25–50 mg	3–8
Piperazine derivatives						
Hydroxyzine	+++	+++	NA	Yes	25–100 mg	20
Cyclizine HCl	+	+++	NA	No	50 mg	NA
Cinnarizine	+	+	NA	No	25 mg	3
Alkylamines						
Chlorphenamine (Chlorpheniramine)	+	++	< 20%	No	4–8 mg (oral), 5–20 mg (IV or IM)	30
Dexchlorphenamine	+	++	NA	No		20–24
Phenothiazines						
Promethazine	+++	+++	75%	No	25–50 mg (oral)	7–14
Mequitazine	0/+	0/+	~99%	No	5 mg	40
Miscellaneous						
Clemastine	+	+	NA	No	2 mg (oral and IV)	4–6

NA, not available; IV, intravenous; IM, intramuscular.

antimuscarinic and moderate antiserotonin actions. Chlorphenamine causes less sedation than some other antihistamines. Transient CNS stimulant effects may be seen when injected intravenously. Chlorphenamine is a racemic mixture, with the antihistamine action residing mainly in the (+) laevo isomer (dexchlorphenamine). This isomer is also commercially available.

Phenothiazines

Promethazine has prominent sedative effects as well as anti-muscarinic and dopamine D_2-blocking effects. These make it useful as an anti-emetic, and it is especially useful for the prevention and treatment of motion sickness. Like other phenothiazines, it has weak α_1-adrenergic blocking effects and can lower blood pressure if injected rapidly intravenously. Intramuscular injection can be painful.

Alimemazine tartrate is a phenothiazine with H_1 antagonist activity that produces marked sedation. It is used mainly for its marked relief of pruritus, and is also popular for the premedication of children (dose 2 $mg \cdot kg^{-1}$).

Mequitazine is a phenothiazine with a greater affinity for peripheral than central H_1 receptors. Although it crosses the blood–brain barrier, its transport into the CNS is complex and animal studies suggest that a threshold concentration gradient exists, below which little passage occurs. This may partly explain the lower incidence of sedation compared with other phenothiazines. It has only weak anticholinergic activity. Mequitazine is only available in oral form. The half-life is long, approximately 40 hours and the apparent volume of distribution is very high, 4000 litres, as a result of extensive protein and tissue binding. It undergoes extensive enterohepatic recirculation and because of this, and its extensive protein binding, its pharmacokinetics may be altered in patients with hepatic disease.

Miscellaneous

Clemastine fumarate is a first-generation H_1-receptor antagonist with a long duration of action. It has high H_1-receptor specificity and only weak antimuscarinic effects. The incidence of CNS side effects is generally low. Sedation is less than with most other first-generation drugs but more than second-generation antihistamines, such as loratadine. It is available in parenteral form, and is useful for the prophylaxis and treatment of acute anaphylaxis. It can be given intravenously in a dose of 2 mg, together with an H_2 antagonist, such as ranitidine, to patients at risk of an allergic reaction, e.g. before giving protamine to a patient undergoing a repeat cardiac operation. The onset is rapid after intravenous administration.

Second-generation (non-sedating) H_1 antagonists

The newer, second generation of H_1-receptor antagonists have greater specificity for the H_1 receptor than the older agents. Most are extensively bound to plasma proteins, mainly albumin (Table 15.4). An exception is acrivastine, which is only 50% protein-bound. They have difficulty in crossing the blood–brain barrier and produce little or no sedation or central anticholinergic symptoms when given in the recommended doses. Higher doses may be associated with some CNS depression, especially if taken in combination with other CNS-depressing drugs. In addition to antagonising the effects of histamine, they have other actions that may contribute to their anti-allergic effectiveness. They interfere with mediator release from mast cells by inhibiting either calcium influx across the cell membrane or intracellular calcium release within the cell. They may also inhibit the late-phase allergic reaction by acting on leukotrines or prostaglandins. *In vitro* a membrane-stabilising action similar to cromolyn sodium has been shown for ketotifen, but this has not been confirmed by *in vivo* studies, and there is little indication for the use of this drug in patients with bronchial asthma.

Most of the second-generation H_1-receptor antagonists are administered orally and are extensively absorbed. Peak plasma drug concentrations are generally reached within 1–3 hours (0.5 h for cetirizine). None is available for parenteral use. Azelastine is generally administered as a nasal spray and levocabastine is only available for intranasal administration or as eye drops. Ebastine, loratadine, mizolastine, and terfenadine undergo extensive presystemic metabolism, mainly by cytochrome P-450 enzymes in the liver and/or the gut. The main metabolic pathway for mizolastine is glucuronidation (66% of the administered dose), but it also undergoes oxidative metabolism by CYP3A4 and CYP2A6. The first pass metabolism of ebastine and terfenadine is virtually complete and the clinical effects with the recommended doses are due to pharmacologically active metabolites, fexofenadine (terfenadine

Table 15.4 Pharmacological characteristics of some second-generation H_1 antagonists (figures in parentheses refer to data for the active metabolite)

Drug	*Presystemic metabolism*	*Active metabolites*	*Protein binding*	*Dose (mg)*	*Half-life (h)*
Acrivastine	Minimal	None	50%	8	1.7 ± 0.2
Cetrizine	< 10%	None	93%	10	7–10
Ebastine	~95%	Yes	(98%)	10	(13–16)
Fexofenadine	< 5%	None	70%	10	14–20
Loratidine	> 90%	Yes	98%	10	8–10 (24 ± 9)
Mizolastine	65%	None	98%	10	13
Terfenadine	~100%	Yes	(70%)	60	(14–20)

carboxylate) and carebastine. Terfenadine is potentially cardiotoxic but fexofenadine is not. Fexofenadine has recently been registered in its own right. The primary pathways of elimination are biliary and renal excretion and there is minimal biotransformation. Neither ebastine nor its metabolite cause clinically significant cardiotoxicity. Cetirizine, the carboxylic acid metabolite of the first-generation H_1-antagonist, hydroxyzine, is eliminated mainly by renal excretion of the unchanged drug.

The incidence of side effects of the second-generation drugs, when given in the recommended doses, is very low. Even after massive overdoses of cetirizine (150–300 mg; recommended dose 10 mg) the only adverse side effect was sedation. In dogs, no evidence of toxicity was observed with oral doses up to 2000 mg·kg^{-1} (450 times the maximum recommended dose for adult humans). Terfenadine and astemizole have been associated with rare but severe cardiac arrhythmias. Both are prodrugs and normally little of the parent compound reaches the systemic circulation after oral administration. Following an overdose, however, or in patients with liver disease or those taking drugs that inhibit cytochrome P-450 enzymes, such as ketoconazole or erythromycin, the parent drug accumulates in the blood. Terfenadine and astemizole, but not their metabolites, inhibit the rapid component of the cardiac delayed rectifer K^+ current and block K^+ channels encoded by the human ether-à-go-go-related gene (HERG), resulting in a quinidine-like delay in cardiac repolarisation and prolongation of the QT interval in the electrocardiogram (ECG). This can develop into the life-threating ventricular arrthythmia, *torsades de pointes*, characterised by prolonged ventricular depolarisation, a prolonged QT interval, and polymorphic ventricular tachycardia. The risk of arrhythmia is also increased in patients with QT pathology or who are taking drugs that increase the QT interval, such as amiodorarone, sotalol, and tricyclic antidepressants. Although the incidence of cardiac toxicity is very low (de Abajo and Rodriguez 1999), astemizole was withdrawn by the manufacturer in 1999, and terfenadine was withdrawn in the US after approval of fexofenadine. Terfenadine is still available in Europe. Ketotifen should not be administered concomitantly with oral antidiabetic agents since the combination can lead to a reversible fall in the platelet count in some patients. The mechanism of this interaction is not known. Ketotifen and azelastine have been reported to stimulate appetite and cause body weight gains.

H_2-RECEPTOR ANTAGONISTS

Cimetidine was the first clinically available H_2 antagonist. Currently, five H_2-receptor antagonists are available, cimetidine, ranitidine, famotidine, nizatidine, and roxatidine. Famotidine and nizatidine have durations of action considerably longer than that of cimetidine, so that a single daily oral dose is sufficient. They all competitively inhibit the actions of histamine at all H_2 receptors. There is some evidence that these drugs may be inverse agonists rather than pure antagonists (Smit and co-workers 1998). A combination of H_1 and H_2 antagonists is more effective than an H_1 antagonist alone in the prevention of reactions to drug-induced histamine release. The value of combined therapy in the prevention and treatment of anaphylactic and anaphylactoid reactions is less well established. Since H_2 antagonists block some of the desirable effects of histamine, such as positive inotropy and coronary artery dilatation, they should be used with caution. In addition, H_2-receptors exert a negative feedback on histamine release and antagonism of this might increase histamine release.

The main clinical use of H_2-receptor antagonists is as inhibitors of gastric acid secretion. They inhibit both basal and stimulated gastric secretion of acid and pepsin, with a reduction in the volume of gastric juice. Acid secretion may be inhibited by 90% or more. All are well absorbed when given orally, but undergo varying presystemic metabolism, from 25% to 50% in the case of cimetidine and ranitidine to less than 10% with famotidine, nizatidine and roxatidine. Adverse reactions to these drugs are rare with the doses used to treat patients with peptic ulcers. Cimetidine binds to androgen receptors, displacing dihydrotestorone, and may cause gynaecomastia and impotence in men. A decrease in oestradiol metabolism induced by cimetidine may also be a factor in these symptoms. The frequency of gynaecomastia is about 1 in 1000 but is dose-related. The incidence is higher in patients given high doses, for instance for the treatment of the Zollinger-Ellison syndrome. None of the other three H_2 antagonists have anti-androgenic effects.

Cimetidine is a potent inhibitor of hepatic cytochrome P-450 enzymes responsible for the phase I metabolism of many drugs, including opioids, benzodiazepines, lidocaine (lignocaine) and warfarin. The P-450 inhibition results from a direct interaction between the P-450 haem iron and one of the nitrogen atoms of the imidazole nucleus of cimetidine. Ranitidine, which contains a furan ring in place of imidazole, does not inhibit P-450, although it does form a complex with hepatic cytochrome P-450, but more weakly than cimetidine. None of the other H_2 antagonists inhibit P-450 enzymes.

These drugs are effective in reducing the volume of gastric secretions and raising the pH in surgical and obstetrical patients requiring urgent operations, and so protect against aspiration damage to the lungs. Of the available drugs, ranitidine is most widely used for this purpose. An oral dose of ranitidine 150 mg, 60–90 min given before surgery will produce a peak effect at the time of induction of anaesthesia, and the effect will last for 5–8 hours. Alternatively, it may be given intravenously (dose 50 mg). For reduction of gastric acidity during prolonged surgery or in intensive care patients, ranitidine can be given as a continuous infusion of 200–400 mg per 24 hours. Intravenous cimetidine should be given slowly (over 10 min) to patients with cardiovascular disease, because of a potential risk for cardiac arrhythmias (bradycardia and atrioventricular dissociation).

FURTHER READING

de Abajo FJ, Rodriguez LA. Risk of ventricular arrhythmias associated with nonsedating antihistamine drugs. *Br J Clin Pharmacol* 1999;47:307–13.

Smit MJ, Timmerman H, Alewijnse AE, Leurs R. From histamine H_2 receptor regulation to reclassification of H_2 antagonists; inverse agonism as the basis for H_2 receptor upregulation. *Receptors Channels* 1998;5:99–102.

16

Antineoplastic and immunosuppressive drugs

JG Bovill

Antineoplastic drugs • Immunosuppressive drugs • Specific immunosuppressive drugs

ANTINEOPLASTIC DRUGS

These drugs, also known as chemotherapeutic or cytotoxic agents, are used for the primary treatment of cancer and as adjuvant therapy to surgery and/or radiation therapy. They interfere with DNA synthesis, replication, or transcription, inhibiting division of the cancer cell. Because they act on actively dividing cells, toxicity is common especially in rapidly dividing normal tissues, such as the bone marrow, gastrointestinal epithelium, hair follicle cells, and the reproductive system. Bone marrow suppression results in decreased leucocyte production and an increased risk of infection. Gastrointestinal toxicity is common, and nausea and vomiting can be extremely severe, especially with the alkylating agents and cisplatin. The rapid destruction of tumour cells can increase purine and pyrimidine breakdown products, with increased uric acid production. Precipitation of uric acid crystals in the distal renal tubules causes nephropathy and renal failure. Many cytotoxic drugs are carcinogenic, and some patients, cured of a primary cancer, subsequently develop a second, treatment-induced cancer. Common secondary cancers include leukaemia, lymphoma and squamous cell carcinomas.

Alkylating agents

These compounds contain alkyl groups that form strong, covalent bonds with the nucleic acid bases of DNA, especially guanine. This interferes with DNA transcription and replication, inhibiting mitosis (Figure 16.1). They have a broad spectrum of antitumour activity and are used in the treatment of lymphoma, breast and ovarian carcinoma, melanoma and multiple myeloma.

Nitrogen mustards

These drugs were developed from 'mustard gas' used during the First World War. In addition to bone marrow suppression they cause pulmonary toxicity, that can lead to fibrosis and death. The fibrosis, which is not reversible, can be detected by pulmonary function studies, which should be included in the pre-operative evaluation of patients receiving these drugs.

Cyclophosphamide is the most commonly used alkylating agents, and is also used as an

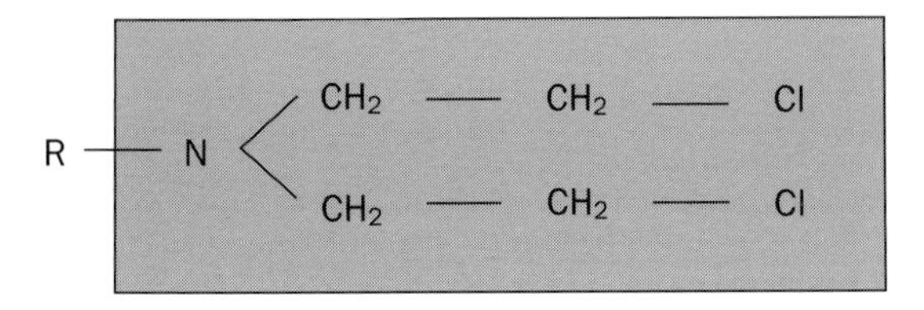

Nitrogen mustards

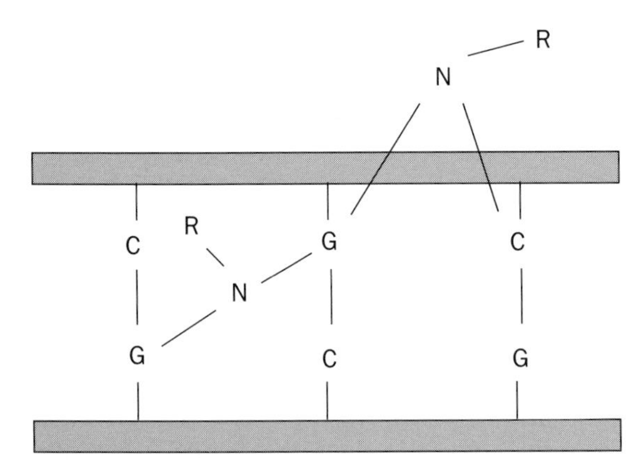

Figure 16.1 *Structure of the nitrogen mustard alkylating agents. The portions of the molecule contained within the shaded box are the nitrogen mustard group. Two of the mechanisms whereby alkylating agents and related compounds act are by interacting with the nucleic acid bases of DNA to form intra- and interstrand cross-links. This interferes with DNA replication and transcription.*

immunosuppressive. It can be administered orally and intravenously. Cyclophosphamide is a prodrug that is metabolised to the active cytotoxic compound, phosphoramide mustard, and acrolein. Acrolein has little cytotoxic activity but is responsible for most of the adverse side effects of cyclophosphamide. The excretion of acrolein in the urine causes haemorrhagic cystitis. Cyclophosphamide can also cause inappropriate water retention due to a direct effect on the renal tubules, and patients should be monitored for hyponatraemia. Cyclophosphamide inhibits plasma cholinesterase synthesis, with a prolonged response to succinylcholine. Other nitrogen mustards are estramustine (a combination of mustine with an oestrogen), melphalan, ifosfamide and chlorambucil. The latter is also used as an immunosuppressive agent.

Nitrosoureas

The main drugs in this group are lomustine, carmustine, semustine and streptozotocin. The nitrosoureas are lipophilic and cross the blood–brain barrier. They are therefore effective against brain tumours. They cause a severe cumulative bone marrow depression that starts within 1–2 months of treatment. Lomustine and carmustine cause direct injury to the pulmonary epithelium leading to alveolar fibrosis. Streptozotocin has little bone marrow toxicity, but destroys the pancreatic β cells, causing diabetes mellitus.

Busulfan

Busulfan has a selective activity on the bone marrow, suppressing granulocyte and platelet formation, and is primarily used in granulocytic leukaemia. Like the nitrogen mustards it can cause pulmonary fibrosis.

Platinum-containing compounds

Cisplatin, and its derivative carboplatin, are used in the treatment of testicular, ovarian and bladder carcinomas as well as head and neck tumours. Cisplatin is a water-soluble compound with a central platinum atom surrounded by two chloride and two ammonia groups (Figure 16.2). Within the cell the chloride ions dissociate, leaving a reactive complex that causes local denaturation of DNA strands. It can cause severe nephrotoxicity and is associated with a high incidence of severe nausea and vomiting, as well as ototoxicity and neurotoxicity. Hydration is a key determinant of the development of renal toxicity and acute renal failure may occur in underhydrated patients. Myleotoxicity is low. Carboplatin causes less nephrotoxicity, ototoxicity and neurotoxicity, and emetic symptoms than cisplatin, but is more myleotoxic. Anaesthetic agents that might be nephrotoxic as a result of free fluoride release, e.g. sevoflurane, should be avoided in

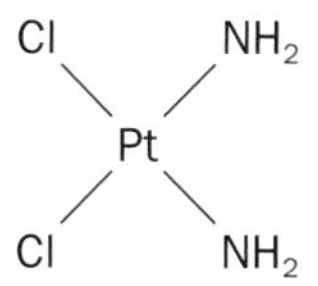

Cl NH$_2$ Pt Cl NH$_2$

Figure 16.2 *The chemical structure of cisplatin.*

patients treated with cisplatin. Non-steroidal anti-inflammatory drugs (NSAIDs) should also be avoided as they may potentiate the nephrotoxicity of cisplatin.

Antimetabolites

Antimetabolites are structural analogues of normal cellular constituents that interfere with the synthesis of purine and pyrimidine, which are essential for DNA synthesis and cell division. They are used in the treatment of gastrointestinal and pulmonary carcinomas as well as sarcomas and some leukaemias. The major toxic effects are bone marrow suppression, mucositis, severe diarrhoea, nausea and vomiting. They have been associated with acute and chronic hepatotoxicity.

Folate antagonists

The main folate antagonist is methotrexate, an analogue of folic acid. Methotrexate competitively inhibits dihydrofolate reductase, the enzyme responsible for the synthesis of purine and pyramidine from folic acid. Trimetrexate, a methotrexate analogue, is useful in treating methotrexate-resistant tumours. It is also used to treat *Pneumocystis carinii* infections. Methotrexate is usually given orally, but may also be given intravenously or intrathecally. In addition to its use in cancer therapy, it is used in the treatment of psoriasis. Methotrexate can cause an obstructive nephropathy due to its precipitation in the renal calyx.

Purine and pyrimidine analogues

The main purine analogues are mercaptopurine, tioguanine, fludarabine, pentostatin and cladribine. They are given orally, although absorption is poor and bioavailability variable. Allopurine inhibits the metabolism of mercaptopurine by xanthine oxidase and increases its bioavailability fivefold. Fluorouracil and cytarabine act primarily by inhibiting pyrimidine synthesis. Fluorouracil may be given orally or intravenously. It readily crosses the blood–brain barrier. Fluorouracil and its derivative deoxifluridine are also administered by intrahepatic arterial infusion in patients with metastases confined to the liver. The high hepatic clearance of these drugs (> 50% for fluorouracil and > 95% for deoxifluridine) allows little drug to escape into the systemic circulation. Their main toxic effects are myelosuppression and gastrointestinal damage.

Cytotoxic antibiotics

The anthracycline antibiotics, which include doxorubicin, daunorubicin, bleomycin, and mitomycin C, inhibit DNA and RNA synthesis. Doxorubicin also interfers with *topoisomerase II* (a DNA gyrase), the activity of which is markedly increased in proliferating cells. Structurally related to doxorubicin are epirubicin and mitozantrone. The cytotoxic antibiotics are used to treat leukaemias and lymphomas and also for solid tumours in the breast, lung, thyroid and ovary. Cardiotoxicity is the major dose-limiting factor, with arrhythmias and myocardial depression (Bacon and Nuzzo 1993). The chronic phase of cardiotoxicity is a dose-dependent cardiomyopathy that leads to congestive heart failure in 2–10% of patients. Myocardial injury is the result of oxygen free radical formation. Children are particularly sensitive to these cardiotoxic reactions and may require a heart transplant in their later years. Epirubicin is less cardiotoxic than doxorubicin.

Bleomycins are a group of glycopeptide antibiotics that degrade preformed DNA. Bleomycin is used in the treatment of testicular carcinoma, sarcomas, and carcinomas of the oesophagus and lung. In contrast to most anticancer drugs, bleomycin causes little myelotoxicity. It is primarily dose-limited by its pulmonary toxicity, occurring in 5–10% of patients. Lung damage is due to formation of superoxide and oxygen free radicals. Lung injury occurs in two phases. The first, occurring one week after treatment, is characterised by interstitial pulmonary oedema, sloughing of the alveolar lining cells, and hyaline membrane formation. The second phase is characterised by interstitial infiltration by inflammatory cells and hyperplasia that eventually lead to pulmonary fibrosis (Goldiner and Shamsi 1993). Symptoms can be delayed up to 4–10 weeks following therapy. A restrictive pattern develops on pulmonary function tests and a decrease in the carbon monoxide diffusion capacity denotes pulmonary compromise. The administration of high-dose corticosteroids may help prevent progression of the fibrosis. In addition to concerns about lung damage prior to surgery, anaesthetists need to be aware of the risk of inducing lung damage by high intraoperative concentrations of oxygen. Exposure to oxygen concentrations greater than 28% increases the incidence of pulmonary toxicity and death after bleomycin.

Mitomycin is used against gastrointestinal, lung and breast cancers. When activated by NADPH cytochrome P-450 reductase within the cell, it acts as an alkylating agent and inhibits DNA function and causes cell death. During this activation process oxygen free radicals are formed, and this can result in lung damage similar to that associated with bleomycin. Once pulmonary toxicity develops there is a very high mortality. The role of increased oxygen concentration in the development of mitomycin-induced pulmonary toxicity has not been proven in humans, but the use of oxygen concentrations less than 28% is recommended, especially in patients with impaired diffusion capacities.

Spindle poisons

Vinca alkaloids

This class of agents, derived from the periwinkle plant *Vinca rosea*, includes vincristine, vinblastine, vinorelbine and vindesine. They bind to and inactivate tubulin, inhibiting microtubule assembly and preventing spindle formation. This arrests the cell in the metaphase of mitosis. The vinca alkaloids are used primarily in the treatment of testicular carcinoma, sarcomas, Hodgkin's and non-Hodgkin's lymphoma, and some leukaemias. The major toxic effect of vinblastine, and to a lesser extent vindesine and vinorelbine, is on the bone marrow. Vincristine is not myelosuppressive but is associated with major neurotoxicity, with a progressive and disabling sensory and motor peripheral neuropathy. Although muscle damage is uncommon, there can be considerable muscle wasting in severely incapacitated patients. Because of the risk of hyperkalaemia, succinylcholine should be avoided in patients with severe neurotoxicity. The vinca alkaloids are administered intravenously, and care is needed to avoid drug extravasation which may cause severe soft-tissue injury.

Taxanes

The taxanes, paclitaxel and docetaxel, derived from the bark of the yew tree, are primarily used in the treatment of breast, lung and ovarian carcinomas. Taxanes enhance tubulin polymerisation, a mechanism that is opposite to that of the vinca alkaloids. Paclitaxel is highly insoluble in water and is emulsified in Cremaphor EL, with an associated risk of anaphylactic reaction. For both drugs, neutropenia is the major dose-limiting side effect, with counts reaching a minimum in 10 days and returning to normal by 21 days. Surgical procedures should, if possible, be scheduled after recovery of the neutropenia. Neurotoxicity can result in a painful peripheral sensory neuropathy. Cardiac toxicity has been observed, causing bradydysrhythmias and second- and third-degree heart block, as well as ventricular tachycardias. Asymptomatic bradycardia occurs in up to 30% of patients during infusion of taxanes and is clinically non-significant.

Immunotherapy and hormones

Interferon and interleukin 2 (IL-2) are used in the treatment of malignant melanoma, renal cell carcinoma, Karposi's sarcoma and various leukaemias and lymphomas. Interferon is synthesized in normal cells as a response to a viral infection. The theory underlying its use is that those malignancies induced by a virally mediated change in DNA may respond to this agent. IL-2 is used to activate naturally occurring killer T cells and tumour-infiltrating lymphocytes. Steroids such as prednisalone are used to treat leukaemias and lymphomas. Tumours derived from hormone-sensitive tissues may be hormone-dependent and their growth inhibited by hormones with opposing actions or hormone antagonists. Oestrogens are used to treat prostate and breast cancers, while progestogens are useful in endometrial cancers and some renal neoplasms. Gonadotrophin-releasing hormone analogues, such as goserelin, are used in the treatment of breast and prostate cancer. The anti-oestrogen, tamoxifen, is very effective in some cases of hormone-dependent breast cancers.

IMMUNOSUPPRESSIVE DRUGS

The main clinical uses of immunosuppressive drugs are suppression of organ and tissue rejection after transplant surgery and the treatment of diseases with an autoimmune component. Thses include renal diseases, e.g. glomerulonephritis, some nephrotic syndromes, connective tissue diseases, such as systemic lupus erythematosus rheumatoid arthritis, and systemic vasculitis.

The immune response

The immune system is an organisation of cells and molecules with specialised roles in the defence against foreign invasion, including infection, transplanted tissues, and tumour cells. It is also involved in a variety of autoimmune diseases. Lymphocytes play a central role in the functioning of the immune system by specifically recognising and responding to different antigenic material (Delves and Roitt 2000). Mature B lymphocytes, when activated by foreign antigens, produce specific antibodies. Antibodies are γ globulins (immunoglobulins) that recognise and interact specifically with antigens, and also activate the host's defence system. They seldom function in isolation but instead marshal other components of the immune system to defend against the invader. T lymphocytes, which mature in the thymus (hence 'T'), are important for the induction phase of the immune response and also cell-mediated immune reactions. Normally, tissue antigens present in the body do not provoke an immune response. However, under certain conditions an immune response will develop against the body's own tissues. This results in an autoimmune disease.

SPECIFIC IMMUNOSUPPRESSIVE DRUGS

Many immunosuppressive drugs act by reducing lymphocyte proliferation during the induction phase of the immune response, but some also have inhibitory actions on the effector phase. They can be classified according to their modes of action:

- Inhibit cytokine gene expression: glucocorticosteroids.
- Inhibition of interleukin-2 (IL-2) production or action: cyclosporin, tacrolimus, rapamycin (sirolimus).
- Cytotoxic mechanisms: cyclophosphamide, chlorambucil.
- Inhibit purine or pyrimidine synthesis: azathioprine, mercaptopurine, myclophenolate mofetil.
- Block surface molecules on T lymphocytes involved in signalling: polyclonal and monoclonal antibodies, immunoglobulins.

Glucocorticosteroids

In humans, the major effect of glucocorticosteroids seems to be to influence lymphocyte traffic. Like cyclosporin, they suppress the clonal proliferation of T cells by inhibiting the transcription of the gene responsible for the expression of IL-2 and possibly other cytokines in both the induction and effector phases of the immune response. The anti-inflammatory actions of steroids are also thought to be involved in their immunosuppressive effect. This may be related to the ability of corticosteroids to block activation of the IL-1 and IL-6 genes in a variety of cells.

Thiopurines

Azathioprine is a cytotoxic inhibitor of purine synthesis effective for the control of tissue rejection in organ transplantation. It is also used in the treatment of autoimmune diseases. Its biologically active metabolite, mercaptopurine, is an inhibitor of DNA synthesis. Mercaptopurine undergoes further metabolism to the active antitumour and immunosuppressive thioinosinic acid. This inhibits the conversion of purines to the corresponding phosphoribosyl-5′ phosphates and hypoxanthine to inosinic acid, leading to inhibition of cell division and this is the mechanism of the immunosuppression by azathioprine and mercaptopurine. Humans are more sensitive than other species to the toxic effects of the thiopurines, in particular those involving the haematopoietic system. The major limiting toxicity of the thiopurines is bone marrow suppression, with leucopenia and thrombocytopenia. Liver toxicity is another common toxic effect.

Cyclophosphamide

Cyclophosphamide belongs to the family of nitrogen mustard alkylating agents also used for their antineoplastic actions. Cyclophosphamide has powerful immunosuppressive properties, with a particular action on lymphocytes, and may induce a profound lymphocytopenia. Life-threating toxicity may occur, particularly myelosuppression, haemorrhagic cystitis and cardiomyopathy. Cyclophosphamide can be used for the treatment of autoimmune diseases and to prevent graft rejection, but its use has significantly decreased with the advent of cyclosporin. It reduces the activity of plasma cholinesterase by 50% and may be associated with prolonged apnoea following succinylcholine (Davis and co-workers 1997). Chlorambucil is another alkylating agent with effects similar to cyclophosphamide used as an immunosuppressive.

Cyclosporin

The introduction of cyclosporin, a peptide derived from a fungus, revolutionised immunosuppressive therapy, and was one of the major influences in the improvement of early graft survival in transplant surgery when introduced in the 1980s. The main action is a relatively selective inhibition of IL-2 production and consequently a decreased proliferation of T cells. A major advantage of cyclosporin is that it does not cause myelosuppression in therapeutic doses. The major side effect is nephrotoxicity, which occurs in about 20% of patients, and about 50% of patients develop moderate hypertension. The other major side effect is hepatotoxicity with cholestasis and hyperbilirubinaemia.

Cyclosporin is metabolised by the hepatic cytochrome P-450 enzyme system, and enzyme induction by phenobarbital, phenytoin, carbamazepine, or rifampicin will drastically increase the clearance of cyclosporin. Concurrent administration of these drugs has caused rejection of transplanted organs. Conversely, the use of enzyme inhibitors, such as erythromycin or the azole antifungal agents, e.g. ketoconazole, will increase the blood concentrations of cyclosporin leading to an increased risk of toxic side effects.

Cyclosporin is usually given orally, although absorption is often unpredictable. The intravenous route is usually restricted to patients who cannot take the drug orally, because of the risk of anaphylactic reactions. Other uses of cyclosporin include psoriasis and severe, active rheumatoid arthritis when these do not respond to conventional treatment, and steroid-resistant nephrotic syndrome.

Tacrolimus

Tacrolimus (previously known as FK506) is a macrolide antibiotic with immunosuppressive properties very similar to cyclosporin. It is more potent than cyclosporin but the side effects are similar. Tacrolimus is a very active immunosuppressive drug both in the prevention and treatment of liver and renal allograft rejection. It is especially valuable for small bowel transplantation.

Rapamycin

Rapamycin, also known as sirolimus, is a new macrolide antibiotic that interacts with cell-cycle regulating proteins and inhibits cell division. The main side effects are thrombocytopenia and hyperlipidaemia. There is also evidence that it causes interstitial pneumonitis, which may resolve on withdrawing the drug or dose reduction. The drug is currently being assessed for combination therapy with tacrolimus or cyclosporin.

Mycophenolate mofetil

Mycophenolate mofetil is a semisynthetic derivative of a fungal antibiotic with a selective effect on immunocompetent cells. It is given in combination with cyclosporin and steroids to prevent graft rejection, especially after kidney transplants. It is converted by plasma esterases to the active metabolite, mycophenolic acid, which is a non-competitive, reversible inhibitor of inosine monophosphate dehydrogenase, an enzyme essential for the synthesis of purine. B and T lymphocytes are particularly dependent on this pathway, since unlike other cells they cannot obtain purine via alternative pathways. Side effects are generally mild, the most common being a dose-dependent gastrointestinal toxicity, although bone marrow depression can also occur. Other new antimetabolite agents with similar actions are mizoribine and brequinar sodium.

Polyclonal antibodies, antithymocyte globulins (ATG)

Polyclonal antibodies or ATG are obtained by injecting animals (horse or rabbit) with human thymocytes and then separating the resulting immune sera to obtain purified γ-globulin fractions. These preparations have been used for organ transplantation since the 1970s and have proved to be more effective than corticosteroids for reversing acute allograft rejection. Each polyclonal immunoglobulin preparation varies in its constituent antibodies. As a consequence, treatment is associated with variable efficacy as well as with adverse reactions. Unwanted antibodies can cause thrombocytopenia and granulocytopenia. Owing to the development of host antibodies to the animal polyclonal immunoglobulin, serum sickness commonly occurs during treatment. There are several possible mechanisms by which ATG may exert its immunosuppressive effect. These include classic complement-mediated lympholysis, clearance of lymphocytes in the mononuclear phagocytic system, and masking of T-cell antigens, resulting in inhibition of lymphocyte function.

Monoclonal antibody anti-CD3, OKT3

OKT3 is a murine monoclonal antibody (moab) directed against the CD3 molecule present on the surface of human thymocytes and mature T cells. OKT3 is a very powerful immunosuppressive agent in renal transplantation. The initial use of OKT3 is accompanied by side effects, which are usually transient and seldom life-threatening. These are partly attributed to the release of cytokines as a result of mononuclear cell activation or lysis, or complement activation. There is an increased incidence of infections and post-transplant lymphoproliferative disease and lymphomas associated with OKT3. Development of human antimouse antibodies represents an important limitation to OKT3 treatment. Because of concerns about the risk of infection and malignancy, OKT3 is not used for the treatment of autoimmune diseases.

FURTHER READING

Bacon DR, Nuzzo RJ. Anthracycline antineoplastic chemotherapy agents: anesthetic implications. *Semin Anesth* 1993;12:74–8.

Davis L, Britten JJ, Morgan M. Cholinesterase. Its significance in anaesthetic practice. *Anaesthesia* 1997;52:244–60.

Delves PJ, Roitt IN. The immune system. *New Engl J Med* 2000;343:37–49; 108–17.

Goldiner PL, Shamsi A. Bleomycin–oxygen interaction. *Semin Anesth* 1993;12:79–82.

17

Drugs acting on the haemostatic system

JG Bovill

Clotting cascade • Heparin • Hirudin • Fondaparinux • Protamine • Oral anti-coagulants • Thrombolytic (fibrinolytic) drugs • Antifibrinolytic agents • Antiplatelet drugs

CLOTTING CASCADE

Haemostasis is a complex interplay between the processes that promote clotting and those that inhibit it. The primary element in the arrest of bleeding after blood vessel injury is the aggregation and disposition of platelets. The second key element is the blood coagulation cascade. This consists of a complex sequence of biochemical events involving various factors that circulate in an inactive form until the *milieu intérieur* is disturbed. The end-point of the coagulation sequence is the cleavage of prothrombin into two fragments, one of which is the enzyme thrombin. Thrombin acts on fibrinogen to produce fibrin which then polymerises to form insoluble fibrin (Figure 17.1). Thrombin also activates factor XIII which catalyses the formation of covalent bonds between the fibrin molecules to form a clot resistent to dissolution.

Clotting activity is critically balanced by the fibrinolytic system, which is activated by the deposition of fibrin. Fibrinolysis is mediated through the activation of plasminogen which is the precursor of the proteolytic enzyme plasmin. Plasminogen binds to lysine residues on the surface of fibrin and is converted to plasmin by tissue plasminogen activator (tPA) which is released from damaged endothelial cells. Plasmin degrades fibrin into soluble fibrin degradation products. Excess plasmin is rapidly removed from the plasma by the protease inhibitor, α_2 antiplasmin. Both the coagulation cascade and the fibrinolytic system can be manipulated by a variety of drugs.

HEPARIN

Heparin is a negatively charged mixture of polysaccharide molecules of different chain lengths. Unfractionated heparin, produced from porcine intestines or bovine lungs, consists of chains of alternating residues of D-glucosamine and either glucuronic acid or iduronic acid. The distribution of molecular weights ranges from 5000 to 30 000 daltons (Da), with an average of 12 000–15 000 Da. Heparin acts as an anticoagulant by binding to antithrombin via a specific pentaseccharide sequence, promoting the interaction of antithrombin with activated plasma coagulation factors, thrombin (factor IIa) and factor Xa. The heparin–antithrombin complex inhibits several clotting factors, including thrombin, IXa and Xa. Antithrombin, like tPA and prostacyclin, is an endothelial-derived factor instrumental in preventing thrombosis. Patients deficient in antithrombin are resistant to the anticoagulant effects of heparin. Acquired antithrombin

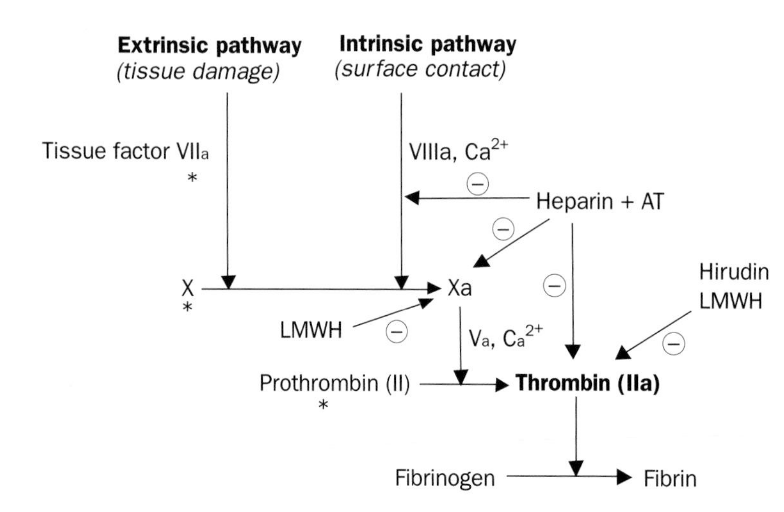

Figure 17.1 *The coagulation cascade. *, Site of action of vitamin K antagonists; LMWH, low molecular weight heparin.*

deficiency occurs due to either a decrease in the amount of antithrombin produced, an increase in the rate at which it is consumed, or an abnormal loss from the circulation. Examples of acquired antithrombin deficiency states include acute liver failure (it is produced by the liver), disseminated intravascular coagulation, sepsis, cardiopulmonary bypass, or prolonged heparin administration, which leads to excessive consumption of antithrombin. This form of heparin resistance can be treated by the administration of human plasma antithrombin, which is approved for clinical use in Europe. A recombinant human antithrombin, produced from the milk of transgenic goats, is undergoing clinical trials. The formation of the heparin–antithrombin complex requires a critical chain length of 18 sugar units and a molecular weight of 5400 Da. This sequence is not required for the inhibition of factor Xa. Because most of the molecules in unfractionated heparin have a molecular weight above 5400 Da, the anti-Xa/anti-IIa activity is approximately 1.

The bioavailability (subcutaneous) and anticoagulant effect of heparin is reduced by binding to plasma and platelet proteins. The plasma half-life is about 90 min (range 30–360 min). Endothelial and reticulo-endothelial uptake is the most important process for termination of the anticoagulant effect with renal clearance being a much slower process. As a result, the pharmacokinetics of heparin is non-linear and low doses are cleared rapidly while higher doses are cleared more slowly. Heparin-induced anticoagulation is monitored by the activated partial thromboplastin time (aPTT) or the activated clotting time (ACT). The anticoagulant effects of standard heparin are rapidly neutralised by equimolar doses of protamine. Because of the heterogenicity of unfractionated heparin, potency is determined by a biological assay and the dose is expressed in units of activity rather than mass (130 units corresponds to approximately 1 mg heparin).

Clinical use of heparin

The main use of unfractionated heparin is the treatment of thromboembolic diseases, e.g. pulmonary embolism, myocardial infarction or established deep venous thrombosis, or the prevention of coagulation during cardiac and vascular surgery. In the past low-dose subcutaneous unfractionated heparin (5000 units every 8–12 hours) was commonly used as prophylaxis against deep venous thrombosis, but low molecular weight heparins are now more often used. Much higher doses are needed for full therapeutic anticoagulation. For the treatment of thromboembolic disease heparin is given as an intravenous loading dose (5000–1000 units) followed by either repeated subcutaneous injections or a continuous IV infusion, adjusted to maintain the aPTT at 1.5–2.5 times the control value. For cardiac surgery the usual initial dose is 300 units·kg^{-1}.

Low molecular weight heparin

Low molecular weight heparins (LMWHs) are fractions of unfractionated heparin with molecular weights ranging from 2000 Da to 10 000 Da, with mean molecular weights of 4000–6000 (Figure 17.2). They also bind to antithrombin (AT), but this results in far less anti-AT activity. LMWHs exhibit higher anti-Xa activity than unfractionated heparin. The different preparations have slightly different molecular weight distributions and this accounts for differences in the anti-Xa/anti-IIa ratios (Table 17.1). Currently, it is not known whether these differences have practical clinical consequences.

Table 17.1 Anti-factor Xa/anti-factor IIa ratio for marketed low molecular weight heparins (LMWHs)

LMWH	*Anti-Xa/Anti-IIa ratio*
Ardeparin	2
Certoparin	4.2
Dalteparin	4.0
Enoxaparin	3.8
Nadroparin	3.6
Parnoparin	1.5–3
Reviparin	5.0
Tinzaparin	1.9

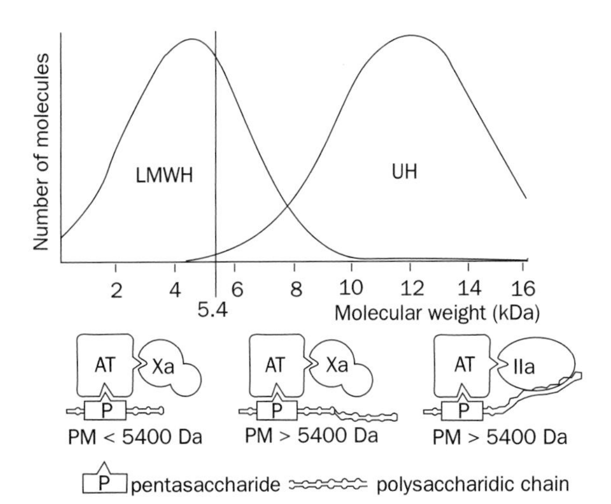

Figure 17.2 *Schematic representation of the molecular weight distribution of unfractionated heparin (UH) and of low molecular weight heparin (LMWH). In the lower part of the figure, the polysaccharide chain of heparin, the pentasaccharide sequence, and the interaction between heparin, antithrombin (AT), thrombin, and factor Xa is represented. (Reproduced from Boneu B. Thrombosis Research 2000;100:V113–20, with permission from Elsevier Science.)*

Activated clotting time (ACT) and activated partial thromboplastin time (aPTT) are relatively unaffected by LMWH. Anti-Xa activity can be used to monitor anticoagulation activity, but this is expensive and time-consuming and is seldom indicated. Although protamine has some effect on LMWH, about 60–80% of the antithrombotic activity will persist. This is because of the reduced protamine binding to these drugs and because only the anti-IIa activity is completely reversed whereas anti-Xa activity is only partially neutralised.

In contrast to unfractionated heparin, LMWHs bind weakly to endothelial cells and are cleared mainly by renal excretion. A consequence of this is that their pharmacokinetics and pharmacodynamics are linear and the pharmacodynamics effect is proportional to the dose. This makes them more predictable than standard heparin, and is the main reason why routine monitoring is not needed. Because of the predominantly renal excretion there is a risk of accumulation in patients with reduced renal function. In this group of patients it may be advisable to monitor the anti-Xa activity.

Side effects of heparin

Bleeding is uncommon with prophylactic doses of unfractionated or LMWH but more likely in patients receiving therapeutic doses. The incidence of major bleeding in fully anticoagulated patients has been estimated as approximately 5%. Unlike warfarin, heparin does not cross the placenta and has not been associated with fetal malformations and heparin is therefore used for anticoagulation during pregnancy. If possible, heparin should be discontinued 24 hours before delivery to minimise the risk of postpartum bleeding. Osteoporosis is an uncommon adverse effect of long-term (6 months or more) treatment with heparin, usually during pregnancy.

Heparin-induced thrombocytopenia (HIT) is relatively common in patients receiving therapeutic doses of intravenous heparin, with an incidence of 1–3%. The incidence is about 2–3 times higher for bovine heparin than for porcine heparin. Two clinically distinct types of HIT have been described, type I and type II (Chong 1995). In Type I, the thrombocytopenia is mild and the platelet count seldom falls below $100 \cdot 10^9 \cdot L^{-1}$, and may return to normal even if the heparin is continued. In contrast, type II HIT is a severe thrombocytopenia with platelet counts often below $60 \cdot 10^9 \cdot L^{-1}$. The onset is delayed, usually appearing 4–14 days after commencement of treatment, and the thrombocytopenia will not recover unless the heparin is stopped. After heparin withdrawal, platelet counts usually rise to normal levels within 5–7 days, although occasionally recovery may take several weeks. Treatment of type II thrombocytopenia is immediate cessation of heparin. Anticoagulation therapy can be continued with oral anticoagulants, but since these take 3–5 days to achieve a full therapeutic effect, an immediate-acting agent should be administered. Alternatives to heparin include the low molecular weight heparinoid, orgaran, ancrod or LMWHs. Orgaran is a mixture of heparan sulphate, dermatin sulphate, and chrondroitin sulphate, all three derived from pig intestinal mucosa after removal of the heparin. Ancrod is a defibrinogenating agent derived from the Malayan pit viper.

The underlying pathophysiology of type I HIT is probably related to the platelet-aggregating effect of heparin itself. The mechanism of type II HIT is likely immune. It has been suggested that binding of heparin to platelet factor 4 stimulates the production of an immunoglobulin (IgG) antibody. This then binds to the heparin-platelet factor 4 molecule, forming an immune complex that binds to platelets causing their activation and increased clearance by the reticuloendothelial system. Activation also releases more platelet factor 4 so that a vicious circle of platelet destruction is established. Possibly because they interact less with platelets, the risk of thrombocytopenia is less with the LMWHs. In some patients, however, there is a cross-reactivity with the heparin-dependent antibody, and in these patients LMWHs should not be used to replace heparin if type II HIT develops. Cross-reactivity can be detected by the platelet aggregation test.

HIRUDIN

Hirudin, originally isolated from the medicinal leach, *Hirudo medicinalis*, is a very potent and specific inhibitor of thrombin. Its anticoagulant activity is independent of antithrombin, and it does not interact with platelets. Hirudin is now produced through recombinant DNA technology (r-hirudin). It has been used in patients with unstable angina pectoris or myocardial infarction, drug-induced thrombocytopenia and deep-venous thrombosis. Hirudin has also been used successfully during cardiac surgery in patients with heparin-induced thrombocytopenia (Latham and co-workers 2000). Conventional monitoring of thrombin activity using aPTT is not suitable for monitoring hirudin because of a very high inter-individual variability. The method of choice is the ecarin clotting time (eCT). Ecarin is a protease isolated from the snake, *Echis carinatus*, which activates prothrombin to form an intermediate that rapidly forms complexes with r-hirudin. Because the eCT relies on measuring prothrombin activity, it is unreliable in patients with low levels of prothrombin.

FONDAPARINUX

Fondaparinux sodium is the first of a new class of direct-acting antithrombin agents. The anticoagulant activity of heparin depends on the binding of ATIII to a critical pentasaccharide sequence within the heparin molecule. This results in a change in the conformation of ATIII. This leads to the inhibitory effect of ATIII on factor Xa, which activates the conversion of prothrombin to thrombin. Fondaparinux is a synthetic pentasaccharide identical to the ATIII-binding site of heparin. It is thus a selective inhibitor of factor Xa. Fondaparinux binds very strongly and exclusively to its ATIII target, with no detectable binding to other plasma proteins. It has no direct activity against thrombin, and no known interactions with other coagulation enzymes. Its effect on routine haemostasis tests is therefore very limited. Unlike heparin, it does not bind to platelets and has no effect on platelet function. It is rapidly and almost completely absorbed after subcutaneous injection. The half-life is 17 hours, allowing once-daily dosing. Fondaparinux is not metabolised and is almost completely excreted by the kidneys as the unchanged compound. Thus, its clearance may be delayed in patients with renal insufficiency. There are no known interactions with other drugs.

PROTAMINE

Protamines are low molecular weight basic proteins synthesised in the sperm of most vertebrate species, including humans. Protamine used clinically is isolated from fish, especially salmon sperm, and is available both as sulphate and chloride salts. Although protamine chloride may have a more rapid onset than protamine sulphate, clinically there is little to choose between either preparation. The main clinical indication is to reverse the anticoagulant effect of heparin, especially following cardiac surgery and other vascular procedures. The recommended dose varies from 1–1.5 mg/100 IU heparin. About 66% of the protamine molecule is composed of positively charged arginine amino acids that bind to the negatively charged heparin, neutralising it. Protamine neutralises the antithrombin effect of heparin much better than the anti-Xa effect. This explains its poor efficacy in neutralising LMWHs.

Adverse effects

Protamine itself is an anticoagulant and when given in excess of that needed to neutralise heparin can increase bleeding. The heparin–protamine complex inhibits thrombin-induced platelet aggregation and protamine binds to thrombin, preventing it from converting fibrinogen to fibrin. It also stimulates the release of tissue plasminogen activator from endothelial cells.

Cardiovascular

When given rapidly, protamine causes hypotension due to a decrease in vascular resistance, possibly linked to the release of nitric oxide from endothelium. Hypotension can be minimised by slow administration over 10–15 minutes. Protamine does not affect myocardial contractility. In some patients, systemic hypotension occurs in conjunction with pulmonary hypertension and, in severe cases, right ventricular failure. The mechanism is activation of the complement pathways by the heparin–protamine complex leading to release of thromboxane A_2, which mediates pulmonary vasoconstriction. Unlike in anaphylaxis, plasma histamine concentrations are not increased. When this syndrome develops protamine administration should be stopped, and some have recommended giving heparin in an attempt to reduce the size of the heparin–protamine complex.

Anaphylactoid/anaphylactic reactions

About 28% of patients develop IgG or IgE antibodies after a single exposure to protamine, but fortunately few develop a catastrophic allergic reaction on subsequent exposure to the drug. Nonetheless, prior exposure does increase the risk for an anaphylactic reaction. Other risk factors are fish allergy and patients with diabetes mellitus treated with neutral protamine Hagedorn (NPH) insulin. After vasectomy, 22%

of men develop IgG antibodies to human protamine which may cross-react with salmon protamine. However, these autoantibodies are usually present in low titres and vasectomy remains only a theoretical risk for protamine allergy. Many patients with prior vasectomy have received protamine during cardiac surgery without adverse effects.

ORAL ANTICOAGULANTS

The discovery of the coumarin oral anticoagulants is one of many examples of serendipity in pharmacology. In 1924, a mysterious haemorrhagic disorder developed in cattle feeding on spoiled sweet clover silage. The haemorrhagic agent was isolated and identified as bishydroxycoumarin (dicoumarol). Dicoumarol was the first oral anticoagulant used clinically, but it is now seldom used because it is absorbed slowly and erratically and frequently causes gastrointestinal side effects. Subsequent research led to the development of warfarin, initially introduced as a rodenticide in 1948 but later as an oral anticoagulant for humans. Warfarin was named as an acronym derived from the name of the patent holder, Wisconsin Alumni Research Foundation, plus the coum*arin*-derived suffix. Several hundred derivatives of coumarin have since been synthesised. Warfarin is the prototypical oral anticoagulant, but the anticoagulant action of all the drugs in this class is similar, differing mainly in potency and duration of action. Warfarin is almost completely (99%) bound to plasma proteins, principally albumin. Concomitant use of drugs that decrease the metabolism of warfarin or displace it from protein binding sites, such as phenylbutazone, sulfinpyrazone, metronidazole, allopurinol, cimetidine, amiodarone, or acute intake of ethanol enhance the risk of hemorrhage in patients taking oral anticoagulants. The half-life of warfarin is 42 hours. Concentrations in fetal plasma approach the maternal values, but active warfarin is not found in milk (unlike other coumarins and indandiones). Oral anticoagulants should not be used during pregnancy, since during the first trimester they are associated with birth defects and abortion. Central nervous system abnormalities have been reported following exposure during the second and third trimesters. Fetal or neonatal haemorrhage and intrauterine death may occur, even when maternal international normalised ratio (INR) values are in the therapeutic range (see below).

Coumarins are competitive inhibitors of vitamin K, which is required for the formation in the liver of the amino acid, gamma-carboxyglutamic acid. This is necessary for the synthesis of prothrombin and factors VII, IX and X (Figure 17.1). After starting treatment the anticoagulant effect is delayed until the concentration of normal coagulation factors falls (36–72 h). The effects can be reversed by vitamin K (slow; maximum effect only after 3–6 h) or by whole blood or plasma (fast). Gut bacteria synthesise vitamin K and thus are an important source of this vitamin. Consequently, antibiotics can cause excessive prolongation of the prothrombin time in patients otherwise adequately controlled on warfarin.

The prothrombin time (PT) is used to monitor anticoagulation. The patient's PT is determined along with that for a control sample of plasma, and the two values are often reported as a ratio. Because this ratio can vary widely between laboratories, the INR system of reporting has been adopted. The INR is the ratio of the patient PT to a control PT obtained by a standard method using a World Health Organisation primary standard (human) thromboplastin. PT measurements are converted to INR measurements by the following equation:

$$\mathrm{INR} = \left(\frac{PT_{\mathrm{pat}}}{PT_{\mathrm{ref}}}\right)^{ISI}$$

where ISI is the international sensitivity index (usually very close to 1). Therapeutic anticoagulation requires an INR between 2.5 and 3.5, although higher values (3.5–5.0) are indicated in patients with artificial heart valves.

THROMBOLYTIC (FIBRINOLYTIC) DRUGS

The body's vascular system has inherent fibrinolytic activity, involving the conversion of the inactive precursor, plasminogen, to the active enzyme plasmin (Figure 17.3). Plasmin hydrolyses key bonds in the fibrin matrix, causing dissolution of the clot. Thrombolytic agents accelerate and amplify the conversion of plasminogen to plasmin. There are well-documented benefits for the use of thrombolytic agents in restoring vascular patency when given within 12 hours after a myocardial infarction. Their use in the immediate management of stroke is still controversial. Streptokinase and urokinase are first-generation thrombolytic drugs. Urokinase is a trypsin-like serine protease that activates plasminogen directly, converting it to the active plasmin. It is prepared from cultures of human embryonic kidney cells. It is less effective than streptokinase and its clinical usefulness is limited. Streptokinase is a non-enzymatic protein produced by β-haemolytic streptococci. It activates the fibrinolytic system indirectly by forming complexes with plasminogen, thereby activating it. Antistreptococcal antibodies develop about 4 days after the initial dose, blocking its action. Streptokinase is cleared rapidly from the circulation, with a half-life of 15 minutes.

Anistreplase is a complex of human plasminogen and streptokinase in which an anisoyl group has been introduced in the plasminogen molecule, protecting it from autodigestion. The half-life of activation is about 100 min. This allows it to be given as an intravenous bolus, whereas streptokinase must be given as an infusion. Newer thrombolytic agents, such as altepase, duplase, reteplase, and lanotreplase, are recombinant versions of the naturally occurring tissue plasminogen activator (tPA). Like the parent tPA, their activity is markedly enhanced in the presence of fibrin. Because they are more active on fibrin-bound plasminogen than on free plasminogen in the plasma, they are referred to as 'clot-selective'. Altepase and duplase have very short durations of action and must be given by infusion. Reteplase and lanotreplase have a longer half-life and can be administered as a bolus. The main adverse effect of all these agents is bleeding, including gastrointestinal and intracerebral haemorrhage. Streptokinase can cause hypotension, thought to be due to generation of kinins secondary to the rapid production of plasmin.

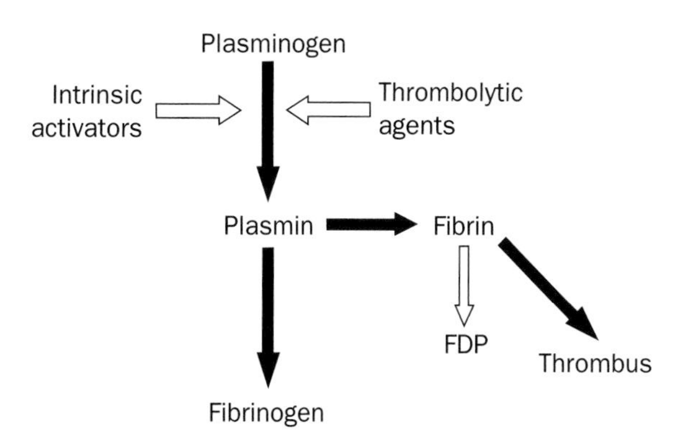

Figure 17.3 *Schematic representation of the fibrinolytic system. FDP, degradation products.*

ANTIFIBRINOLYTIC AGENTS

Epsilon-aminocaproic acid and tranexamic acid are lysine analogues that inhibit the breakdown of cross-linked fibrin by plasmin. Epsilon-aminocaproic acid has a structure closely related to the amino acid, lysine. In tranexamic acid, the 4-carbon chain of aminocaproic acid is substituted by a cyclohexane molecule producing a compound with 7–10 times greater potency. Both molecules bind to the lysine-binding sites of plasminogen and plasmin, which are then unable to bind to the C-terminal lysine residues of fibrin or fibrinogen (Figure 17.4). In addition to its greater potency, tranexamic acid is able to cross the blood–brain barrier and has a much wider tissue distribution. Both ε-aminocaproic acid and tranexamic acid may improve haemostasis by a combination of inhibition of fibrinolysis, reduced release of tPA, and preservation of platelet function. Tranexamic acid is more potent and has the same low toxicity as ε-aminocaproic acid and the latter is now seldom used and is no longer registered for clinical use in many countries.

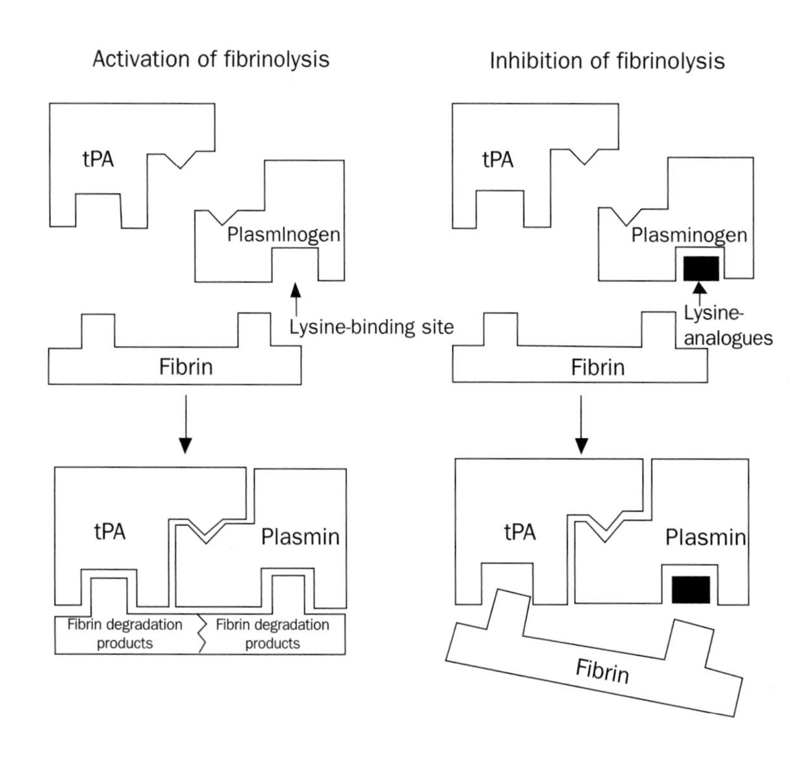

Figure 17.4 *Antifibrinolytic action of the lysine analogues. Normally, plasminogen binds to fibrin at a lysine-binding site and is converted in the presence of tissue plasminogen activator (tPA) to plasmin. The lysine analogues block the lysine-binding site and prevent access of plasminogen to the fibrin molecule. (Reproduced from Dunn CJ, Goa KL.* Drugs *1999;57:1005–32, with permission.)*

Concern about adverse effects of these compounds has centred on their potential to produce or potentiate abnormal thrombus formation. Significant upper urinary tract bleeding is regarded as a contraindication to ε-aminocaproic acid treatment because of the formation of insoluble clots resulting in urinary obstruction. There are also case reports of cerebral thrombosis during ε-aminocaproic acid therapy for subarachnoid haemorrhage and similar reports linking tranexamic acid with intracranial thrombosis. However, prospective studies have not shown clear evidence of acceleration of thrombosis by short-term administration of either drug.

Aprotinin

Aprotinin, a highly basic polypeptide, is a naturally occurring inhibitor of proteolytic enzymes. Its main physiological function is inhibition of plasmin and kallikreins although it also inhibits the tissue factor VIIa complex. The concentration and activity of aprotinin are given as KIU (kallikrein inactivator units); 100 000 KIU are equivalent to 14 mg of the pure polypeptide or 2.15 $\mu mol \cdot L^{-1}$ aprotinin. Aprotinin is only active by the intravenous route and is largely excreted by the kidney. The key activity of aprotinin in reducing surgical blood loss is reduction of fibrinolytic activation, although there is also clear evidence of an anticoagulant effect and reduced activation of coagulation. The inhibition of both plasmin and thrombin production is probably responsible for the preservation of platelet function and reduction in peri-operative haemorrhage. Aprotinin also appears to be effective in reducing transfusion requirements in patients on aspirin. High-dose aprotinin appears to reduce bleeding by around 50% in open heart surgery, the effect being more prominent in redo surgery and more prolonged procedures.

Desmopressin

Desmopressin (1-deamino-8-D-arginine vasopressin; DDAVP) is a synthetic analogue of vasopressin. The substitution of D-arginine for L-arginine gives desmopressin both greater potency and a more prolonged duration of action than vasopressin. There are two classes of vasopressin receptors; V_1 receptors mediate smooth muscle contraction in the peripheral vasculature, while V_2 receptors regulate water reabsorption in the collecting ducts of the kidney. Desmopressin is a strong V_2 receptor agonist with no effect on V_1 receptors. Its haemostatic effects are also mediated via low affinity, extrarenal V_2 receptor. Activation of V_2 receptors by desmopressin increases circulating levels of procoagulant factor VIII, von Willebrand factor, and tPA, and it has been successfully used in the treatment of type I von Willebrand's disease, mild factor VIII deficiency (haemophilia A), and intrinsic platelet function defects for almost three decades. It increases platelet adhesiveness by mechanisms that are not fully understood, but may involve platelet von Willebrand factor and platelet glycoprotein (GP) IIb/IIIa receptors. Desmopressin reduces bleeding time in a variety of disorders, such as congenital or drug-induced platelet dysfunction, uraemia, and liver dysfunction. It shortens the bleeding time prolonged by drugs such as aspirin or ticlopidine. It can be administered intravenously, subcutaneously or by intranasal spray.

Because it does not interact with V_1 receptors desmopressin has virtually no vasoconstrictive effect and does not contract the uterus or gastrointestinal tract. Rapid injection will cause hypotension due to a decrease in vascular resistance. It is not known whether this is secondary to the known action of desmopressin to induce prostacyclin release or by stimulation of V_2 receptors. Although desmopressin is of minor value in reducing blood transfusion requirements in cardiac surgery, it may have some role, together with correction of the haematocrit and/or cryoprecipitate transfusion, in correcting the bleeding tendency in uraemic patients, which is in part due to acquired platelet dysfunction. Desmopressin is a potent antidiuretic agent but water retention rarely occurs in clinical practice, and no problems with fluid overload or congestive heart failure have been reported in uraemic patients. It should, however, be used with caution in patients with congestive heart disease because of its antidiuretic effect.

ANTIPLATELET DRUGS

Aspirin

Platelets occupy a primary role in haemostasis, maintaining vascular integrity and contributing to the complex process of coagulation. All NSAIDs interfere with platelet function by mechanisms involving inhibition of cyclooxygenase. This blocks the formation not only of platelet-activating eicosanoids, such as PGG_2, PGH_2, and thromboxane A_2, but also of the platelet inhibitors PGD_2 and PGI_2. For all NSAIDs, except aspirin, the inhibition of cyclooxygenase is reversible and the antiplatelet effect is present only while the drug is present in the body in sufficient concentration. In the case of aspirin, the effect lasts for the 5–11 days of the life of the platelet because of the irreversible acetylation of platelet cyclooxygenase, coupled with the inability of platelets to synthesise new enzyme. Aspirin is the only NSAID that is used therapeutically for its antiplatelet effects. Aspirin in low doses is widely used in patients with cardiovascular disease to reduce the incidence of myocardial infarction and stroke. Doses as low as 40 mg per day can produce maximum inhibition of thromboxane and prostacyclin synthesis. The use of aspirin can reduce the risk of myocardial infarction by 25% and reduce the risk of a fatal infarction significantly. The effectiveness of aspirin is, however, limited since it fails to block platelet activation by other important agonists such as shear stress, thrombin, collagen and ADP (adenosine 5′-diphosphate).

Dipyridamole

Dipyridamole, a phosphodiesterase inhibitor, is a vasodilator that interferes with platelet function by increasing the cellular concentration of adenosine monophosphate (cAMP). This effect is mediated by inhibition of cyclic nucleotide phosphodiesterase and/or by blockade of uptake of adenosine. Adenosine acts at A_2 receptors to stimulate platelet adenylyl cyclase. Dipyridamole alone is no better than aspirin in preventing intravascular thrombosis, but the combination with aspirin appears to confer advantages when compared to aspirin alone, at least for the prevention of stroke.

Ticlopidine

Ticlopidine, a thienopyridine derivative, is an antiplatelet drug that, unlike aspirin, does not affect the cyclooxygenase pathway, but acts by inhibition of ADP-dependent activation of the glycoprotein (GP) IIb/IIIa receptor. It is a prodrug, working through an active metabolite, and the onset of action is slow, taking 3–7 days to reach maximum effect. Neutropenia occurs in 1–2% of patients and this has limited its long-term use. There is also an approximately 0.2% incidence of thrombocytopenia, a condition that is fatal in 25–50% of patients. Because of these two blood dyscrasias patients receiving ticlopidine must undergo regular serial blood counts. Gastrointestinal side effects and rashes are also common. The main indication is in the management of patients who continue to experience cerebrovascular events, despite adequate aspirin therapy, or who cannot tolerate aspirin. The combination with aspirin may also benefit patients with coronary artery disease. *Clopidogrel* is structurally related to ticlopidine, but with a more favourable side effect profile (Quinn and Fitzgerald 1999). Recovery is slow after drug withdrawal, and these drugs should be stopped at least 7 days before major surgery to prevent excessive intra- and postoperative bleeding.

Platelet glycoprotein IIb/IIIa receptor antagonists

The adhesion and aggregration of platelets is mediated by surface membrane GP IIb/IIIa receptors, which interact with the distal ends of fibrinogen. This enables a bridge to be formed between two adjacent platelets. Several compounds that act as antagonists of this receptor and so prevent platelet aggregation and to some extent adhesion have been developed. The GPIIb/IIIa inhibitors in clinical use and under development are antibody- and peptide-based antagonists given intravenously, and non-peptides with parenteral or oral routes of administration. Abciximab, the first drug of this class to be tested and used extensively in man, is the Fab fragment of a murine monoclonal antibody to GPIIb/IIIa attenuated by generating a chimeric molecule of human and murine protein to reduce immunogenicity. Large phase III trials are currently underway assessing their efficacy and safety for the management of patients with coronary artery disease or acute myocardial infarction (Quinn and Fitzgerald 1998; Becker 1999).

FURTHER READING

Becker RC. New thrombolytics, anticoagulants, and platelet antagonists: the future of clinical practice. *J Thromb Thrombolysis* 1999;7:195–220.

Chong BH. Heparin-induced thrombocytopenia. *Br J Haematol* 1995;89:431–9.

Latham P, et al. Use of recombinant hirudin in patients with heparin-induced thrombocytopenia with thrombosis requiring cardiopulmonary bypass. *Anesthesiology* 2000;92:263–6.

Quinn MJ, Fitzgerald DJ. Long-term administration of glycoprotein Iib/Iia antagonists. *Am Heart J* 1998;135:S107–12

Quinn MJ, Fitzgerald DJ. Ticopidine and clopidogrel. *Circulation* 1999;100:1667–72.

18

Adverse drug reactions and drug interactions

W McCaughey

Introduction • Definitions • Adverse reactions • Drug interactions • Pharmacokinetic • Pharmacodynamic • Clinically important interactions

INTRODUCTION

Drugs act, in the majority of cases, by interfering with the complex intercellular and intracellular signalling mechanisms by which the body maintains its functions. Drug action has been described as 'selective toxicity'. In practice, of course, selectivity is only partial, and most drugs have a spectrum of side effects which may give rise to toxicity. Thus, the concept of *therapeutic ratio*—the ratio of dose or concentration of the drug causing the desired effect, to that causing toxic effects. In addition to such adverse reactions, where two or more drugs are given simultaneously, either or each may modify the action of the other, giving rise to a *drug interaction*.

How common are these problems? Forty years ago a study showed that: '18 to 30 percent of all hospitalised patients have a drug reaction, and the duration of their hospitalisation is about doubled as a consequence.' Despite awareness, this has changed little—the recent publication *To Err is Human* (2000) by the Institute of Medicine in the US quoted a 2% incidence of preventable adverse drug reactions in hospitalised patients, with—apart from the human cost—a financial implication of £2000 million per year in that country.

Patients in developed countries are increasingly more elderly, and with more serious acute illnesses and chronic comorbidity. Polypharmacy is the rule rather than the exception. An audit by the author of 100 surgical patients found that medication on discharge included some 450 separate items (excluding analgesics). Of these the majority were cardiovascular drugs (150), drugs acting on the gastrointestinal (GI) tract (75), psychoactive drugs (53), and drugs acting on the respiratory tract (48). There is obviously considerable potential for both adverse reactions to and interaction between these drugs—yet physician awareness is low. Another recent study showed that almost half patients attending a hospital emergency department received additional medication, and that even though their drug history was recorded and available to prescribing doctors, in 10% of cases the new medication added a potential adverse interaction.

Withdrawal of medication is also a risk, and during the peri-operative period is associated with an increase in complications—a doubling in the case of cardiovascular drugs. However, there are often problems with continuing such therapy, e.g. continuing ileus (intestinal obstruction), and the unavailability of many preparations in parenteral form.

DEFINITIONS

Overdosage or underdosage. These may occur because of error, or because of a change in the formulation of a drug. This is a potential problem with generic prescribing, where in a small number of cases there are significant differences between preparations from different manufacturers. Relative over- or underdose may also occur because of a change in the pharmacodynamic or pharmacokinetic profile of the patient (see below for some examples).

Intolerance. Here, a patient shows a qualitatively normal response to the drug, but at an abnormally low dose. This may simply be a response at the extreme of the normal range of variation. The Gaussian distribution of response to a drug includes individuals who are unusually sensitive as well as those who are resistant. On the other hand, the response to some drugs shows two or more genetically determined populations, e.g. the response to suxamethonium in normal persons and in those with abnormal variants of cholinesterase.

Idiosyncrasy. This is a response that is qualitatively different from the action of the drug in normal individuals, again often genetically determined. Of importance to anaesthetists are abnormal responses to several drugs in patients with acute intermittent porphyria, and in those susceptible to the malignant hyperpyrexia syndrome.

Allergy and hypersensitivity. These responses are not dose-related, and are not related to the usual mechanisms of action, effects, and sided effects of the drug.

Direct organ toxicity. Some substances may directly damage cells of a particular organ or system, either because they or their metabolites are specifically toxic to these cells, or because they are concentrated in one area, e.g. the renal fluoride ion toxicity of methoxyflurane, or the liver damage that occurs in paracetamol overdose because of a toxic intermediate product binding to hepatocytes.

Secondary effects. Some effects are only indirectly related to the action of the drug, e.g. vitamin deficiency in patients whose gut flora have been modified by broad-spectrum antibiotics.

Drug interaction. When more than one drug is given, one may modify the action of the other in some manner. Predictable drug interactions form the basis of the drug combinations used in anaesthesia. However, with the increasing number of drugs being used in different facets of the patient's management, there is a considerable risk of unexpected interactions occurring before, during or after anaesthesia and surgery. Improved knowledge of the modes of action and pharmacokinetic disposition of drugs is gradually making more of these interactions understandable and thus predictable. Overall, drug interactions form only a small proportion of all adverse reactions to drugs (6.9% in one large study), but some are important. The number of reported interactions is enormous, and only those of relevance to anaesthesia and intensive care are discussed in this chapter.

ADVERSE REACTIONS

Pharmacogenetic

Genetically determined differences in drug metabolism may result in up to a sixfold difference in the rates of metabolism in different individuals. Much of this difference can be seen as the normal Gaussian distribution of any property between individuals. However, in a number of instances this variability is due to variant alleles resulting from mutations in genes encoding enzymes responsible for the metabolism of a drug. This manifests as a bimodal distribution of activity within a population.

A different type of problem arises when there are genetically determined defects in enzyme activity, as in porphyria (described below), or defects at receptor or intracellular level as in malignant hyperpyrexia.

Most drug metabolism occurs in hepatic microsomes, although biotransformation also occurs elsewhere in the body including the plasma, gastrointestinal tract, lungs, and non-microsomal systems in the liver. However, in this context the most important variation is in activity of phase 1 processes in the liver, by cytochrome P-450 enzymes. (The cytochrome P-450 system consists of a large number of genetically related enzymes, named systematically as CYP, followed by a numeral indicating family, a letter indicating subfamily, and a numeral for individual form, e.g. P-450 3A4 or CYP3A4.) There is a large inter-individual variation in the levels of expression of the enzymes, which is a major factor in differences in individual patients' responses to drugs. The best studied cause of important variability in drug metabolism, which affects many cardiovascular, psychotropic, and other drugs, is the existence of poor and good metabolisers, due to polymorphism of CYP2D6 (debrisoquine 4-hydroxylase). This may lead to either relative underdosage with inadequate effect, or relative overdosage and toxicity. There is a correlation between blood concentrations of antidepressants and measured CYP2D6 activity. Volatile anaesthetic drugs are metabolised mainly by CYP2E1, which also oxidises alcohol. This enzyme is also genetically polymorphic.

In addition to the cytochrome P-450 iso-enzymes, other enzymes carrying out phase I processes also show considerable polymorphism and thus variation in activity.

Genetic polymorphism is clinically important e.g. in the CAST (Cardiac Arrhythmia Suppression Trial), serious problems were identified with encainide and flecainide, because of polymorphic metabolism by CYP2D6.

Porphyria

A number of drugs used in anaesthetic practice are highly dangerous in patients suffering from one of the three 'acute' porphyrias—acute intermittent porphyria, variegate porphyria or hereditary coproporphyria—as they may precipitate an acute attack. Chronic porphyrias, such as porphyria cutanea tarda are not relevant. The mechanism involved is induction of hepatic δ-aminolaevulinic acid synthase, in patients who have inherited (mostly by an autosomal dominant pattern) a deficient enzyme for a later stage of the porphyrin pathway, leading to accumulation of porphyrin intermediates. The status of many drugs is uncertain, and the reader is referred for details to a review by James and Hift (2000). Barbiturates are the classic example of drugs dangerous in porphyrics. Propofol is the best choice at present for intravenous induction, although there is some doubt about its use as an infusion. Halothane from long use has proven safe, isoflurane is probably so; enflurane should be avoided and information on seroflurane and desflurane is insufficient. Opioids, such as morphine and fentanyl, are safe, whereas there is insufficient data on some other analgesics to be sure of their position. All muscle relaxants are probably safe, although there are insufficient data about most to be completely sure; atropine and neostigmine are safe. Drugs which are unsafe or probably unsafe include barbiturates, etomidate, enflurane, alcuronium, mepivacaine, pentazocine, some benzodiazepines (temazepam is safe, other benzodiazepines less certain), calcium channel blockers and aminophylline.

DRUG INTERACTIONS

Classification

Drug interactions are normally considered as *pharmacokinetic* or *pharmacodynamic*, or they may be grouped according to the site at which the interaction takes place. Many drug interactions can be predicted from the knowledge of the principles of pharmacokinetics and of the mode of action of the drugs concerned, and so this chapter should be read in conjunction with the chapters which describe these principles.

Pharmacokinetic interactions occur when one drug interferes with the absorption, distribution, metabolism, or excretion of another drug so as to increase or decrease the concentration of 'free' drug in the plasma (and at its site of action). Such interference may be two-way and may involve more than one mechanism. These may augment or counteract each other.

Pharmacodynamic interactions on the other hand lead to a change in the activity of the drug at the site of action itself. This may be by competition for receptor sites, or by other mechanisms related to the mode of action of the drug at cellular level. The complex interplay between different ion channels and second messenger systems is slowly becoming better understood, but interactions here are less easy to predict.

Definitions

When drugs interact, there may be an increased action of one or both, a decreased action, or an effect qualitatively different from either. A number of specific terms are used to describe these.

When the combined effect of the two drugs is simply the sum of each (2 + 2 = 4): allowing for the fact that it is generally the 'log' dose which is proportional to effect—this is an *additive* effect (or *summation*). In this case, there is in fact no real interaction between the drugs. Where the combined effect is greater than this (2 + 2 = 5) the effect is *supra-additive* (or *synergism),* or if less (2 + 2 < 4) it is *infra-additive or sub-additive*. The term *potentiation* is used where one agent shows no appreciable effect on the biological system, but causes an increased response from the second substance (2 + 0 = 3). Comparison of dose–response curves (see Chapter 1) is used to determine the type of interaction occurring, often using an isobologram, a graphical technique. Isoboles are iso-effect curves, curves that show dose combinations that result in equal effect. The combination of two doses (d1 and d2) can be represented by a point on a graph, the axes of which are the dose axes of the individual drugs (Figure 18.1). The isobole connects isoeffective doses of the two drugs when administered alone, D1 and D2. If the isobole is straight (A), then the relation is additive. If the isobole bows toward the origin (B), then smaller amounts of both drugs are needed to produce the drug effect when administered together, so the relation is supra-additive or synergistic. If the isobole bows away from the origin (C), then greater amounts of both drugs are needed to produce the drug effect when administered together, so the relation is infra-additive.

Where one drug opposes all, or part, of the action of another, the term *antagonism* is used. Antagonism at receptor sites may be *competitive* or *non-competitive*. Non-competitive antagonism (or potentiation) can also occur for pharmacokinetic reasons, if a drug modifies the absorption, transport, biotransformation, or excretion of another. Another non-competitive mechanism is *physiological* or *functional* antagonism, where two drugs have directly opposing effects, but at different sites. If the two drugs form an inactive complex, this is 'chemical antagonism'.

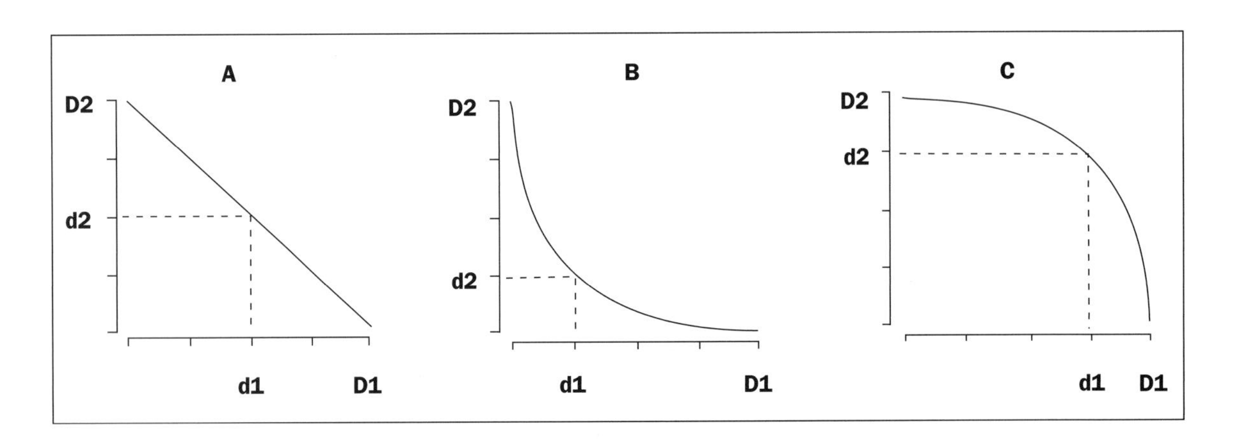

Figure 18.1 *An isobologram: A, additive; B, supra-additive; C, infra-additive.*

Mechanisms

The mechanisms of drug interactions are:

Pharmaceutical
Physical or chemical incompatibility

Pharmacokinetic
1. Modified drug metabolism
2. Modification of renal or biliary excretion
3. Changes in drug disposition
4. Interference with absorption

Pharmacodynamic
1. Physiological antagonism or antagonism
2. Competition at receptor site
3. Changes at intracellular level

Miscellaneous
1. Changes in fluid and electrolyte balance
2. Interference with antibacterial drugs

PHARMACOKINETIC

Pharmaceutical interactions and *modified absorption* will not be described here, as they are relatively unimportant in anaesthetic practice, where few drugs are given by the oral route. However, it should be noted that the absorption of drugs from the jejunum may be delayed by drugs, such as opioids or atropine, which reduce gastric motility.

Modified drug metabolism

The hepatic cytochrome P-450 system is particularly subject to *enzyme induction*—exposure to environmental substances or drugs can increase the level of expression of the gene coding for the enzyme, and thus the amount of the enzyme present—one of the most important mechanisms of drug interaction. Induction may be of one or several of the CYP subtypes, and may increase metabolism of the inducing substance, or of another drug, thus increasing its excretion and reducing its effect. There are several examples of relevance to anaesthetic practice. The toxicity of pethidine may be enhanced by barbiturates, increasing metabolism to the toxic metabolite norpethidine. Monoamine oxidase inhibition and alanine (Ala) synthase induction in porphyria are other examples.

Inhibition of metabolism may also occur. It may be due to inhibition of enzymes, or more commonly to competition between drugs for the same metabolic pathway. With most drugs which are eliminated by processes obeying first order kinetics, competition rarely causes significant inhibition of metabolism, but competition is more important in those eliminated by zero order kinetics, where the enzyme system is easily saturated.

Modified excretion

Two main effects occur here. First, change in the pH of urine—weak bases, such as pethidine, are more easily excreted in an acid urine while alkalinisation promotes excretion of weak acids, such as salicylates and phenobarbital. Second, drugs that compete for an active excretion mechanism will reduce each other's elimination—probenecid was used in the early days of penicillin to conserve the drug, while less desirable interactions also occur, e.g. chlorpropamide and phenylbutazone interact to give increased levels of chlorpropamide and a danger of hypoglycaemia.

Transport and distribution

Most drugs are carried by the circulation from their site of administration to their sites of action and elimination. Competition for protein binding sites and other factors have been described in Chapter 2, and some relevant examples are given in Table 18.1.

PHARMACODYNAMIC

These are defined here as interactions that take place at or near the site of action of the drug at cellular level, and thus represent some modification of the drug–receptor association, or

Table 18.1 Drug reactions and interactions and some special risk situations with anaesthetic drugs

Drug	*Secondary drug or clinical situation*	*Site and pharmacology*	*Potential interaction or risk*
Inhalational anaesthetics			
Halothane and other halogenated volatile anaesthetics	Adrenaline (epinephrine) and other sympathomimetics	(S) Anaesthetic sensitises myocardium to adrenaline, (epinephrine) risk of severe ventricular arrhythmias	Adrenaline (epinephrine) solutions should be dilute and not given IV Avoid hypercarbia
Methoxyflurane Enflurane Sevoflurane?	Renal disease	(M) Renal toxicity from inorganic fluoride	Avoid prolonged exposure in patients with pre-existing renal disease
	Tetracycline	(S) Increased risk of renal toxicity	
Diethyl ether Enflurane	β-adrenergic blockers	Blockade of normal compensation for cardiodepressant effects	Risk of myocardial depression and hypotension
Diethyl ether Enflurane	Epilepsy	(S)	Risk of convulsions
All volatile anaesthetics	MHS patients	(S) May trigger malignant hyperthermia	
Intravenous anaesthetics			
Thiopentone	Renal failure Cirrhosis	(B) Decreased protein binding of thiopentone may enhance its activity	Reduced rate of administration
	Metabolic acidosis	(B) Enhanced activity	
Thiopentone Methohexitone	Acute intermittent porphyria	(M) Induction of Ala synthase by barbiturates	Precipitation of attacks
Methohexitone	Epilepsy	(S)	Risk of convulsions
Thiopentone Methohexitone	Allergy Asthma	(S) Hypersensitivity	Increased risk of anaphylactic response and bronchospasm
Etomidate	Prolonged use	Blockade of corticosteroid synthesis	Impaired stress response Especially in ICU patients

Table 18.1 continued

Drug	*Secondary drug or clinical situation*	*Site and pharmacology*	*Potential interaction or risk*
Local anaesthetics			
All local anaesthetics	Metabolic acidosis	(B)	Increased risk of toxicity
Amethocaine Procaine	Low serum cholinesterase activity	(M)	Prolonged activity
Prilocaine	Large or repeated doses Neonates and infants	(M) Methaemoglobinaemia	Care with dosage
Muscle relaxants			
Suxamethonium Mivacurium	Severe liver disease Anticholinesterases	(M) Reduced serum cholinesterase levels	Prolonged block
	Procaine Metoclopramide	(M) Competition for plasma Cholinesterase	Prolonged block
Non-depolarising relaxants	Diuretics Hypokalaemia	(S) Potentiation of neuromuscular block	Danger of prolonged paralysis
	Antibiotics: Aminoglycosides Polymyxins Tetracyclines Lincomycin Clindamycin	(?S) Depending on group, either or both pre- and postganglionic block and potentiation of non-depolarising muscle relaxants	Prolonged neuromuscular block Rarely, muscle weakness caused by antibiotic alone
	Calcium channel-entry blockers	(S) Preganglionic block	Potentiation of block
Analgesic drugs			
Opioids			
Morphine, etc.	Diazepam and other CNS depressants	(S) Additive effect	Titrate doses carefully
	Antagonist and agonist-antagonists	(S) Competitive antagonism	Precipitation of abstinence syndrome in addicts

Table 18.1 continued

Drug	*Secondary drug or clinical situation*		*Site and pharmacology*	*Potential interaction or risk*
Pethidine (Meperidine)	MAOI drugs		(see text)	Dangerous interaction (see text)
	Phenobarbital and other enzyme inducers	(M)	Increased production of norpethidine	Increased sedation, danger of convulsions
Alfentanil	Erythromycin	(M)	Reduced clearance of alfentanil	Prolonged action of alfentanil
*NSAID*s	Surgery	(S)	Inhibition of prostaglandins:	
			• in platelets	Risk of bleeding
			• in kidney	Risk of acute renal failure
Antidepressants				
MAOIs	Pethidine (Meperidine)	(?)	Possibly due to increased 5-HT level in brain; a certain critical level may have to be reached	Severe, potentially fatal reaction in some patients
	Indirectly acting sympathomimetics	(S) (M)	Inhibition of metabolism of noradrenaline (norepinephrine) which accumulates at sympathetic nerve endings Release leads to overstimulation and adrenergic crisis	
Antihypertensive drugs				
β-adrenergic blockers	Diethyl ether Enflurane	(S)	Additive cardiovascular depressant effects	β-blockade not normally a problem during anaesthesia but avoid drugs that are myocardial depressants
	Calcium channel-entry antagonists	(S)	Additive negative inotropic Effect on the heart	Severe bradycardia possible Use cautiously together
ACE inhibitors	General anaesthesia	(S)	Renin-angiotensin system blockade	Intra- and postoperative Hypotension
Clonidine	Withdrawal of treatment	(S)		Rebound hypertension
Angiotensin II receptor antagonists	General anaesthesia	(S)	(see text)	

M, metabolism; S, at or near site of action; IV, intravenously; MHS, malignant hyperthermia syndrome; ALA, alanine; ICU, intensive care unit; CNS, central nervous system; MAOI, monoamine oxidase inhibitor, NSAID, non-steroidal anti-inflammatory drug; ACE, angiotensin-converting enzyme; 5-HT, 5-hydroxytryptamine.

change in the events which occur after the drug acts on its receptor. The complexity of the intracellular signalling mechanisms and the interdependence of many pathways—relationships that are only gradually being worked out—gives opportunities for a wide range of possible interactions between drugs at this level. The simplest concepts to understand are those of competition for attachment to receptor sites, and augmentation of adenylate cyclase activity by phosphodiesterase inhibition, but other interactions occur, involving both G protein-coupled and inositol 1,4,5-triphosphate (IP_3) pathways, as well as the effects of modifying the opening of different ion channels.

Many of the pharmacodynamic interactions of most interest to the anaesthetist occur in pathways associated with the various divisions of the nervous system, central and autonomic, and thus influence the control of the cardiovascular system.

In the rest of this chapter, the drugs discussed will be grouped by drug class or by body system, as many may have both a pharmacodynamic and a pharmacokinetic element to their spectrum of interactions, and these will be described together.

CLINICALLY IMPORTANT INTERACTIONS

Psychoactive drugs

A growing number of drugs are used that affect the many neurotransmitters in the brain: benzodiazepines and others act on GABAergic transmission; antidepressants, such as monoamine oxidase inhibitors and tricyclic antidepressants, are thought to increase the concentration of transmitter amines in the brain and so elevate mood—these will also act at peripheral nerve terminals, so interactions with them are a combination of peripheral and central actions. Levodopa (L-dopa) increases central as well as peripheral dopamine, and the newer class of psychoactive drugs, the selective serotonin reuptake inhibitors (SSRIs) of which the ubiquitous fluoxetine (Prozac) is best known, act in a similar way on serotonergic pathways.

Monoamine oxidase inhibitors (MAOIs)

Newer MAOI drugs are selective for the MAO-A subtype of the enzyme, and are less likely to interact with foods or other drugs. Monoamine oxidase (MAO) inactivates monoamine substances, many of which are, or are related to, neurotransmitters. The central nervous system mainly contains MAO-A, whose substrates are adrenaline (epinephrine), noradrenaline (norepinephrine), metanephrine, and 5-hydroxytryptamine (5-HT), whereas extraneuronal tissues, such as the liver, lung, and kidney, contain mainly MAO-B which metabolises β-phenylethylamine, phenylethanolamine, *o*-tyramine, and benzylamine.

MAO inhibition has been thought to act by increasing levels of transmitter substances such as noradrenaline (norepinephrine) in the brain. However, the results of their administration are complex. Central nervous system (CNS) levels of monoamine do increase, but this leads to reduced rates of synthesis. By-products, such as the false transmitter octopamine, accumulate, and slowly displace noradrenaline (norepinephrine) from storage vesicles. Inhibitory presynaptic α-adrenergic and dopamine receptors may be stimulated. With longer treatment there are reduced numbers and sensitivity of α_1, α_2 and β receptors, 5-HT_1 and 5-HT_2 receptors but not dopamine receptors. Apart from behavioural changes, the main effect of MAO inhibition is a generalised reduction in sympathetic tone, with lower resting blood pressure and a reduced ability to respond to stresses, such as postural change. The classic (type I) reaction with MAOIs, although complex, can be regarded as extreme overstimulation of the sympathetic nervous system. Tyramine, one of the main culprits in the 'cheese' reaction, has been shown to act by inhibiting the inhibitory α_2-adrenergic pathways in the locus coeruleus.

Should it occur, treatment is largely symptomatic: chlorpromazine 50–100 mg may control the central excitatory symptoms, and contribute to control of others, while more specific antihypertensive therapy may be required; labetalol, a combined α- and β-adrenoceptor antagonist, has been used successfully. Arrhythmias may require β blockade.

There are no serious interactions with the commonly used anaesthetic agents, but problems have occurred with pethidine—a reaction characterised by hypertension, hyperthermia, decreased level of consciousness or coma, and even convulsions. This is unlikely to occur with other opioids unrelated to pethidine, although data are scarce, and there has been only one report implicating fentanyl. Indirectly acting sympathomimetics, i.e. those that work by stimulating catecholamine release, such as ephedrine, may have an augmented action. Local analgesic solutions that contain adrenaline (epinephrine) are unlikely to cause problems, but it may be wise to use a solution containing felypressin instead. It is less well recognised that in addition to this excitatory response, a 'depressive' type of reaction (type II) can occur due to reduced metabolism, resulting occasionally in an increased and prolonged response to drugs, such as morphine.

Withdrawal of monoamine oxidase inhibitors can result in severe anxiety, agitation, pressured speech, sleeplessness or drowsiness, hallucinations, delirium, and paranoid psychosis, and thus should not be undertaken lightly. The older drugs caused irreversible inhibition of MAO, and it was advisable to stop treatment at least 1 week before operation. Newer MAO-A selective inhibitors should be reversible in 24–48 hours, although, with careful selection of anaesthetic management it should usually be possible to avoid drugs likely to interact. Patients receiving these newer MAOIs should, however, omit the drug on the morning of operation.

Tricyclic antidepressants

These act by blocking the re-uptake of noradrenaline (norepinephrine) into nerve terminals. As would be expected, they enhance the action of noradrenaline (norepinephrine), adrenaline (epinephrine), and other directly acting sympathomimetic compounds. They also exhibit anticholinergic activity that potentiates the activity of atropine-like drugs and can induce sinus tachycardia, atrial ectopic beats, or—more dangerously—arrhythmias. Tricyclic antidepressants have a high affinity for cardiac muscle and have a negative inotropic effect. They exert a quinidine-like, membrane-stabilising action on the heart that causes delayed conduction, manifest on the electrocardiograph as prolonged PR, QRS, and QT_c times, the latter increasing the risk of sudden ventricular fibrillation. At therapeutic doses, orthostatic hypotension may occur, but severe cardiovascular side effects are usually only a feature in overdose.

Levodopa (L-dopa)

In parkinsonism the basal ganglia are depleted of dopamine. As dopamine does not cross the blood–brain barrier, its precursor levodopa (L-dopa), which does, is used in treatment. About 95% of orally administered levodopa is rapidly decarboxylated in the periphery to dopamine, although this is reduced by giving with a dopa-carboxylase inhibitor. Cardiovascular effects occur due to increased circulating levels of dopamine. In particular, increased myocardial irritability, maximal about 1 hour after taking levodopa, may lead to the development of arrhythmias, especially in the presence of halogenated volatile anaesthetics. Sudden withdrawal of levodopa carries the danger not only of worsening of the control of parkinsonism, but also a small risk of the development of hyperthermia or neuroleptic malignant syndome—a syndrome that clinically resembles the malignant hyperthermia syndrome (MHS), and may be due to imbalance in central dopaminergic pathways.

Anticonvulsants

Anticonvulsants, such as the barbiturates and phenytoin, are well-known inducers of hepatic enzymes and may increase the dosage requirements of many drugs including fentanyl. They also cause resistance to non-depolarising muscle relaxants (excepting atracurium) but the mechanism of the interaction is unclear, and may be pharmacodynamic, perhaps due to a change in the sensitivity of acetylcholine receptors. There are no clinically significant interactions between the benzodiazepines and drugs used in anaesthesia.

Alcohol

Chronic long-term alcohol intake leads initially to induction of hepatic enzymes, and enhances the metabolism of alcohol itself together with other drugs. Later, the picture may change with the development of cirrhotic damage to the liver. In contrast, acute intake of alcohol tends to inhibit microsomal drug metabolism and enhances the effects of drugs. However, if the toxicity of a drug, e.g. paracetamol, depends on the formation of toxic metabolites, the acute intake of alcohol may, paradoxically, reduce the toxicity whereas chronic alcohol intake may increase it. Pharmacodynamic alterations may also occur with chronic alcohol abuse, perhaps related to adaptive changes in cell membrane lipids or proteins, leading to tolerance. Note that the alcoholic shows tolerance to the CNS effects of anaesthetic drugs, but not to their cardiovascular depressant effects.

Cardiovascular drugs

Aspirin is increasingly prescribed for prophylaxis of cardiovascular events—being taken by up to a fifth of the patients. Confusion still reigns as to the risks of low-dose aspirin in the peri-operative period, in particular in relation to neuraxial block.

Care should be taken with all patients taking non-steroidal anti-inflammatory drugs (NSAIDs) to be aware of their potential to cause acute renal insufficiency, especially in patients stressed by major surgery, or by sepsis.

Nitrates either isosorbide or glyceryl trinitrate, are the second most common group of cardiovascular drugs prescribed. Although patients taking these will by definition have significant cardiovascular disease, the drugs themselves have no adverse interactions during anaesthesia. Inadvertent withdrawal may slightly increase the risks of ischaemic episodes, but this is less likely than on withdrawing other antianginal treatment such as calcium channel blockers.

Antihypertensive drugs

Antihypertensive drugs act by many different mechanisms. Over the past two decades, there has been a consensus that hypertensive patients are in general at less risk if treatment is continued throughout the peri-operative period; adequate pre-operative antihypertensive treatment may be the most important prophylaxis against postoperative hypertension with its attendant risks of myocardial ischaemia and infarction. The spectrum of drugs used in the treatment of hypertension has changed. Currently, diuretics, β-adrenoceptor antagonists, and calcium channel blocking drugs (see below), angiotensin-converting enzyme (ACE) inhibitors, angiotensin II receptor antagonists, and drugs acting on α-adrenergic receptors are first-line treatment, with some differences in prescribing patterns between different countries.

ACE inhibitors

The ACE inhibitors, captopril, enalapril, etc., act on the renin-angiotensin system, inhibiting the formation of the powerful vasoconstrictor angiotensin II. In addition to its systemic effects angiotensin II causes changes in local, end-organ renin-angiotensin systems that control local perfusion to the kidney, adrenal gland, heart, etc. Thus, the effects of ACE inhibitors are complex.

It is usually recommended that ACE inhibitors be continued peri-operatively in common with other antihypertensives. There is some evidence that postoperative haemodynamic stability is improved and renal function protected. Pretreatment with ACE inhibitors may reduce tachyphylaxis to sodium nitroprusside and help to prevent rebound hypertension. On the other hand, there is evidence that ACE inhibitors may predispose to hypotension during anaesthesia and that they reduce cerebral blood flow during any period of systemic hypotension. Furthermore, the response to and recovery from hypotensive episodes due to blood loss or circulatory depletion may be impaired. At present, the advice concerning these drugs would be to continue therapy up to and including the day of operation. Another rare side-effect of ACE inhibitors is angioneurotic oedema, which has occasionally been seen complicating intubation.

New classes of drugs are being introduced. *Angiotensin II inhibitors* are increasingly used, and may be associated with hypotension following induction of anaesthesia which can be resistant to conventional vasopressor therapy, such as ephedrine or phenylephrine (although responding to a vasopressin system agonist). In contrast to most other antihypertensives, cardiovascular stability appears to be improved by discontinuation of the angiotensin II inhibitor therapy on the day before surgery.

Clonidine

Clonidine is an antihypertensive agent which acts by multiple and complex mechanisms, including a prominent central α_2-agonist action combined with some reduction of peripheral adrenergic transmission. It reduces the incidence of hypertensive episodes during anaesthesia, such as the response to laryngoscopy and intubation, but at the expense of an increased incidence of hypotension and bradycardia at other times peri-operatively, with the latter being somewhat resistant to atropine. In contrast, pressor responses to indirectly acting vasopressors, such as ephedrine, may be increased. These factors must be considered in deciding in individual cases whether to continue clonidine treatment up to the day of operation. If it is discontinued abruptly, the release of catecholamines from stores in nerve terminals may lead to a potentially fatal syndrome of rebound hypertension, anxiety, tremor, and cardiac arrhythmias. Alternative antihypertensive treatment must be substituted to avoid this danger, preferably well in advance of surgery.

Calcium channel-entry blockers

Calcium channel-entry blockers are used principally in the management of hypertension or ischaemic heart disease. Generally, when a patient is taking one of these drugs, it should be continued peri-operatively. They have three main effects:

1. Depression of cardiac conduction, with slowing of the rate of SA node discharge, prolongation of AV node refractoriness, and slowing of AV conduction.
2. A direct negative inotropic effect.
3. Vasodilatation of both coronary and systemic arteries and arterioles.

The potential for depression of cardiac function is thus usually offset by afterload reduction, especially in the case of nifedipine, which actually has the most marked negative inotropic effect.

Serious side effects are rare and result from improper use of these agents, as when intravenous verapamil (or diltiazem) is given to patients with sinus or atrioventricular nodal depression from drugs or disease, or nifedipine to patients with aortic stenosis.

Calcium channel blockers with vasodilator effects, such as nifedipine, nicardipine, and nimodipine, will potentiate the effect of vasodilator effects of, e.g. halothane or isoflurane, potentiating any hypotension. This is especially obvious in hypertensive patients and when combined with similarly acting agents, such as sodium nitroprusside or nitroglycerin. Similarly, they also enhance the tendency of volatile anaesthetics to reduce hypoxic pulmonary vasoconstriction, which might exacerbate ventilation/perfusion mismatching during anaesthesia.

Halothane and enflurane have direct cardiac inhibitory effects similar to verapamil and diltiazem and these effects may summate. Interaction may also cause an additive effect on conduction with, e.g. isoflurane or halothane.

Drug interactions involving calcium antagonists occur with other cardiovascular agents, such as α- and β-adrenergic antagonists, digoxin, quinidine, and disopyramide. Some of these interactions are pharmacokinetic. For example, plasma concentrations of carbamazepine or phenytoin may rise when calcium channel blockers are given concurrently. Verapamil can cause an increase in the plasma concentrations of other cardiovascular drugs and digoxin levels may be raised by 50–80%, although the change is relatively small with other calcium channel blockers. With β-adrenergic antagonists the interaction can be mutual (see below).

Combined therapy using calcium channel blockers with β-adrenoceptor antagonists is increasingly common, and is probably safest with the dihydropyridines. Synergy occurs that can lead to marked interference with conduction, leading to bradycardia or even sinus arrest. Caution is needed during anaesthesia in patients receiving such a combination, as conduction disturbances can occur, although very careful monitoring of the electrocardiograph will usually forestall any problems. Some of the depressant effects of the combination may be antagonised by amrinone or glucagon.

There is some evidence that the cardiotoxicity of bupivacaine may be intensified in patients who are receiving either calcium channel blockers or β-adrenergic antagonists.

β-Adrenoceptor antagonists

These drugs are widely used for a number of medical indications, including hypertension, angina and migraine. Adverse effects can include bronchospasm, heart failure, prolonged hypoglycaemia, bradycardia, heart block, intermittent claudication and Raynaud's phenomenon. Neurological reactions include depression, fatigue and nightmares.

Bradycardia (in particular after neostigmine which is best given *after* an anticholinergic), hypotension, and bronchospasm are the main hazards in β-blocker treated patients undergoing anaesthesia. However, continuation of β-blockade up to and including the day of operation results in improved peri-operative haemodynamic stability and avoids the rebound effect which can result from abrupt withdrawal.

Bronchospasm is not a direct action of these drugs but blockade of β-receptors increases the reactivity of the airway and increases the likelihood of bronchospasm during laryngoscopy and tracheal intubation. It is also possible that the severity, and possibly the incidence of acute anaphylaxis is increased in patients on large doses of β blockers and that resuscitation may be hampered in these circumstances.

Digoxin remains a first-line treatment. Although the risks of digoxin toxicity have long been known, current dosing guidelines are still based on a nomogram published in 1974. A recent survey found high levels in 8% of patients, of which about two-thirds showed signs of toxicity. Most cases were associated with reduced renal function or a drug interaction. There can be an important interaction with clarithromycin (very commonly used in triple therapy for *Helicobacter*), which may lead to an acute rise in digoxin concentrations to toxic levels. This is believed to be due to reduced presystemic elimination because of modification of bowel bacteria which metabolise digoxin.

The neuromuscular junction

Several different classes of drug given pre-operatively or during anaesthesia may affect the duration of neuromuscular blockade. Muscle weakness is not a common result of the use of these drugs, except when function is also compromised by another factor, a neuromuscular disease, for example, or the presence of clinical or subclinical doses of other drugs acting in this region. A number of antibiotics possess neuromuscular-blocking activity. The aminoglycoside, polymyxin, lincosamide and tetracycline groups are those most commonly involved, while penicillins, cephalosporins and erythromycin have not caused clinical problems. They have their action at different sites, the aminoglycosides mainly prejunctional, the polymyxins, tetracyclines and lincosamides mainly postjunctional. Clinically, it is usually safer to continue ventilation until adequate muscle power has returned. Less difficulty might be expected with the newer non-depolarising drugs, such as atracurium and vecuronium, but clinical concentrations of aminoglycosides (gentamicin, tobramycin) can prolong blockade.

Calcium channel blockade interferes with prejunctional calcium flux at the neuromuscular junction, and verapamil (but probably not nifedipine) can thus potentiate neuromuscular blockade. Magnesium sulphate, used in management of pre-eclampsia, has a similar effect, and the two drugs in combination may themselves cause neuromuscular block.

Suxamethonium breakdown may be delayed by drugs that reduce plasma cholinesterase levels or compete as substrates. Many of the drugs that do this, such as procaine or propanidid, are mainly of historical interest, but metoclopramide, which is often given before obstetrical anaesthesia, prolongs the duration of action of suxamethonium and mivacurium by as much as 50%.

Herbal medicines

Patients do not reliably normally volunteer what over-the-counter or herbal remedies they are taking. This may have relevance, as a number of these have significant toxicity or potential for interaction, and the American Society of Anesthesiologists has issued a guidance leaflet. Warnings have been circulated of renal toxicity from *Aristolochia* in some Chinese medicines, and of hepatic enzyme induction by hypericins in St John's wort, which has been shown to be an effective antidepressant. Closer to home, alkaloids from solanaceous plants can significantly inhibit human BuChE and prolong mivacurium action at concentrations similar to those found in serum of individuals who have eaten a standard serving of potatoes!

Hypersensitivity reactions

Definitions

These are adverse reactions resembling the effects of histamine liberation ('histaminoid') and unrelated to the mode of action of the drug itself. Histamine release appears to be the main factor involved in all types of hypersensitivity reactions and its release explains most of the manifestations. The term 'anaphylactoid' may equally be used to describe these reactions, meaning simply that they resemble anaphylactic reactions, while the term anaphylactic is used specifically for *immune-mediated* phenomena involving previous sensitisation of the patient. It is often difficult to determine the true nature and cause of the reaction.

Mechanisms

Most anaphylactoid reactions are due to a direct or 'chemical' release of histamine, and other mediators, from mast cells and basophils. Immune-mediated hypersensitivity reactions have been classified as types I–IV. Type I, involving IgE or IgG antibodies, is the main mechanism involved in most anaphylactic or immediate hypersensitivity reactions to anaesthetic drugs. Type II, also known as antibody-dependent hypersensitivity or cytotoxic reactions are, for example, responsible for ABO-incompatible blood transfusion reactions. Type III, immune complex reactions, include classic serum sickness. Type IV, cellular responses mediated by sensitised lymphocytes, may account for as much as 80% of allergic reactions to local anaesthetic.

In type I reactions, the first exposure to the antigen results in the formation of specific IgE antibodies which are firmly fixed to mast cells and basophils. Subsequent exposure results in rapid degranulation of these cells and liberation of vasoactive substances, particularly histamine, but including a number of peptides, leukotrienes, prostaglandins, kinins, etc. Histamine levels are raised, and correlate closely with the severity of the reaction, concentrations above $10\ ng{\cdot}mL^{-1}$ indicating a severe reaction and above $100\ ng{\cdot}mL^{-1}$ usually being fatal. However, histamine concentrations decrease rapidly and are thus difficult to estimate, particularly in the emergency situation, and are not useful in diagnosis. Levels of mast cell tryptase, released at degranulation, remain high for 1–6 hours. Raised tryptase levels are a valuable and sensitive indicator of an anaphylactic reaction during anaesthesia. Their presence favours an IgE-mediated cause but does not always distinguish between anaphylactoid and anaphylactic reactions, and patients in whom mast cell tryptase concentrations are not increased still require skin testing.

Predisposing factors

A history of atopy (asthma, hay fever or eczema) or of allergy to any injected substance is frequently seen in patients reacting to anaesthetic drugs and this association can be confirmed statistically. In most of these cases there is probably a raised IgE level, but this is not an essential feature in patients having true hypersensitivity reactions. Repeated exposure to particular drugs is not a predisposing factor to reactions as judged by the drug history of thiopentone reactors and others. In general, reactions are most common with substances of high molecular weight, but smaller molecules can attach themselves to plasma proteins or polypeptides and become antigenic.

Frequency of reactions

In the field of anaesthesia, hypersensitivity reactions occur in between 1:10 000 and 1:20 000 anaesthetics, most frequently with muscle relaxants (70%), induction agents, plasma substitutes, and antibiotics, as well as to latex, and it is often difficult to identify the causative drug. Among muscle relaxants, suxamethonium is most often incriminated, and the lowest number of reactions occurs with pancuronium and vecuronium. The incidence for muscle relaxants is probably higher than for intravenous barbiturates, while the safest of the induction agents appears to be etomidate. Reactions to plasma substitutes are also relatively frequent. A recent French study found rates of 1/300 for gelatins, 1/400 for dextrans, 1/1000 for albumin, and 1/1700 for starches, of which about 20% were serious. Figures for penicillin are about 1 in 5000. The mortality in published reactions to thiopentone is approximately 10% and the same figure applies to penicillin reactions, but this is much lower with other agents.

Clinical features and management

Cutaneous

The majority of clinically definite and immunologically confirmed reactions have erythema as a main feature. Erythema is, however, a common accompaniment to the administration of many drugs, often as a result of directly mediated histamine release, and it should not be regarded as part of a life-threatening reaction unless there are changes in other systems of the body. In addition, most reactors have oedema, particularly of the eyelids.

Cardiovascular

Hypotension is the other common feature of hypersensitivity reactions. Its basis is hypovolaemia from extravasation of protein-containing fluid through the capillary wall, together with arteriolar and capillary vasodilatation. Both these are classical features of histamine liberation. There is usually a marked tachycardia which is both histamine-induced and compensatory for the hypotension. Plasma loss of up to 35% of circulating blood volume may occur within 10 minutes, due to capillary permeability, and rapid replacement, using colloid for preference, is indicated. Adrenaline (epinephrine), infused intravenously with electrocardiographic monitoring, is the drug treatment of choice. When adrenaline (epinephrine) and adequate volume do not produce improvement, noradrenaline (norepinephrine) may be lifesaving. Antihistamines and corticosteroids have little effect in the acute stages, although they are worth trying as second-line drugs.

Respiratory

Bronchospasm occurs in more than half of the more severe hypersensitivity reactions, either on its own or as an accompaniment to other changes. It is more common, as one would expect, in asthmatic patients and in patients receiving muscle relaxants (where tracheal intubation may be a factor). It should, however, only be regarded as indicative of a reaction if other forms of airway obstruction and other causes of tracheal irritation have been excluded.

Confirmation of reaction

Measurement of plasma tryptase levels immediately (1–4 h) following an episode may be useful to confirm that a histaminoid reaction has occurred. Some four weeks later, intradermal skin tests and specific antibody tests (radioallergosorbent; RAST, enzyme-linked immunosorbent; ELISA) may help to identify the causative drug, although these tests do produce false-positive and false-negative results.

Prevention of reactions

At further anaesthetics, prevention obviously involves attempts to identify the causative agent, and avoidance of this where possible. There can be cross-reactivity between muscle relaxants. Pre-emptive histamine (H_1 and H_2)

blockade and corticosteroids may attenuate a reaction. It has been suggested that morphine may be suitable to block second reactions to neuromuscular blocking drugs by hapten inhibition. Morphine is monoquaternary and avidly binds to neuromuscular blocking drug-specific IgE, without IgE bridging, which is a prerequisite for allergic mediator release.

FURTHER READING

James MF, Hift RJ. Porphyrias. *Br J Anaesth* 2000;85: 143–53.

Kohn LT, Corrigan JM, Donaldson MS (eds). To err is human: Building a safer health system. Washington DC, National Academy Press 2000.

19

Drugs in special circumstances

JG Bovill

Pregnancy • Anaesthetic drugs • Lactation • Neonates and infants • Renal disease • Liver disease

PREGNANCY

Because of the potential detrimental effects on the fetus, in particular teratogenicity, extreme caution must be exercised with administration of drugs during pregnancy, especially during the first trimester. After delivery, drugs given to the mother may also reach the infant via breast milk.

Drug transfer across the placenta

The placenta is unique among all membrane systems, separating the blood of two distinct individuals, mother and fetus. The maternal to fetal diffusion distance decreases from 50–100 μm in the second month of pregnancy to only 4–5 μm at term. Because the fetal capillary endothelium has loose intercellular connections, it does not pose a significant barrier to nutrient or drug transport. Diffusion is by far the most important mechanism of drug distribution across the placenta, although other mechanisms apply to some drugs.

Drug transfer by simple diffusion is the primary mechanism for drug transfer across the placenta, and represents the free passage of a drug down its concentration gradient (Garland 1998). Only unionised molecules with a molecular weight < 500 Da that are not bound to circulating proteins can transfer by passive diffusion. The rate of diffusion (dQ/dt) is governed by the Fick equation:

$$\frac{dQ}{dt} = \frac{\mathrm{K} \cdot A\,(Cm - Cf)}{D}$$

where K is the diffusion constant (which depends on the physicochemical characteristics of the drug), A is the surface area of the membrane, D its thickness, and Cm and Cf are the maternal and fetal concentrations of the drug. The average exchange area ranges from ~4 m^2 at 28 weeks gestation to 11–12 m^2 at term.

Facilitated diffusion is a carrier-mediated mechanism of transplacental transfer. It is important for endogenous substances, such as glucose. It is also the mechanism for some drugs, e.g. the antibiotic cefalexin. Active transport is a carrier-mediated process that requires energy against an electrochemical or concentration gradient. Amino acids and calcium are transported by this mechanism. Only a few drugs, such as α-methyldopa and 5-fluorouracil, are transferred by active transport.

Factors affecting transplacental transfer

Lipid-soluble drugs diffuse easily across the placenta, whereas water-soluble ones pass through at slower rates. Although the placenta is relatively impermeable to polar compounds, some transfer will occur if a sufficiently high maternal–fetal concentration gradient exists and sufficient time is allowed (Pacifici and Nottoli 1995).

Drugs cross biological membranes most readily in the unionised state, and placental transfer is influenced by the pH of the maternal and fetal blood. The pH of the fetal blood is usually 0.1–0.15 pH units lower than that of maternal blood. Basic drugs therefore cross from the maternal to the fetal circulation where they become more ionised, and can accumulate in the fetus (ion trapping). This becomes more marked during fetal acidosis (Figure 19.1). The opposite is true for acidic drugs, such as propofol or thiopentone; fetal concentrations are lower than in the maternal blood. The increased blood flow as pregnancy progresses also increases delivery of drugs to the fetus from the maternal circulation. Conversely, delivery will decrease in pathological states associated with a reduction in placental blood flow, e.g. pre-eclampsia.

Protein binding in the maternal circulation inhibits transfer and highly bound compounds will not cross the placenta readily. Maternal plasma albumin is lower during pregnancy so that unbound drug concentrations are higher than in non-pregnant individuals. This makes more drug available for placental transfer. Fetal plasma proteins have a lower binding affinity than those of adults and this results in a higher fraction of the free drug in the fetus.

ANAESTHETIC DRUGS

Of the intravenous agents, ketamine and thiopentone undergo complete placental transfer. Propofol is also rapidly transferred across the placenta, and propofol infusions should be used with caution during Caesarean section when a prolonged induction to delivery time is anticipated. However, neonates clear propofol rapidly and residual effects in healthy newborn are usually negligible.

The placental transfer of most local anaesthetics, with the exception of prilocaine, is incomplete. Local anaesthetics are highly protein-bound, and binding to maternal proteins may influence the extent of placental transfer.

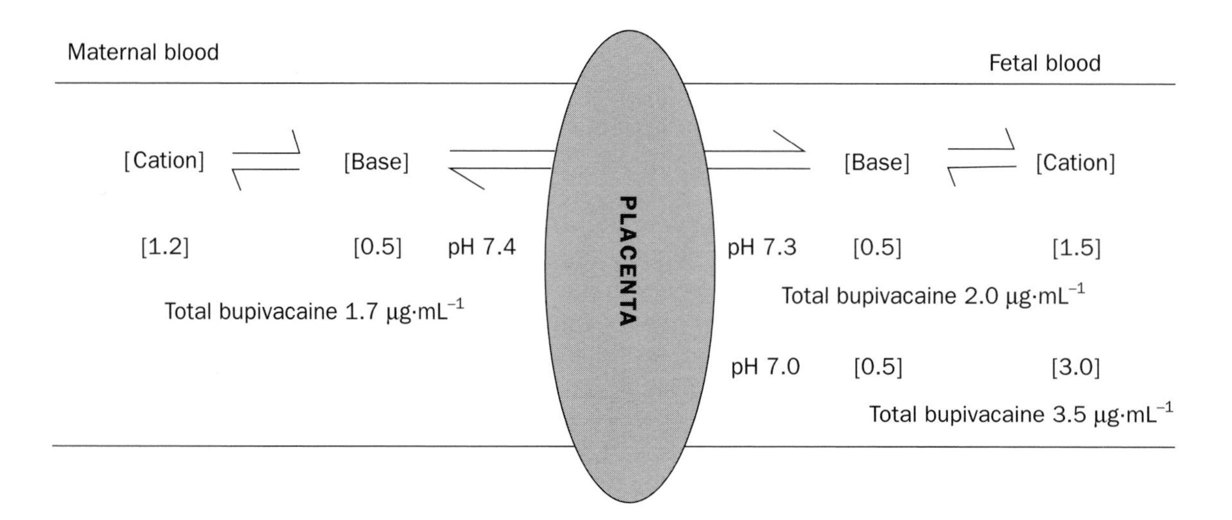

Figure 19.1 *Schematic of the influence of fetal pH on the maternal–fetal distribution of bupivacaine across the placenta. With fetal acidosis (pH 7.0) the total amount of drug increases due to an increase in the amount of ionised drug (cation).*

Caution is required with a paracervical block because the amount of local anaesthetic reaching the fetus may be high enough to produce fetal bradycardia, hypoventilation, and hypotonia. The myocardial toxic effects resulting from hypoxic acidosis may be increased by the high concentrations of local anaesthetics. This will be most likely for bupivacaine, which binds tightly to myocardial sodium channels, causing a block that is slow to reverse. There is evidence from animal models that the myocardial cells are more sensitive to the toxic effects of bupivacaine during pregnancy. Cardiotoxicity induced by an excessive dose of bupivacaine to the mother will also be reflected in the fetus. Maternal hypoxia will lead to increased fetal hypoxia and acidosis, which will further increase ion-trapping of bupivacaine in the fetus. This in turn will lower the toxic threshold for cerebral and cardiac toxicity in the fetus. Since systemic toxicity of local anaesthetics is directly related to blood concentrations, the selected dose should be administered in a manner that will allow identification of unintentional intravascular injection and minimise the volume of drug injected.

Opioids, such as fentanyl, alfentanil and sufentanil, are basic, lipophilic drugs that readily enter the fetal circulation. The magnitude of the maternal–fetal transfer is fentanyl > alfentanil > sufentanil. Pethidine, a popular analgesic in obstetrics, can be detected in the fetal plasma within 2 minutes of maternal administration. The average cord to maternal ratio for pethidine and its main metabolite, norpethidine, is 0.81 and 0.87, respectively.

Non-depolarising neuromuscular blocking drugs are mostly distributed to the extracellular volume with minimal binding to tissues. They also have relatively high molecular weights that vary from 573 for pancuronium and 633.7 for vecuronium to 1243 for atracurium. These characteristics limit their transfer across the placenta. The umbilical/maternal venous concentrations are thus low, 0.07–0.12 for atracurium, 0.1–0.14 for vecuronium, and 0.19–0.26 for pancuronium. Because of its higher transfer, pancuronium given to the mother during Caesarean section may induce partial neuromuscular block in the newborn infant (Guay and co-workers 1998). Plasma pseudocholinesterase concentrations are decreased by approximately 35% during normal pregnancy, and remain low for 2–7 days after delivery. Despite this, the clinical duration of succinylcholine is unchanged in term pregnant women.

LACTATION

Most drugs enter breast milk by passive diffusion so the concentration in milk is directly proportional to the maternal blood concentration. As milk is slightly more acidic than the plasma, lipophilic weak bases with limited protein binding are most likely to be secreted in the milk, although virtually all drugs have the potential to cross into breast milk. Even when the milk concentration approaches that in the mother's plasma, the amount ingested is rarely sufficient to reach therapeutic, let alone toxic, concentrations. A number of drugs are contraindicated, however, during breast feeding. Bromocriptine and the ergot analogues suppress prolactin activity and amiodarone can cause iodine-induced hypo- or hyperthyroidism. Lithium, which has a low toxicity threshold, passes freely into milk and significant plasma concentrations may occur in nursing infants.

Drugs that are not absorbed from the gastrointestinal tract of the baby, such as warfarin, are safe for the mother to take. The administration of antibiotics to a breast-feeding mother usually poses no concern for the newborn infant. However, metronidazole, which has mutagenic properties, reaches concentrations in milk that equal or exceed maternal plasma levels. Caution is also advised with sulphonamides, nitrofurantoin, or naladixic acid since these can cause haemolysis in infants with glucose-6-phosphate dehydrogenase deficiency.

NEONATES AND INFANTS

Because of differences in their physiology, children handle drugs differently from adults. The largest differences occur in the neonatal period. In neonates, 80% of body weight is water compared with only 60% in adults, and a greater proportion of the water is extracellular. This increases the distribution volumes of water-soluble drugs such as muscle relaxants and digoxin. The concentrations of many protein fractions, in particular albumin, γ-globulin and α_1-acid glycoprotein are reduced and, in the neonate, fetal albumin has a lower affinity for some drugs. This results in lower protein binding and thus higher concentrations of the active unbound drug. Higher concentrations of unconjugated fatty acids and bilirubin also compete with acidic drugs for protein binding sites. These differences are most important for drugs that are highly protein-bound, such as fentanyl, diazepam, and most local anaesthetics. The increased concentration of free drug will facilitate transfer to the brain, enhancing the effect and increasing the risk of side effects.

While the neonate possesses the ability to metabolise some drugs, such as paracetamol, as efficiently as adults, for most drugs metabolism is much slower since many enzymes are immature at birth. The activity of cytochrome P-450 enzymes, responsible for phase I metabolism of most drugs, is only half that in adults. The activity of plasma and other cholinesterases is also reduced, as are the enzymes responsible for conjugation. Morphine, which is eliminated by conjugation, has a prolonged half-life in neonates. Poor renal excretion of the active metabolite, morphine-6-glucuronide, will further prolong the action of morphine. Renal function in the newborn is only about 20% of the adult value, and is even less developed in the premature infant born before 34 weeks gestation. The clearance of drugs, such as gentamycin and pancuronium, which are eliminated largely by glomerular filtration, will be markedly reduced in these infants.

Changes in pharmacodynamics further complicate the pharmacology of many drugs in the neonate and infant. The blood–brain barrier is poorly developed, allowing more rapid transfer of drugs into the central nervous system (CNS). However, the response to higher brain concentrations may be tempered by an inadequate response due to lack of receptor maturation.

RENAL DISEASE

The kidneys are important for the excretion of the water-soluble metabolites of many drugs, and are the primary eliminating organ for others. As glomerular filtration and intrinsic renal function deteriorates the renal clearance of drugs that depend on this route, e.g. gentamycin, digoxin, and some neuromuscular blocking agents, decreases. The renal excretion of unchanged pancuronium is 50–60%. Even though only 20–30% of vecuronium is excreted by this route, the half-life is prolonged by 50% in patients with end-stage renal failure. Although the renal excretion of morphine is minimal, renal failure leads to accumulation of morphine-3-glucuronide and morphine-6-glucuronide. The latter is pharmacologically active and its accumulation can markedly prolong the action of morphine and increase the risk of adverse side effects. Similar problems can occur with diazepam and midazolam, both of which have active glucuronide metabolites.

Patients with renal disease often have hypoalbuminaemia, which reduces the protein binding of acidic drugs, such as phenytoin, thiopentone or paracetamol, with an enhanced pharmacological effect. This will be particularly marked for drugs that are highly bound since a small change in protein binding will lead to a marked increase in the free (active) concentration. Conversely, the plasma concentrations of α_1-acid glycoprotein, which binds basic drugs, such as local anaesthetics, opioids, and benzodiazepines, may be increased up to three times normal in uraemic patients. For many basic drugs, however, the free concentration changes little because of concomitant increases in their volume of distribution. For some drugs the picture is further complicated by displacement of the drug from protein-binding sites by endogenous products of uraemia. This is the case for digoxin, for which loading and maintenance doses should be reduced by 50–70%.

In patients with end-stage renal failure standard doses of many drugs commonly used in the pre-operative period may have exaggerated or prolonged effects. Thus, it is best to individually titrate sedatives, analgesics, and muscle relaxants to effect rather than rely on a standard dosing schema. Increased plasma levels of magnesium are common and can potentiate the effects of depolarising and non-depolarising muscle relaxants. Suxamethonium should be avoided if possible because of the increase in potassium that it causes. Atracurium or cisatracurium are probably the best choice for muscle relaxation. Inhalational agents that have the propensity for free fluoride ion release (enflurane and sevoflurane) are probably best avoided to minimise the risk of further renal damage. Non-steroidal anti-inflammatory drugs (NSAIDs) should be used with extreme caution, because they suppress renal prostaglandin synthesis and interfere with renal vascular homeostasis.

Patients with end-stage renal failure are often on renal dialysis, which by removing drug from the bloodstream can alter the pharmacokinetics of some drugs. The extent to which drugs will be removed in the dialysate depends on a number of factors. Drugs that are water-insoluble are poorly dialysed, as are those that are highly protein-bound. The volume of distribution (V_D) is an important rate-limiting factor in the removal of a drug by dialysis. Drugs with a high V_D will be slowly removed from the body. Even if the dialysis is very efficient in extracting drug from the blood, the fraction of drug in the blood will be very small relative to the total amount in the body. For example, digoxin has a V_D of 300 litres and only about 5% of the body store of the drug will be removed during a 4-hour dialysis. In contrast drugs with a $V_D < 1\,L{\cdot}kg^{-1}$, e.g. most non-depolarising muscle relaxants, are readily dialysed.

LIVER DISEASE

Liver disease is a continuum, ranging from abnormalities of liver function tests found on routine biochemical screening, with no adverse clinical consequences, to severe end-stage liver failure. Severe liver disease can result in marked, and often unpredictable, changes in the pharmacokinetics and dynamics of drugs. Changes in pharmacodynamics are partly due to disease-induced changes in the blood–brain barrier potentiating the action of centrally acting drugs. Some patients are particularly sensitive to the effects of sedative drugs, especially benzodiazepines. Drug disposition may be altered by disease-induced morphological and functional changes in the liver, although these changes are not as consistent as in patients with renal impairment. They do not always correlate with biochemical indices of hepatic function.

The liver receives 80% of its blood supply from the splanchnic circulation via the portal system and 20% from the systemic circulation via the hepatic artery. Because of its position between the enteric sites of absorption and the systemic circulation, the liver has a profound influence on the proportion of a drug given orally that reaches the systemic circulation (bioavailability). Disease-induced changes in liver blood flow, protein binding, and hepatocellular functioning can alter the hepatic metabolism of a drug. Decreases in blood flow, portosystemic shunting, and impaired metabolic capacity have the greatest influence on the elimination of drugs with a high hepatic extraction ratio (ER), since these are dependent on hepatic blood flow, e.g. fentanyl and propofol. Hepatic blood flow is reduced in patients with liver disease, and portosystemic shunting allows blood draining the splanchnic area to bypass the liver. This leads to high peak drug concentrations after oral administration with less effect on elimination half-life, and the first pass effect may be reduced by 50%. For high-extraction drugs, the oral doses should be reduced by at least 50%. Greater reductions in the oral dose may be indicated in patients with cirrhosis, because of the high degree of intrahepatic and extrahepatic shunting.

The disposition of poorly extracted drugs, e.g. thiopentone (ER 0.16) and diazepam (ER 0.02), is more sensitive to changes in the metabolic capacity of the liver than to blood flow, and the influence of hepatic disease on these drugs is highly variable. In general, the half-life of low-extraction drugs is prolonged and the frequency rather than the dose should be reduced. When the drug is given by intravenous infusion, the time to reach steady state concentrations will be prolonged since this depends only on half-life.

Most drugs used in anaesthesia are metabolised in the liver by phase I reactions, mediated by cytochrome P-450 enzymes. These are susceptible to destruction by cirrhosis, so that the biotransformation of drugs, such as opioids (except morphine), benzodiazepines, barbiturates, and inhalational agents, may be markedly altered in severe liver disease. These enzymes are found in the centrilobular areas, which are more prone to hypoxia. In contrast, the enzymes responsible for phase II reactions, found predominantly in the peripheral areas, often function normally even in advanced disease. The disposition of benzodiazepines that are eliminated primarily by glucuronidation, e.g. lorazepam and oxazepam, are unaffected by chronic liver disease. For drugs with low hepatic extraction, advanced hepatocytic dysfunction decreases phase I and II biotransformation with a reduced clearance and prolongation of the elimination half-life. This is often partially offset by an increased free fraction due to decreased protein binding.

Liver disease is often associated with sodium and water retention and an increased extracellular fluid volume. For highly polar drugs, such as neuromuscular blocking agents, this results in an increased volume of distribution and lower concentrations compared to the same dose given to healthy patients. This is part of the explanation why patients with liver disease need higher doses of these drugs. There is an association between liver and renal disease, and NSAIDs should be used with extreme caution in patients with liver disease. Some NSAIDs, e.g. salicylates, are hepatotoxic and even low doses can precipitate fulminant liver failure in patients with pre-existing cirrhosis.

FURTHER READING

Garland M. Pharmacology of drug transfer across the placenta. *Obstet Gynecol Clin North Am* 1998;25:21–42.

Guay J, Grenier Y, Varin F. Clinical pharmacokinetics of neuromuscular relaxants in pregnancy. *Clin Pharmacokinet* 1998;34:483–96.

Pacifici GM, Nottoli R. Placental transfer of drugs administered to the mother. *Clin Pharmacokinet* 1995;28:235–69.

20

Plasma volume expanders and artificial blood substitutes

JG Bovill and CP Henney

Introduction • Crystalloids • Colloids • Artificial blood substitutes

INTRODUCTION

Various fluids for intravenous infusions are used in the clinical management of surgical and critically ill patients, to replace insensible water and electrolyte loss and to maintain circulating blood volume. The normal insensible water loss during normothermia is about 1–2 $ml \cdot kg^{-1} \cdot h^{-1}$, but can increase to 5–12 $ml \cdot kg^{-1} \cdot h^{-1}$ during abdominal and thoracic surgery. This is best replaced by crystalloid solutions, which are isotonic solutions containing electrolytes in concentrations similar to that in plasma (Table 20.1). While in an emergency crystalloid solutions can also be used to replace blood loss and rapidly expand the circulating blood volume, this can be more effectively achieved with colloid solutions.

CRYSTALLOIDS

Crystalloids are solutions of substances with molecules of relatively small size, e.g. NaCl. Even though crystalloids can exert an osmotic pressure that may be several hundred times greater than that exerted by colloids, their contribution to plasma osmotic pressure is small since their concentration differences across the capillary membrane are also small. Crystalloid solutions used clinically include physiological saline (NaCl 0.9%), balanced salt solutions, such as Ringer-lactate or Hartmann's solution, and glucose- or dextrose-containing solutions. They are used for maintenance of water and electrolyte homeostasis to replace insensible or other losses. Because they equilibrate rapidly within the extracellular space their volume-expanding effects are relatively short-lived, about 20 min (Table 20.2). There has been much debate about the pros and cons of using crystalloids versus colloids for fluid resuscitation, but no consensus has been reached (Choi and coworkers 1999).

COLLOIDS

Colloids (from the Greek *kollae*, glue) are large molecules with molecular weights above 30 kDa. Because of their size they cannot easily pass through biological membranes, such as the walls of capillaries, and thus can exert substantial osmotic pressure in the vascular space. The plasma proteins, especially albumin, are the most important colloids responsible for maintaining plasma osmotic pressure.

Table 20.1 Electrolyte composition ($mmol \cdot L^{-1}$) and osmolality ($mosmol \cdot kg^{-1}$) of some intravenous fluids*

Solution	*Na^+*	*Cl^-*	*K^+*	*Ca^{2+}*	*Lactate*	*Osmolality*
0.9% NaCl	154	154	–	–	–	308
Ringer's solution	147	156	4	2.2	–	281
Ringer's Lactate	131	111	5	2	29	273
Modified gelatin (Gelofusine®)	154	120	–	–	–	310
Urea-linked gelatin (Haemaccel®)	145	145	5.1	6.25	–	310

* The normal osmolality of plasma is 280–310 $mosmol \cdot kg^{-1}$.

Table 20.2 Volume expansion data for available intravenous fluids

Solution	*Mean MW (kDa)*	*Volume expansion (%)*	*Intravascular persistence (h)*
0.9% NaCl	–	~25	~0.2
Ringer's lactate	–	~25	~0.25
4% albumin	60	70–80	6–8
Modified gelatin	35	60–80	2–3
Urea-linked gelatin	35		2–3
Dextran 40 (10%)	40	170–180	4–6
Dextran 70 (6%)	70	100–150	6–8
HES 200/0.5 (6%)	200	103	3–4
HES 200/0.5 (10%)	200	145	3–4
HES 200/0.62	200	160	~8
HES 130/0.4	130	100	4–6

Albumin

Human plasma has a colloid osmotic pressure of 3.6 kPa, of which 2.8 kPa is contributed by albumin. Volume-for-volume, 4.5% albumin is approximately four times more effective in expanding the plasma volume than crystalloid solutions, and the effect lasts 6–8 hours, compared to only 15–20 min with crystalloids. Although popular in the past as volume expanders, albumin solutions have fallen into disfavour. They are prepared from pooled human plasma, with all the inherent risks of pooled blood products. Albumin can cause adverse reactions, similar to other transfusion reactions, such as chills, urticaria, and vasodilatation. These may be caused by organic or inorganic substances formed during the processing (heating at 60° C for 10 h). There is also a 0.01–0.02% incidence of allergic reactions. It has been suggested that the use of albumin in critically ill patients was associated with a 5% excess mortality (Cochrane Injuries Group 1998). This meta-analysis generated considerable media attention and also much criticism from the medical profession (Horsey 2002a, b). Indeed, more recent studies suggest that albumin is associated with improved, not reduced, patient survival (Wilkes and Navickis 2001).

Dextrans

Dextrans are glucose polymers produced by bacterial digestion of sucrose. Dextrans with different average molecular weights are available. Dextran 70 (6%, 70 kDa) and dextran 40 (10%, 40 kDa) are the most widely used solutions. Because dextran solutions are polydisperse, i.e. they consist of molecules with a wide range of molecular weights, the initial volume expansion is relatively short. The smaller molecules are rapidly lost from the circulation, by diffusion into the interstitial space, and excretion by the kidneys. The larger molecules are more slowly eliminated by enzymatic degradation. For dextran 40, about 50% of the infused molecules disappear from the vascular compartment within 3 hours and 60% within 6 hours. Dextran 70, because of its larger molecules, remains much longer in the circulation; approximately 35% of the molecules are cleared within 12 hours. The popularity of dextrans as volume expanders has markedly decreased because of the frequency and severity of anaphylactic reactions. In addition to their use as volume expanders, dextrans affect blood viscosity. This is dependent on the molecular weight of the dextran. The lower molecular weight solutions, such as dextran 40, decrease viscosity by reducing erythrocyte aggregration, while dextrans with molecular weights above 60 kDa tend to aggregate red cells. Dextran 40 has in the past been popular for preventing deep venous thrombosis, particularly after orthopaedic and plastic surgery.

Gelatins

Two types of gelatin products are currently used clinically, both derived from bovine gelatin. Urea-linked gelatins (e.g. Haemaccel®) are produced by cross-linking polypeptide chains with hexamethyl di-isocyanate. Haemaccel® has an average molecular weight of 35 kDa. Gelofusine® (average 30 kDa) is a succinylated gelatin produced from polypeptide chains treated with succinic acid anhydrase. This replaces amino groups with a negatively charged COO– group. Haemaccel has a higher content of calcium (6.3 mmol·L^{-1}) and potassium (5.1 mmol·L^{-1}) than Gelofusine, and the high calcium concentration can lead to clotting if infused together with blood. The volume-expanding effect of both solutions lasts 2–3 hours (Table 20.2). Gelofusine is almost totally eliminated by the kidneys within 24 hours, and 50% of Haemaccel is excreted unchanged in the urine within 12 hours. Modified gelatins may interfere with coagulation by inhibition of platelet aggregation. This effect is more pronounced with Haemaccel than Gelofusine, possibly due to the higher concentration of calcium in Haemaccel (de Jonge and co-workers 1998, Evans and co-workers 1998). They are also associated with allergic reactions, with an incidence of 0.07% for Gelofusine and 0.15% for Haemaccel.

Because they are derived from cattle, there is a concern that gelatins might be vehicles for the transmission of the prion agent responsible for bovine spongiform encephalopathy (BSE) in cattle and variant Creutzfeldt-Jakob disease (vCJD) in humans. There is at present no evidence that these products have contributed to the transmission of BSE or vCJD. However, the incubation period may be up to several years, and due prudence is warranted when such products are used.

Hydroxyethyl starch

Hydroxyethyl starch (HES) is a derivative of the highly branched starch, amylopectin, in which the anhydroglucose residues are substituted by hydroxyethyl groups to reduce metabolic degradation by plasma α-amylase. The

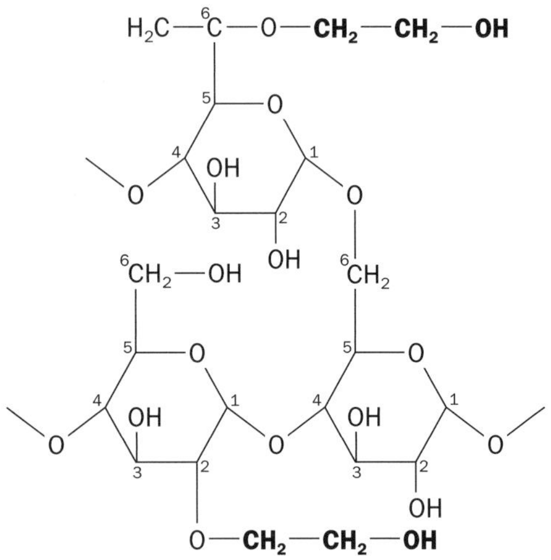

Figure 20.1 *Basic structure of hydroxyethyl starch (HES), showing HES (–CH_2–CH_2–OH) substitution at positions C_2 and C_6.*

hydroxyethyl groups can be introduced at three positions, C_2, C_3 and C_6, on the glucose molecules (Figure 20.1). The degree of substitution and the substitution site, expressed as the C_2/C_6 ratio, determine the extent of enzymatic degradation. Although the maximum possible substitution per glucose molecule is 3, the molar substitution of HES used clinically ranges from 0.4 to 0.7. A molar substitution ratio of 0.5 means that on average 5 hydroxyethyl groups are substituted per 10 glucose groups.

As with other synthetic colloid solutions, HES solutions are polydisperse. They are characterised by the average molecular weight (MW), the degree of substitution and the C_2/C_6 ratio. There is an arbitrary classification into low (< 100 kDa), medium (100–250 kDa), and high (> 250 kDa) molecular weight solutions. In comparison to other colloids, the larger MW of HES contributes to a prolonged intravascular retention. In Europe, only low and medium MW HES are used. These are sometimes referred to as pentastarch, since most have a substitution ratio of 0.5 (EloHaes® has a substitution ratio of 0.62). In the US, only medium and high molecular weight products are available. High molecular weight products, with an average MW of 450 kDa and a substitution ratio of 0.7, are known as hetastarch. The most recently introduced HES solution, HES 130/0.4, has an average MW of 130 kDa (15–380 kDa), a molar substitution of 0.32–0.4, and a C_2/C_6 ratio of 9. The MW distribution is much narrower than with other HES products. The lower molar substitution results in a more rapid metabolism, but this is counteracted by the high C_2/C_6 ratio. This results in a duration of action comparable to that of HES 200/0.5 but with a more favourable pharmacokinetic profile and less accumulation in the tissues. HES 130/0.4 is claimed to cause less interference with coagulation and fewer renal problems than HES 200/0.5, when infused in large quantities.

When HES is infused, the smaller molecules are excreted by the kidneys, while the larger molecules are metabolised by α-amylase, and taken up by the reticuloendothelial system (RES) and the skin. Even though HES molecules disappear from the blood within 10–72 hours, dependent on their molecular weight, they can be detected in the RES for at least one month. Anaphylactic reactions to HES are lower than with other colloids and they have minimal effects on coagulation. Controversy exists regarding the use of HES in patients with renal insufficiency, and dose recommendations are based on the risk of renal tubular overload and the influence on haemostasis (possible decrease in factor VII/von Willebrand factor). The risk is greater with the higher MW solutions, and appears to be lower with the new HES 130/0.4.

ARTIFICIAL BLOOD SUBSTITUTES

One of the most important functions of blood is the binding of oxygen by haemoglobin and its transport to the tissues. Administration of blood and blood products, however, carries with it a number of risks (Table 20.3) and are not always the initial choice to replace blood or plasma loss. Blood and blood products are also expensive, have a limited availability, and a very limited shelf life. A number of alternative oxygen-carrying fluids have been developed, and some are close to release for clinical use.

They can be classified into three main groups, haemoglobin solutions in which the haemoglobin molecule has undergone a modification, liposome-encapsulated haemoglobin, and perfluorocarbons. All of them have intravascular half-lives that are relatively short in comparison to that of transfused erythrocytes.

Stroma-free haemoglobin solutions

The rationale behind the development of these solutions was to separate the oxygen-carrying capacity of haemoglobin from the antigenic determinant present on the membrane of the erythrocyte. When the haemoglobin molecule comes free from the erythrocyte the tetramer structure dissociates into α- and β-chain dimers or haemoglobin monomers. This results in a reduction in molecular weights from about 64 kDa for the tetramer, to 32 kDa for the dimers, and 16 kDa for the monomer. These smaller molecules are excreted by the kidneys, increasing the risk of kidney damage. Another problem is the reduced ability of the dimer to deliver oxygen to the tissues. In the dimer oxygen binding is no longer influenced by 2,3-diphosphoglycerine (2,3-DPG) and this shifts the oxygen dissociation curve to the left. This lowers the dissociation of oxygen in the tissues. It is also difficult to completely remove all stromal material, and these remnants can cause further renal damage as well as systemic toxicity due to activation of the complement cascade. Some of these problems have been reduced by better purification techniques.

There are four classes of haemoglobin solutions, polymerised haemoglobin, intramolecular cross-linked haemoglobin, conjugated haemoglobin, and haemoglobin surrounded by a synthetic membrane. They all contain modified haemoglobin, intended to increase the intravascular retention times, decrease renal excretion and maintain the normal P_{50} of haemoglobin. Several of these haemoglobin solutions are undergoing phase I and phase II clinical trials. These have demonstrated the absence of acute toxicity and of serious adverse events, but have also shown a dose-dependent vasopressor effect attributed to the scavenging of nitric oxide (NO) (Remy and co-workers 1999; Winslow 1999).

A recent development is that of haemoglobin microspheres. These are produced by high-intensity ultrasound, which forms a 'skin' of about 1 million cross-linked haemoglobin molecules. *In vitro*, these microspheres have an oxygen-carrying capacity greater than blood, an oxygen affinity approximately equal to that of normal haemoglobin, and a long shelf life at 4°C. Encapsulation of natural or modified haemoglobin with microvesicles (liposomes or biodegradable nanocapsules) is an elegant solution to some of the problems mentioned above. They do, however, carry the risk of adverse effects due to the vehicle particles and the uptake of the microvesicles by the reticuloendothelial system. The latter decreases the resistance to infection, which in a number of studies has resulted in fatal infections. At the time of writing there are no encapsulated haemoglobin solutions undergoing clinical trials.

Table 20.3 Potential adverse effects of homologous blood transfusions*

Potential adverse effects
Transmission of infections
Hepatitis B (1:100 000 to 1:400 000)
Hepatitis C (1:200 000)
Human immune deficiency virus (HIV) (1:4 000 000)
Human T cell lymphotropic virus
Malaria
Cytomegalovirus and Epstein-Barr virus
Acute haemolytic reactions
Alloimmunisation
Immunosuppression

* Where known, risk (as estimated frequency per unit infused) is shown in parentheses.

Perfluorocarbons

Perfluorocarbons (PFCs) are chemically inert hydrocarbons with 8–10 carbon molecules,

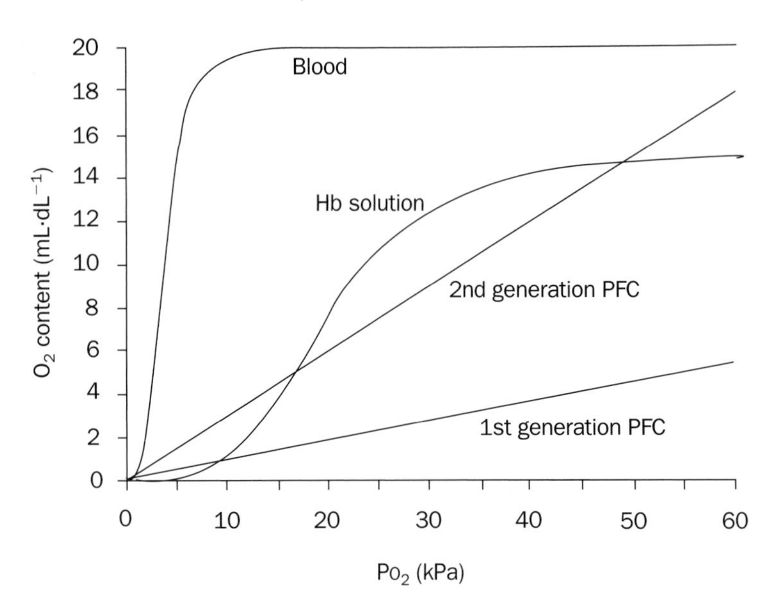

Figure 20.2 *Oxygen-carrying capacity of whole blood, Hb-solution, and first- and second-generation perfluorocarbon (PFC) emulsions.*

where the hydrogens have been replaced by fluorine. Because they are immiscible in water they are prepared as emulsions. All gases, including oxygen and carbon dioxide, are about 20 times more soluble in PFC than in water. Like plasma, but unlike haemoglobin, the quantity of oxygen carried is linearly related to the oxygen partial pressure, and they require a high P_{O_2} (> 40 kPa) to be effective (Figure 20.2). However, although they do not carry large amounts of oxygen, most of this is available for release in the tissues. Experimental work with PFCs began in the 1960s. The first-generation PFCs, however, had several problems. The PFC concentration was low, the emulsion was unstable and had a very short intravascular retention time. In addition, the emulsifying agent triggered a number of complement-mediated side effects. These problems have been much reduced in the second-generation products. A recent large European study has demonstrated that using PFC can decrease transfusion requirements during high-blood-loss non-cardiac surgery (Spahn and co-workers 2002). Like all synthetic oxygen-carrying compounds, PFCs are eliminated partly by phagocytosis and uptake in the reticuloendothelial system (RES), and partly by excretion via the lungs. The half-life in the blood is 12–18 h. Once out of the vascular space, however, they remain in the liver and spleen for several weeks. This limits the use of repeated doses over a short period of time. Currently, PFCs are only licensed for procedures such as coronary artery angioplasty.

FURTHER READING

Choi PT, Yip G, Quinonez LG, Cook DJ. Crystalloids versus colloids in fluid resuscitation: A systemic review. *Crit Care Med* 1999;27:200–10.

Cochrane Injuries Group Albumin Review. Human albumin administration in critically ill patients: Systematic review of randomised controlled trials. *BMJ* 1998;317:235–40.

de Jonge E, Levi M, Berends F, et al. Impaired haemostasis by intravenous administration of a gelatin-based plasma expander in human subjects. *Thromb Haemost* 1998;79:286–90.

Evans PA, Glenn JR, Heptinstall S, Madira W. Effects of gelatin-based resuscitation fluids on platelet aggregration. *Br J Anaesth* 1998;81:198–202.

Horsey PJ. The Cochrane 1998 Albumin Review—not all it was cracked up to be. *Eur J Anaesthesiol* 2002a;19:701–4.

Horsey PJ. Albumin and hypovolaemia: Is the Cochrane evidence to be trusted? *Lancet* 2002b;359:70–2.

Remy B, Delby-Dupont G, Lamy M. Red blood cell substitutes: Fluorocarbon and haemoglobin solutions. *Br Med Bull* 1999;1:277–98.

Spahn DR, Waschke KF, Standl T, et al. Use of perflubron emulsion to decrease allogeneic blood transfusion in high-blood-loss non-cardiac surgery: Results of a European phase 3 study. *Anesthesiology* 2002;97:1338–49.

Wilkes MM, Navickis RJ. Patient survival after human albumin administration: a meta-analysis of randomised controlled trials. *Ann Intern Med* 2001;135:149–64.

Winslow RM. New transfusion strategies; Red cell substitutes. *Annu Rev Med* 1999;50:337–53.

21

Statistics and clinical trials

JG Bovill

Introduction • Probability • Sensitivity, specificity, odds ratio, and relative risk • Types of data and scales of measurement • Measures of central tendency and dispersion • Inferential statistics • Students's *t*-distribution • Comparing means • Comparing more than two means • Regression and correlation • Non-parametric tests • The χ^2-test • Clinical trials

INTRODUCTION

Statistics is concerned with the treatment of numerical data where there is an associated uncertainty or chance. Many situations contain some element of chance, e.g. the outcome from throwing a die or the response of a patient to a drug. Even though it may be impossible to predict a particular outcome with certainty, its probability can often be quantified. Knowledge of statistical principles is essential in designing clinical trials and in the interpretation and evaluation of the results.

PROBABILITY

The probability of an event A, denoted by $P(A)$, is a number between 0 and 1 that gives the long-run proportion of occasions on which event A occurs. If we toss a die a large number of times we would score 1 in 1/6 of the throws (provided the die is true), so $P(1) = 1/6$. An impossible event never occurs, so its probability is 0, and a certain event always occurs, so its probability is 1. The probability that event A does not occur, written as $P(\bar{A})$, is given by $P(\bar{A}) = 1 - P(A)$, since A must either occur or not occur. Events A and $\bar{A}$ are termed **mutually exclusive** since it is impossible for them to occur simultaneously. When the probability that an event A occurs is dependent on whether or not event B has occurred, we speak of the conditional probability of A given B, denoted by $P(A \mid B)$.

SENSITIVITY, SPECIFICITY, ODDS RATIO AND RELATIVE RISK

The diagnosis of a disease is often based on the results of laboratory or other tests, which are never 100% reliable. They may give a positive result when the disease is absent (false positive) or a negative result when the disease is present (false negative) (Table 21.1).

The probability of a true positive is called the **sensitivity**. Sensitivity answers the question: If the condition is present, how likely is it to obtain a positive test for the condition? The greater the sensitivity the less is the likelihood of a false negative. **Specificity** is the chance of ruling out a disease when it is absent. The higher the specificity the less is the likelihood of

Table 21.1 Possible outcomes of a diagnostic test

	Disease	
	Present	*Absent*
Positive test	True positive ($1 - \beta$)	False positive (α)
Negative test	False negative (β)	True negative ($1 - \alpha$)

a false positive. Specificity is a measure of how often a test correctly identifies the absence of a condition when the condition is not present. Note that a test can have high sensitivity but low specificity, so that it will detect the disease in a high proportion of patients with the disease but also give a high number of false positives in patients without the disease.

The **odds ratio** indicates how much more likely an individual given a particular treatment is to have a specific outcome than someone who is not given the treatment. The odds of an event, E, is the ratio of the probability that the event occurs to the probability that it does not occur, i.e. $P(E)/(1 - P(E))$. Table 21.2 shows the incidence of postoperative vomiting in patients given droperidol or saline. In the droperidol group $P(\text{vomiting}) = 37/200 = 0.185$, and $P(\text{no vomiting}) = 163/200 = 0.815 = 1 - 0.185$. The corresponding probabilities for saline are 0.227 and 0.584. Thus, the odds of vomiting in the droperidol group are $0.185/0.815 = 0.227$, and for the saline group the odds are 0.584. The odds ratio is $0.584/0.227 = 2.57$. In other words, the risk of vomiting is 2.57 times higher in patients given saline than in those given droperidol. Had the odds ratio been close to 1 we would conclude that there were no differences between the treatments.

Table 21.2 Number of patients treated with droperidol or saline who vomited

	Droperidol	*Saline*
Vomiting	37	73
No vomiting	163	125
Total	200	198

Relative risk is a measure of the increased or decreased risk of an outcome associated with exposure to the factor of interest, which could be a disease or a drug treatment. A relative risk of one indicates that the risk is the same in the exposed and unexposed groups. If greater than one the risk is higher in the exposed group. The **number-needed-to-treat** indicates how many patients have to be treated in order to observe a specific outcome (Cook and Sackett 1995).

The **likelihood ratio** (LR) is the ratio of the chance of a particular response (positive or negative) when a disease or condition is present to the chance of the same response when the disease or condition is absent. For example, a LR of 2.5 for a positive result for a disease indicates that a positive result is 2.5 times more likely in a patient with the disease than in one without it. For a positive result, LR is related to sensitivity and specificity as follows:

$$LR\ (\textit{for a positive result}) = \frac{\textit{sensitivity}}{1 - \textit{specificity}}$$

TYPES OF DATA AND SCALES OF MEASUREMENT

A **parameter** is some characteristic of a population or model that describes or characterises that population or model. A **variable** is a characteristic that varies from one individual to another. If the relationship between height and age in children is given by *height* = C × *age* + D, then the constants C and D are parameters in the model and height and age are variables.

Variables can be continuous or discrete, quantitative or categorical. Height and blood pressure are continuous variables, while the number of children in a family is a discrete variable. The second distinction is between **quantitative** and **categorical variables**. Quantitative variables assign meaningful numerical values to observations. They can be further subdivided into data on a ratio scale of measurement and data on an interval scale. A **ratio scale** has a constant size interval between any adjacent units on the measurement scale, and there is a true zero point with physical significance. Thus, we can say that an individual weighing 80 kg is twice as heavy as one weighing 40 kg. In contrast, an **interval scale** possesses a constant interval size but not a true zero, e.g. temperature in degrees centigrade (°C). Although the difference in temperature between 15°C and 30°C is the same as that between 45°C and 60°C (i.e. equal intervals) we cannot say that a temperature of 60°C is twice as hot as a temperature of 30°C, since the zero point is arbitrary. However, if temperature is measured in Kelvin (K) then, because this measurement scale has a physically meaningful zero, we can say that 300 K is twice as hot as 150 K.

Categorical variables, subdivided into nominal and ordinal, assign observations to categories. In a **nominal scale** (from the Latin for 'name') a variable is classified by some quality it possesses rather than a numerical measurement. Nominal variables lack any obvious order, e.g. hair colours (black, brown, grey, etc.). In an **ordinal scale**, the categories have an ordered relationship one with another, going from 'least something' to 'most something' (or vice versa). Thus, adverse reactions to a drug might be classified as mild, moderate or severe. Ordinal variables are often assigned numerical values and these respect the ordering, e.g. mild = 1, moderate = 2, severe = 3, but the precise values attached remain arbitrary (we could equally well have assigned values of 0, 1, 2 or 5, 6, 7).

MEASURES OF CENTRAL TENDENCY AND DISPERSION

A characteristic of biological systems is variability, with most values of a variable clustered around the middle of the range of observed values, and fewer at the extremes of the range. The measure of location or central tendency gives an indication where the distribution is centred, while a measure of dispersion indicates the degree of scatter or spread in the distribution. The most widely used measure of central tendency is the arithmetic **mean** or average of the observed values, i.e. the sum of all variable values divided by the number of observations. Another measure of central tendency is the **median**, the middle measurement in the data (if n is odd) or the average of the two middle values (if n is even). The median is the appropriate measure of central tendency for ordinal data. Less commonly used is the **mode**, the most frequently occurring value in the dataset. The mode is the appropriate measure of central tendency for nominal data. Other measures of location (but not of central tendency) are percentiles or quartiles. The **percentile** of x is the percentage of the total cases that falls at or below x in value. Commonly used percentiles are the 25th and 75th percentiles (or 1st and 3rd quartiles). The median is the 50th percentile. The distance between the first and third quartile is the **interquartile range** (Figure 21.1).

The mean summarises only one aspect of a distribution. We also need some measure of spread or dispersion, the tendency for observations to depart from the central tendency. The standard measure of dispersion is the **variance**:

$$Variance = \frac{1}{n}\sum_{i=1}^{n}(x_i - \bar{x})^2$$

When dealing with samples rather than whole populations, it is common to divide by $n - 1$ rather than n, since this gives an unbiased

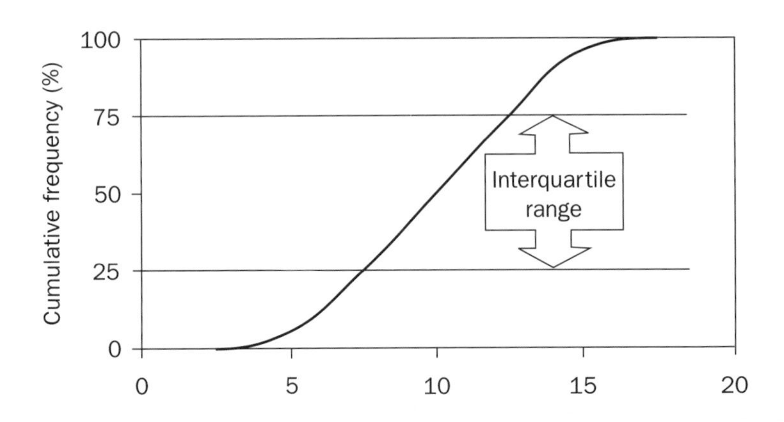

Figure 21.1 *Cumulative frequency plot illustration 25th, 75th percentiles, and the interquartile range.*

estimate of the population variance. Population means and variances are by convention denoted by the Greek letters μ and σ^2, respectively, while the corresponding sample parameters are denoted by $\bar{x}$ and s^2.

Because variance is a quantity in squared units, the square root of the variance, the **standard deviation** (SD), is usually taken as the measure of dispersion since it provides a measure in the original units. Another useful measure of dispersion is the **coefficient of variation** (CV) defined as:

$$CV = \frac{SD}{\bar{x}} \times 100\%$$

The CV is independent of the units of measurement, and thus is particularly useful for comparing the variability in datasets of very different magnitudes. Mice have much faster heart rates than humans, but one could use CV to compare the relative variability in heart rate between these species.

Probability distributions and statistical inference

A very important probability distribution is the **normal** or **Gaussian distribution** (after the German mathematician, Karl Friedrich Gauss, 1777–1855). The normal distribution has the same value for the mean, median and mode. The equation describing this distribution (the probability density function) is:

$$f(x) = \frac{1}{\sigma\sqrt{2\pi}} e^{-\frac{1}{2}\left(\frac{x-\mu}{\sigma}\right)^2}$$

This is quite imposing (and does not need to be memorised!) but illustrates that the distribution is completely characterised by two parameters, the mean (μ) and the standard deviation (σ). The normal distribution has a symmetrical, bell-shaped curve. Two normal distributions with the same mean (10) but different variances are shown in Figure 21.2.

If a variable X is distributed normally with mean μ and variance σ^2, then the variable Z, defined as:

$$Z = \frac{x - \mu}{\sigma}$$

is also normally distributed with mean 0 and variance 1. This distribution is called the **standard normal distribution** (Figure 21.3).

The probability that the variable x takes a value between a and b is given by the area under the graph of the probability distribution between $x = a$ and $x = b$. This is illustrated in Figure 21.3, where the shaded area gives the probability that the standard normal variate, Z, lies between z and infinity, i.e. the probability $P(Z \geq z)$. The total area under the graph is equal to 1, and because of the symmetry of the normal distribution it follows that the area of any one half is equal to 0.5. For any normal

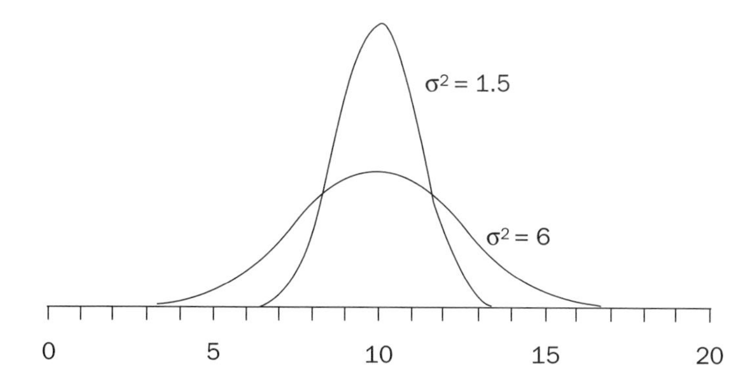

Figure 21.2 Two normal distributions with the same mean (10) but different variances.

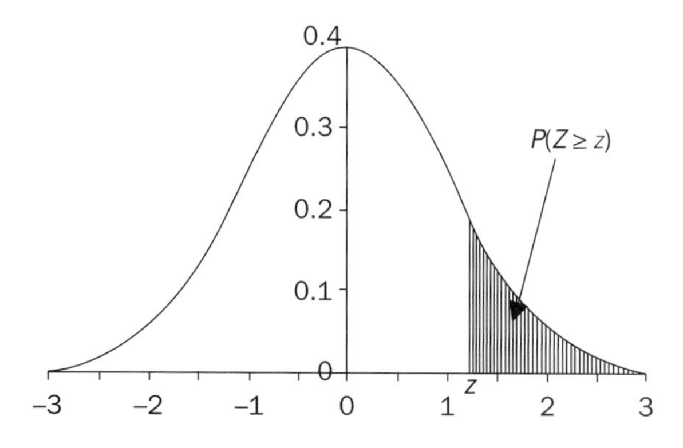

Figure 21.3 The standard normal distribution curve. The shaded area gives the probability that the standard normal variate, Z, lies between z and infinity, i.e. $P(Z \geq z)$.

distribution, 90% of the area (and thus 90% of the values in the distribution) will fall within ± 1.64 standard deviations of the mean, 95% within ± 1.96 standard deviations, and 99% within ± 2.58 standard deviations.

While it is possible, using advanced mathematical techniques, to determine the area under any normal distribution curve, it is obviously impractical to do so for the infinite combinations of μ and σ^2. However, it is possible to normalise a variable to the standard normal deviate, Z, using the formula given above. Tables of areas under the standard normal distribution curve (AUC) are given in standard statistical textbooks. The use of the Z-transformation is illustrated in the following example. In healthy men aged between 20–30 years the mean percentage of lymphocytes in blood cells is 35% with a standard deviation of 13%. What is the probability of an individual having 50% or more lymphocytes. Here, $\mu = 35$, $\sigma = 13$, $x = 50$, so:

$$Z = \frac{x - \mu}{\sigma} = \frac{50 - 35}{13} = 1.154$$

From a table of Z-values (this gives $P(Z \geq z)$), the required probability is 0.1243. Thus, $P(\text{count} \geq 50\%) = P(Z \geq 1.154) = 0.1243$. To put this another way, about 12.5% of healthy mean will have 50% or more lymphocytes.

There are many other distributions used in statistics besides the normal distribution. Common ones are the χ^2 and the F-distributions (see later) and the binomial distribution. The **binomial distribution** involves binomial events, i.e. events for which there are only two possible outcomes (yes/no, success/failure). The binomial distribution is skewed to the right, and is characterised by two parameters; n, the number of individuals in the sample (or repetitions of a trial), and π, the true probability of success for each individual or trial. The mean is $n\ \pi$ and the variance is $n\pi(1 - \pi)$. The **binomial test**, based on the binomial distribution, can be used to make inferences about probabilities. If we toss a true coin a large number of times we expect the coin to fall heads up on 50% of the tosses. Suppose we toss the coin 10 times and get 7 heads, does this mean that the coin is biased. From a binomial table we can find that $P(x = 7) = 0.117$ for $n = 10$ and $\pi = 0.5$. Since $0.117 > 0.05$ ($P = 0.05$ is the commonly accepted level of significance) we conclude that there is no evidence for bias and that the outcome is due purely to chance.

INFERENTIAL STATISTICS

Up to now we have been discussing descriptive statistics. Inferential statistics uses statistical techniques to make inferences about wider populations from that from which our data are drawn. This involves making estimates and hypothesis testing.

Hypothesis testing

Much of medical research involves the testing of hypotheses, for instance, is drug A more or less effective than drug B. The first step in hypothesis testing is to state the **null hypothesis** (given the symbol H_0) that, e.g. drug A is not different from drug B. The opposite of the null hypothesis is the **alternative hypothesis**, denoted by H_1. There can be two types of alternative hypothesis, a two-sided alternative, leading to a two-tailed test, and a one-sided alternative, leading to a one-tailed test. In the first case we would have *H_1: drug A is different from drug B*, without specifying the directions of the difference, i.e. we accept H_1 if either A is more effective or less effective than B (Figure 21.4). In the second case the alternative hypothesis, H_1, is considered true if A is more effective (or less effective) than B (Figure 21.5). Depending on the type of data we are dealing with a variety of tests is available to allow us to decide whether we can accept H_0 (and thus reject H_1) or vice versa.

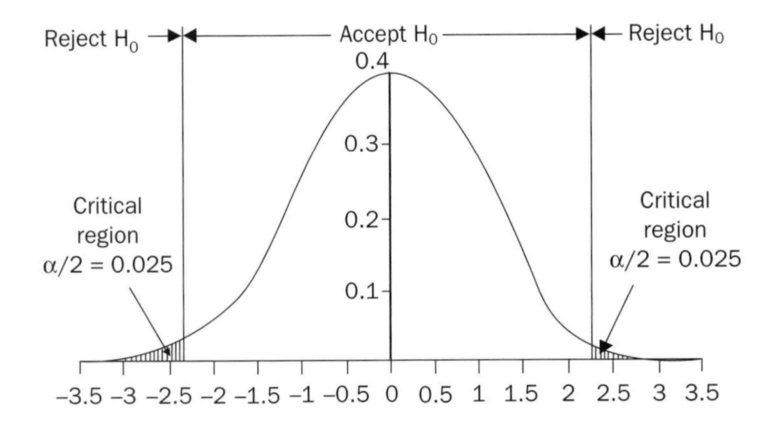

Figure 21.4 *The two-tailed or two-sided test.*

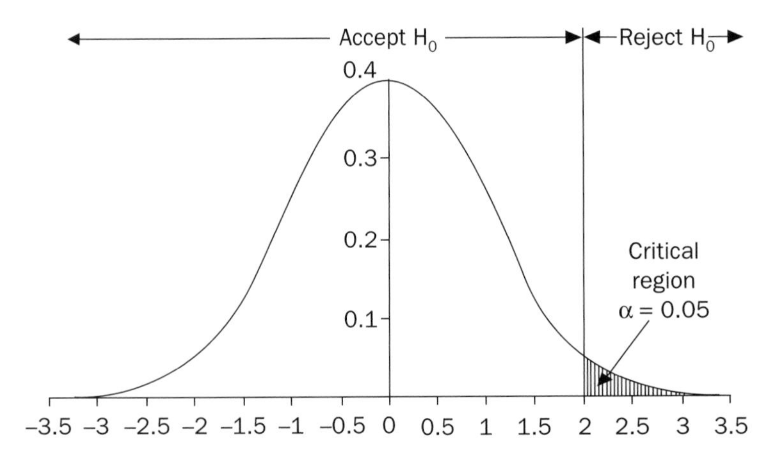

Figure 21.5 *The one-tailed or one-sided test, with a normal distribution curve for comparison.*

Statistical significance

Recall that areas under probability density functions are related to probabilities. In the case of a standard normal distribution, a *Z*-score of 1.96 cuts off 5% of the total area of the standard normal curve (this is equivalent to putting z = 1.96 in Figure 21.3) and a *Z*-score of 2.58 cuts off 1% of the total area. If the *Z*-score for the difference between drugs A and B (measured on some appropriate scale) is > 1.96 then the probability that this difference has arisen by chance is less than 5% (or < 1% if $Z > 2.58$). This is referred to as the significance of the observed difference, often called the *P*-value. A common way of expressing this is to say that the difference was significant at the 5% level ($P \leq 0.05$) or at the 1% level ($P \leq 0.01$). The *P*-value is the probability, assuming the null hypothesis is true, that an event as extreme or more extreme than that observed would occur. In the two-sided case the probability is in both 'big' and 'small' directions and in just one direction in the one-sided case. Often, but not always, there is symmetry in the distributions, resulting in the *P*-value in the two-sided (or two-tailed) case being twice the one-sided *P*-value. The Greek letter α is often used when referring to the probability of accepting H_0, e.g. $\alpha = 0.05$ or $\alpha = 0.01$.

Type 1 and Type 2 errors

The smaller the *P*-value the less likely it is that, under the null hypothesis, i.e. H_0 is true, we would have obtained the observed value of the test statistic. So, a small value of *P* is likely to mean that H_0 is untrue, in which case we should prefer H_1. However, it is possible that H_0 is true but a rather unlikely event has taken place. Thus accepting the 5% level of significance ($P \leq 0.05$) in rejecting H_0 means that 95 times out of 100 we are probably correct in our decision, *but* 5 times out of 100 we run the risk of rejecting H_0 when in fact it is true. Rejecting the null hypothesis when it is actually true is referred to as a Type 1 error. Accepting H_0 when it is not true is a Type 2 error. The probability of a Type 1 error is given the symbol α; the probability of a Type 2 error the symbol β (Table 21.3).

Populations and samples

Consider that we wanted to compare the height of adult males and females in the Netherlands. It would obviously be impractical to measure the heights of the whole population. We would take representative samples from both sexes and use these data to draw conclusions about the larger population. Population characteristics have to be inferred or estimated from measures taken from samples. If the sample is not truly representative of the population from which it is drawn, i.e. if it is a biased sample, then it is virtually impossible to make accurate predictions about the population. For example, choosing our sample of males from a basketball team would introduce considerable bias—basketball players are usually very tall! The way to minimise bias of this type is to take random samples, where each member of the population under study has an equal chance of being selected.

If repeated samples are taken from the same population it is unlikely that they all will have identical characteristics, either to each other or the population. This is a consequence of the randomisation process and the variability in the

Table 21.3 Relationship between Type 1 (α) and Type 2 (β) errors and accepting the null hypothesis (H_0) and rejecting the alternative hypothesis (H_1)

		True	
		H_0	H_1
Accept	H_0	$1-\alpha$	β
	H_1	α	$1-\beta$

population. However, if n independent random samples are drawn from any population with mean μ and variance σ^2, then for large n the distribution of the sample means is approximately normal with mean μ and variance σ^2/n. This is the Central Limit Theorem, which is largely responsible for the ubiquity of the normal distribution in statistics.

STUDENT'S *t*-DISTRIBUTION

When we are dealing with samples rather than populations, we cannot use the standard normal deviate, Z, to make predictions since this requires knowledge of the population mean and variance or standard deviation. In general, we do not know the value of these parameters. However, provided the sample is a random one, its mean $\bar{x}$ is a reliable estimate of the population mean μ, and we can use the central limit theorem to provide an estimate of σ. This estimate, known as the **standard error of the mean**, is given by:

$$s.e.m = \frac{s}{\sqrt{n}}$$

where s is the sample standard deviation. For samples, the standard deviation corresponding to Z is the t-statistic, defined as:

$$t = \frac{\bar{x} - x}{s/\sqrt{n}}$$

The t-statistic follows what is known as the Student's t-distribution, after the statistician William Sealy Gosset (1876–1937) who published under the pseudonym 'Student'. The shape of the t-distribution is similar to that of the normal distribution, but forms a family of curves distinguished by a parameter known as the 'degrees of freedom'. The 5% critical point in the t-distribution always exceeds the normal value of 1.96, but is nevertheless close to 2.0 for all but quite small values of degrees of freedom.

The term '**degrees of freedom**' has many applications in statistics. Suppose we have a set of 10 observations (numbers) where we have complete freedom of choice to select what the numbers are. Then we have 10 degrees of freedom. If, however, the numbers must average 20, we have complete freedom in selecting the first 9 numbers, but for the tenth one we have no choice—the number of degrees of freedom has been reduced by 1. If, in addition, the standard deviation must be 5, then we have lost yet another degree of freedom. After selecting 8 numbers, we will have no freedom in selecting the last 2—we now have only 8 degrees of freedom.

A particular use of the t-statistic is calculating **confidence intervals** (CI). When we calculate the mean of a sample we do not expect that it will be exactly equal to the mean of the population from which the sample was drawn. Nonetheless, we can expect that it will be reasonably close to the population mean. A confidence interval provides an estimate as to how close. The 95% confidence interval is a random interval such that, in 95% of hypothetical replications of the sampling process, the confidence intervals obtained will include the true value of μ. The confidence interval for μ is of the form $\bar{x} \pm$ multiples of s.e.m. The multiple used is $t_{1-\alpha/2}$ $(n-1)$, which is the $100(1-\alpha/2)$ percentage point of the t-distribution with $n-1$ degrees of freedom. Thus, the 95% CI ($\alpha = 0.05$) is given by:

$$\bar{x} \pm [t_{0.975}\,(n-1)]\,\frac{s}{\sqrt{n}}$$

The appropriate value of t can be obtained from standard statistical tables.

COMPARING MEANS

The paired *t*-test

When we wish to test for a zero mean difference in matched paired data the appropriate test is a one-sample or paired t-test. For such data the values of two quantities whose comparison is of interest are both made on the same individual, and both measurements are repeated on many individuals. For example, in an experiment heart rate was measured in 20 patients before and after administration of a drug. The mean heart rate was 76.5 b.p.m. before the drug and 69.0 b.p.m. after giving the drug. To test whether the difference between these means is statistically significant, we work not with the individual heart rates but with the mean difference in heart rates averaged over all 20 individuals. The mean difference ($\bar{d}$) was 7.5 with a standard deviation of 11.64. The null hypothesis to be tested is H_0: $\bar{d} = 0$, against H_1: $\bar{d} \neq 0$. This is a two-tailed test:

$$t = \frac{\bar{d}}{SD/\sqrt{20}} = \frac{7.5}{11.64/\sqrt{20}} = 2.88 \text{ on 19 d.f.}$$

For this value of t we obtain $P = 0.00956$, so we conclude that the drug has a highly significant influence on heart rate.

The unpaired *t*-test

When comparing the means from two independent samples we use the unpaired or two-sample t-test. If the number of observations, means and standard deviations in the respective samples are n_1, $\bar{x}_1$, s_1 and n_2, $\bar{x}_2$, s_2, then:

$$t = \frac{\bar{x}_1 - \bar{x}_2}{\sqrt{\frac{s^2_1}{n_1} + \frac{s^2_2}{n_2}}}$$

with $(n_1 - 1) + (n_2 - 1)$ degrees of freedom. In a study comparing the effects of nitrous oxide and alfentanil on the baroreceptor responses in two groups of 10 patients, the mean ± SD slope for the pressor was 1.8 ± 0.8 ms/mmHg in the nitrous oxide (N_2O) group and 3.1 ± 1.4 ms/mmHg in the alfentanil group. The calculated value for t is 2.5495 on 18 degrees of freedom. From statistical tables the critical value of t for a two-tailed test at the 0.05 level of significance and 18 degrees of freedom is 2.101. Since 2.5495 > 2.101 we conclude that the slope in the N_2O group is significantly less ($P < 0.05$) than that in the alfentanil group.

Use of confidence intervals in comparing means

If the 95% confidence interval for the mean difference ($\bar{d}$) in the paired case contains zero, then one can accept the null hypothesis at the 0.05 level of significance. If zero is not included, then we reject the null hypothesis and accept the alternative hypothesis that the means are different. Similarly, in the unpaired case, if the 95% confidence interval for the difference of the means contains zero, then one can accept the null hypothesis; if not the means are considered different at the 0.05 level of significance.

COMPARING MORE THAN TWO MEANS

When comparing the means of more than two samples we cannot test each pair using the t-test for the following reason. The probability of a Type 1 error, using $\alpha = 0.05$, is 0.05 or 5% for each comparison. However, the probability of making at least one Type 1 error in k comparisons is $1-(1-\alpha)^k$. If we are comparing 4 means ($k = 6$ possible comparisons) the risk of making a Type 1 error when $\alpha = 0.05$ is $1 - 0.95^6 = 0.26$, more that 5 times as large as the probability of making such an error in a single test. With 6 groups the probability is $1 - 0.95^{15}$, or about 0.53, for at least one Type 1 error.

Analysis of variance

The appropriate test when comparing more than two means is analysis of variance (ANOVA). The essential process in ANOVA is to split up, or decompose, the overall variance in the data. This variability is due to differences between the means due to the treatment effect (between-group variance) and that due to random variability between individuals within each group (within-group variance, sometimes called unexplained or residual variance), hence the name 'analysis of variance'. If the group means were all equal the between-group variability would be zero.

The test statistic for ANOVA is the ratio, F, of the between-group and within-group variances. If H_0 is true and the means do not differ, then the between-group and within-group variances will be similar and the F ratio will be close to 1. If there are differences between the groups then the between-group variance will be larger than the within-group variance, the F-ratio will be much greater than 1. The F ratio follows the F-distribution with $k-1, n-1$ degrees of freedom, where n is the total sample size and k the number of groups. Critical values of F for different values of α are reproduced in statistical tables.

When the ANOVA shows that the means are not equal, there are several *post hoc* that can be used to determine where the differences lie, such as the Tukey or the Student-Newman-Keuls test. However, the use of these tests is beyond the scope of this chapter. In addition to simple one-way or one-factor ANOVA described above, other types are available to analyse more complex situations involving several factors. Again, these are beyond the scope of this chapter.

REGRESSION AND CORRELATION

There are many circumstances where the magnitude of one variable (the dependent or response variable) is assumed to be determined by the magnitude of a second variable (the independent variable). We use regression to define the relationship between two such variables. Often complex types of regression, involving multiple variables and non-linear relationships arise in medical statistics, but in this chapter we will only consider simple linear regression, in which only two variables are considered. In linear regression, as the name suggests, the relationship between the variables can be represented by a straight line. This can be written as:

$$\bar{Y}_i = \alpha + \beta x_i$$

where α and β, the intercept and slope of the regression line, are unknown constants that have to be determined in the regression analysis. They are known collectively as the regression coefficients.

We want an estimate of the regression coefficients α and β. If we graph the data using the ordinate (y-axis) for the response variable and the abscissa (x-axis) for the explanatory variable, the data will appear as a scatter of points. What we seek are the values of α and β that will produce the 'best fit' line through the data. The principle that is generally used is that of *least squares*. The idea is to look at the differences, or *residuals*, between the observed values of the response variable and the values predicted by the estimated regression line (Figure 21.6).

We want to choose estimates of the regression coefficients (α and β) to make the sum of the squared residuals, that is the quantity:

$$\sum_{i=1}^{n} [y_i - (\alpha + \beta x_i)]^2$$

as small as possible (this explains the term *least squares*). The least squares estimate of the slope is:

$$\beta = \frac{n\Sigma x_i y_i - \Sigma x_i \Sigma y_i}{n \Sigma x_i^2 - (\Sigma x_i)^2},$$

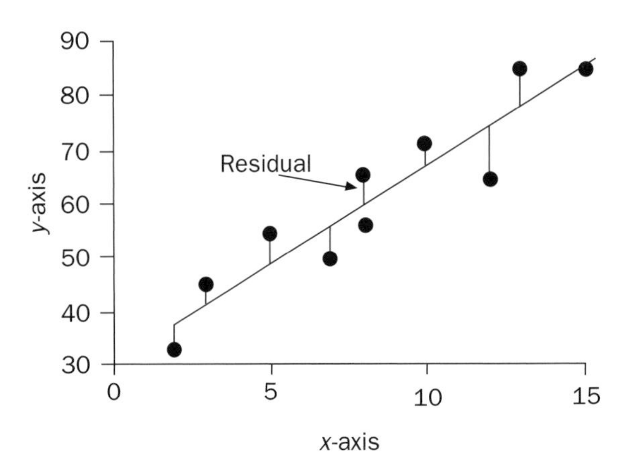

Figure 21.6 *Regression line for the data given by the closed circles. The vertical lines joining each data point to the regression line are the individual residuals.*

and of the intercept:

$$\hat{\alpha} = \bar{y} - \hat{\beta}\,\bar{x}$$

where $\bar{x}$ and $\bar{y}$ are the means of the x- and y-values. The above calculations are tedious to carry out by hand, but are easy to implement on a computer.

The proportion of the total variation in the response variable Y that is explained or accounted for by the fitted regression line is termed the *coefficient of determination*, r^2, which can take values only between 0 and 1. Obviously the higher r^2 is the better the fitted line. The value of r^2 is related to the slope coefficient, $\hat{\beta}$. If $\hat{\beta}$ is close to zero obviously the prediction of Y for any value of X will be very poor. Another way to express the accuracy of the regression is to compute confidence intervals for predicted values of Y.

Regression analysis defines the mathematical relationship between the response variable Y and the explanatory variable X. We cannot, however, automatically assume that there is an underlying biological cause-and-effect relationship between these variables. Conclusions about causal relationships can only be drawn based on some insight into the natural phenomenon being investigated, backed up where possible by statistical testing.

Correlation

In regression there is a dependence of one variable on another. In correlation we also consider the relationship between two variables, but neither is assumed to be functionally dependent on the other. The strength of the association or correlation between the variables is given by the *correlation coefficient* r, also known as the *'Pearson product-moment correlation coefficient'*:

$$r = \frac{\Sigma\,(x_i - \bar{x})(y_i - \bar{y})}{\sqrt{\Sigma\,(x_i - \bar{x})^2\,\Sigma\,(y_i - \bar{y})^2}}$$

The value of r always lies between –1 and +1. When $r = 0$ there is no correlation between the two variables. When $r > 0$ there is a positive correlation, i.e. for a positive increase in one of the variables the value of the other also increases. A negative correlation ($r < 0$) indicates that an increase in one variable is accompanied by a decrease in the value of the other. Note that correlation always requires the assumption of a straight line relationship (this is not necessarily true for regression).

The Bland-Altman test

When comparing two methods of measurement, neither of which is a 'gold standard', e.g. cardiac outout measured by two devices, it is not appropriate to use correlation analysis, since high correlation does not necessairly imply that the two methods agree. Instead, one should use the Bland-Altman limits of agreement (Bland and Altman 1986). This is based on a graphical approach, plotting the difference between the methods and their mean. Agreement is assessed by calculating the bias, estimated by the mean difference, and the standard deviation (SD) of the differences (Figure 21.7).

NON-PARAMETRIC TESTS

The statistical methods discussed up to now have required certain assumptions about the populations from which the samples were obtained. Among these was that the population could be approximated by a normal distribution and that, when dealing with several populations, these have the same variance. There are many situations where these assumptions cannot be met, and methods have been developed that are not concerned with specific population parameters or the distribution of the population. These are referred to as *non-parametric* or *distribution-free* methods. They are the appropriate methods for ordinal data and for interval data where the requirements of normality cannot be assumed. A disadvantage of these methods is that they are less efficient than parametric methods. By less efficient is meant

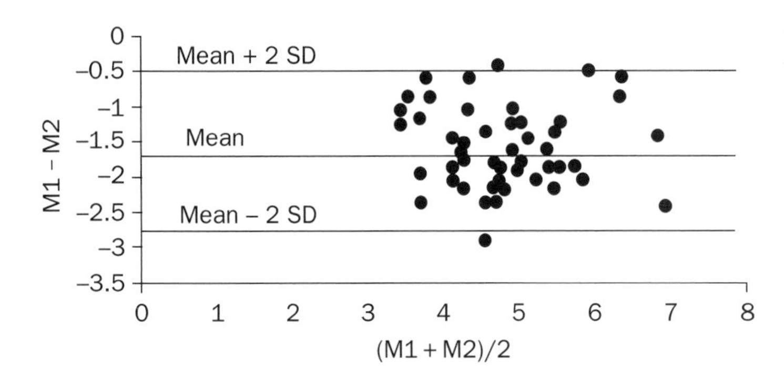

Figure 21.7 An example of a Bland-Altman plot. The bias is –1.5 and the limits of agreement –0.5 to –2.8. There is poor agreement in this case.

that in tests of hypotheses there is a greater risk of committing a Type 2 error, i.e. wrongly accepting the null hypothesis.

In general many of the standard parametric tests have non-parametric equivalents. The **Mann-Whitney test** corresponds to the parametric unpaired *t*-test. This test is based on *rank sums*. The combined data are ranked, usually low to high. If the null hypothesis, that the two samples come from identical populations, is true the sum of the ranks assigned to the observations from the two samples will be close. The null hypothesis is tested using the *U*-statistic:

$$U = n_1 n_2 + \frac{n_1(n_1 + 1)}{2} - R_1$$

where n_1 and n_2 are the sizes of the two samples and R_1 is the sum of the ranks assigned to the values of the first sample. In practice, it is immaterial which sample is referred to as the 'first'. Having calculated *U*, the level of significance can be obtained from appropriate tables. The **Wilcoxon signed rank test** is the non-parametric equivalent of the paired *t*-test. The **Kruskal-Wallis test** is another *rank sums* test that is used to test the null hypothesis that *k* independent samples come from identical populations against the alternative that the means of the populations are unequal. It provides a non-parametric alternative to the one-way analysis of variance.

THE χ^2-TEST

Categorical data are not measured on a scale, but are placed into distinct categories. The basic statistic for categorical data is the count, the number of events per category. When the data can fall into more than one category they can be displayed in a contingency table, so called because the count in each cell is the number in that category of that variable, contingent upon it also belonging to a category of the other variable. These tables are usually laid out in such a way that the rows correspond to the values of one of the variables and the columns to the others. When there are only two variables under consideration we speak of a 2 × 2 contingency table. In general, *r* rows and *c* columns yield an $r \times c$ table. Table 21.4 shows the number of times a double-lumen endobronchial tube was correctly placed when used with or without a stylet.

The analysis of contingency tables involves looking for evidence of association between the variables involved, in the example above whether the use of a stylet influenced correct placement. For this we use the χ^2 (pronounced '*khi*-squared') test. To test the null hypothesis, that correct placement was not associated with use of a stylet, we compare the number of times placement was correct with the number we would expect if there was no association. If there was no association we would expect correct placement in (25/65) × 30 = 11.5 cases when the stylet was used, and (25/65) × 35 = 13.5 cases when no stylet was used. In a similar

Table 21.4 An example of a 2 × 2 contingency table. The number expected in each cell under the null hypothesis is shown in parentheses

	Correct placement		
	Yes	*No*	*Row totals*
Stylet	18 (11.5)	12 (18.5)	30
No stylet	7 (13.5)	28 (21.5)	35
Column totals	25	40	65

way we can obtain the other expected values. The formula for calculating χ^2 is:

$$\chi^2 = \frac{\Sigma (O-E)^2}{E}$$

where O and E are the observed and expected numbers, respectively. Like the t-statistic the distribution depends on a *degree of freedom* parameter. For a contingency table with r rows and c columns the number of degrees of freedom is $(r-1) \times (c-1)$. In the example we have:

$$\chi^2 = \frac{(18-11.5)^2}{11.5} + \frac{(12-18.5)^2}{18.5} + \frac{(7-13.5)^2}{13.5} + \frac{(28-21.5)^2}{21.5} = 11.05$$

The significance of $\chi^2 = 11.05$, with 1 degree of freedom, obtained from a χ^2 table, is large ($P < 0.001$). There is, therefore, strong evidence for an association between use of a stylet and correct placement of a double-lumen tube.

Probabilities given by χ^2 tables are always approximate, but the larger the sample sizes the better the approximation. Two methods are available for improving the accuracy of the probability for small sample sizes when using 2 × 2 contingency tables. *Yate's correction* involves reducing the absolute discrepancy, $|O-E|$, by 0.5 before calculating χ^2. It is recommended when the total sample size, N, is less than 20 or if $20 < N < 40$ and the smallest expected value is < 5. The *Fisher's exact test*, which only applies to 2 × 2 contingency tables, calculates exact probabilities of obtaining the observed table. It should be used for any table with an expected value < 5.

CLINICAL TRIALS

Clinical trials are planned experiments involving human subjects, designed to answer a clinically relevant question concerning treatment. Many involve the evaluation of drugs. In a clinical trial one uses results from a limited sample of subjects to make inferences about the general population. Drug trials are by convention classified into four phases:

Phase 1, concerned with clinical pharmacology and toxicity studies in man (usually healthy volunteers). The goal is to define an acceptable dose range not associated with serious side effects. Phase I trials may also investigate aspects of drug metabolism and disposition.

Phase 2, the initial trials looking for treatment efficacy. They usually involve a limited number of patients.

Phase 3, full-scale clinical evaluations of treatment efficacy. These will involve quite large numbers of patients, and nowadays are often multicentre and multinational trials. They are usually double-blind, placebo-controlled, comparing the new treatment with an existing proven one.

Phase 4, post-marketing surveillance studies. Often organised by drug manufacturers, they can provide valuable additional information from large numbers of patients.

Today, clinical trials must adhere to nationally and internationally agreed codes of good clinical practice, which define ethical and scientific standards. Good clinical trial design and conduct should apply scientific methods. Skilful analysis can never correct for poor design. The purpose of the trial should be defined and specific hypotheses stated in the written study protocol, which will also include details of how the trial will be conducted. Errors in the data have two components, purely random errors and systemic errors or bias, which are not a consequence of chance alone. Randomisation of subjects is important both to avoid observer bias and to prevent or minimise the influence of unknown factors that might influence the results.

Power analysis

The number of subjects required for a trial (sample size) should be determined at the time of design using techniques of power analysis. With too few subjects the trial may not be able to detect an important effect. Apart from a waste of resources it is also unethical, since subjects have been exposed to a trial drug when there was little chance of a useful result. On the other hand, using too many subjects is also unethical and wasteful. The optimal sample size can be calculated in a variety of ways, although exact techniques are beyond the scope of this chapter. In essence, power analysis requires some knowledge about the variability in the population being studied, and an estimate of the smallest effect of clinical interest, i.e. some idea of the results to be expected. These data may come from published studies, or a pilot study. The investigator then needs to decide on the significance level (α), the cut-off level below which the null hypothesis will be rejected, and the required power of the trial. Power is defined as the chance of detecting a specified effect if it exists. Power is often given as $(1 - \beta)$, where β is the chance of falsely accepting the null hypothesis. Commonly used values are $\alpha = 0.05$ and power of 80% ($\beta = 0.02$). Note that the sample size is the number of subjects who complete the trial, not the number who are entered. To allow for drop-outs the planned sample size should be larger than that suggested by power analysis.

FURTHER READING

Bland JM, Altman DG. Statistical methods for assessing agreement between two methods of clinical measurement. *Lancet* 1986;1:307–10.

Cook RJ, Sackett DL. The number needed to treat. A clinically useful measure of treatment effect. *BMJ* 1995;310:452–4.

Index

Page numbers in *italics* indicate figures or tables.